Continued on back

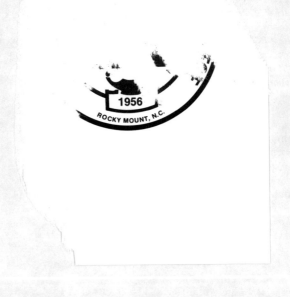

1956
ROCKY MOUNT, N.C.

HANDBOOK FOR
THE PRACTICE OF
PEDIATRIC PSYCHOLOGY

HANDBOOK FOR THE PRACTICE OF PEDIATRIC PSYCHOLOGY

Edited by

JUNE M. TUMA

Louisiana State University

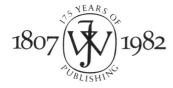

1807 1982

A WILEY-INTERSCIENCE PUBLICATION

JOHN WILEY & SONS
New York • Chichester • Brisbane • Toronto • Singapore

Library of Congress Cataloging in Publication Data:

Main entry under title:

Handbook for the practice of pediatric psychology.

(Wiley series on personality processes,
ISSN 0195-4008)
"A Wiley-Interscience publication."
Includes bibliographical references and index.
Contents: Pediatric psychology / June M. Tuma—
Psychological effects of physical illness and its
concomitants / Diane J. Willis, Charles H. Elliott,
and Susan Jay—Assessment techniques in pediatric
psychology / Phyllis R. Magrab and Ellen Lehr—
[etc.]
1. Pediatrics—Psychological aspects. 2. Sick
children—Psychology. 3. Child psychology
I. Tuma, June M. II. Series.
RJ47.5.H36   618.92′0001′9   81-11567
ISBN 0-471-06284-7   AACR2

Printed in the United States of America

10 9 8 7 6 5 4 3 2 1

To members and friends of the
Society of Pediatric Psychology

Contributors

PAULINE BENJAMIN, Department of Pediatrics and Psychiatry, Case Western Reserve School of Medicine

ROBERT CHWAST, Department of Pediatrics and Psychiatry, Case Western Reserve School of Medicine

DENNIS DROTAR, Department of Pediatrics and Psychiatry, Case Western Reserve School of Medicine

CHARLES H. ELLIOTT, Department of Pediatrics and Behavior Science, University of Oklahoma Health Sciences Center

ELAINE S. ELLIOTT, Department of Psychology, San Diego State University

JAMES S. HENNESSEY, Department of Psychology, San Diego State University

SUSAN JAY, Department of Pediatrics, University of Oklahoma Health Sciences Center

MELISSA R. JOHNSON, Department of Psychiatry, University of North Carolina at Chapel Hill

VRINDA S. KNAPP, Social Services Division, Children's Hospital, Los Angeles

ELLEN LEHR, Department of Pediatrics, Georgetown University Medical Center, Washington, D.C.

CAROLE LITT, Department of Pediatrics and Psychiatry, Case Western Reserve School of Medicine

PHILLIS R. MAGRAB, Department of Pediatrics, Georgetown University Medical Center, Washington, D.C.

GARY B. MESIBOV, Department of Psychiatry, University of North Carolina at Chapel Hill

MICHAEL C. ROBERTS, Department of Psychology, University of Alabama

DONALD K. ROUTH, Department of Psychology, University of Iowa

JOHN P. SHEPOSH, Department of Psychology, San Diego State University

STEVEN N. SPARTA, Children's Hospital and Health Center, San Diego

JOHN J. SPINETTA, Department of Psychology, San Diego State University

RICHARD P. SPRIGLE, Department of Psychology, San Diego State University

JUNE M. TUMA, Department of Psychology, Louisiana State University at Baton Rouge

PAUL VAJNER, Department of Pediatrics and Psychiatry, Case Western Reserve School of Medicine

DIANE J. WILLIS, Department of Pediatrics, University of Oklahoma Health Sciences Center

LOGAN WRIGHT, Institute on Health Psychology for Children, Oklahoma City

Series Preface

This series of books is addressed to behavioral scientists interested in the nature of human personality. Its scope should prove pertinent to personality theorists and researchers as well as to clinicians concerned with applying an understanding of personality processes to the amelioration of emotional difficulties in living. To this end, the series provides a scholarly integration of theoretical formulations, empirical data, and practical recommendations.

Six major aspects of studying and learning about human personality can be designated: personality theory, personality structure and dynamics, personality development, personality assessment, personality change, and personality adjustment. In exploring these aspects of personality, the books in the series discuss a number of distinct but related subject areas: the nature and implications of various theories of personality; personality characteristics that account for consistencies and variations in human behavior; the emergence of personality processes in children and adolescents; the use of interviewing and testing procedures to evaluate individual differences in personality; efforts to modify personality styles through psychotherapy, counseling, behavior therapy, and other methods of influence; and patterns of abnormal personality functioning that impair individual competence.

IRVING B. WEINER

University of Denver
Denver, Colorado

Preface

The pediatric psychologist has emerged from the ranks of clinical and developmental psychology with a strong role in the health care of children as it becomes increasingly apparent that children are particularly susceptible to psychological concomitants to illness-related events. Although psychologists and others working in mental health disciplines enjoy a long history of consultation with pediatricians when specific and persistent problems with a child patient occur on an occasional basis, it has only been in recent years that the extent and complexity of that role has come under scrutiny. As appreciation of the enormity of the prevalence of the need for psychological activities is achieved in the medical and psychological community, more psychologists are given the opportunity to become involved in the screening, evaluation, and treatment of these children. In addition, research on the disorders themselves, the nature and the impact of the illness, its procedures, hospitalization, and all the variants thereof are particularly in the realm of the research-trained psychologist.

The term pediatric psychologist was coined in 1967, and today an identifiable specialty within psychology is embraced with enthusiasm by an ever-increasing number of psychologists. The role of the pediatric psychologist is as yet evolving, but the strong activity both in practice and research during more than a decade has yielded a body of knowledge which describes the functions and potentials of this specialty. It is the purpose of this book to present the most up-to-date accumulation of knowledge about that role. The psychological impact of physical illness and medical treatment in all of its manifestations, the developmental status of the child, the degree of severity of the illness with its consequent incapacities, and the setting in which the child is treated determine the role of the pediatric psychologist. The issues inherent in the practice of pediatric psychology are herein addressed along with the most established and innovative techniques of assessment, intervention, and consultation. Throughout the presentations, and in a special chapter, research in this area is presented in authoritative and comprehensive detail. Finally, in an effort to further define the role, the training of the pediatric psychologist is considered in all its variants and in the context of the relevant issues.

This volume will be invaluable to pediatric psychologists concerned with the practice of psychology which interfaces with medical care of children, and, in addition, to all those concerned with health care of children—pediatricians, psychiatrists, nurses, social workers, child care workers, teachers, and other professionals in fields related to health care—will find the scholarly review of information on all aspects of the psychological impact of physical illness on the child illuminating. Students in psychology will be particularly interested in the comprehensive development of the variables influencing the roles of the pediatric psychologist and in the information concerning appropriate training for the specialty.

JUNE M. TUMA

Baton Rouge, Louisiana
December 1981

Contents

CHAPTER 1

Pediatric Psychology: Conceptualization and Definition

June M. Tuma

Pediatric psychology represents the professional group of psychologists who were among the first to expand psychological/behavioral principles to nonpsychiatric health settings. The earliest conceptualization of pediatric psychology appeared in 1967 in Logan Wright's article "Pediatric Psychology: A Role Model," which appeared in the *American Psychologist*. Wright defined a pediatric psychologist as "any psychologist who finds himself dealing primarily with children in a medical setting which is nonpsychiatric in nature" (p. 323). In 1968, an interest group, the Society of Pediatric Psychology, was formed and it soon became an affiliate of Section I (Section on Clinical Child Psychology) of Division 12 of the American Psychological Association.

Another statement concerning the definition of pediatric psychology appeared in the *Newsletter* of the Society in 1974 following its drafting at the midwinter Executive Committee meeting. The statement was as follows: "The Society of Pediatric Psychology is a professionally oriented group of psychologists who deal with children in interdisciplinary settings such as hospitals, pediatric practices and developmental centers. The purpose of the group is to exchange information on clinical procedures and research and to define training standards for the pediatric psychologist" (p. 8). In this same issue, President Tom Kenny (1975) made note of increasing awareness of the extent of pediatric psychology. He observed that pediatric psychology dealt with the process of child development rather than with the emotionally disturbed child, with teaching normal development to parents as preventive measures of mental health, the effects of physical illness on the development of the child, the reactions of children to hospitalization. "The whole group seems to be synthesizing a developmental based, interdisciplinary model that will concentrate its efforts on providing professional assistance to a broad range of children and their parents" (Kenny, 1975, p. 8).

These early attempts at definition of the role of psychology in pediatric settings were not reflective of the major thrust of development in psychology. It was not until more recent years when growing attention by the public, professionals, and government to issues and problems arising from increasing costs and deficiencies in delivery of health care services that general acceptance of psychologists in medical settings occurred. As interest gained momentum, greater efforts were made to conceptualize the nature of psychological involvement in medical settings.

Perhaps the single most influential factor responsible for psychology's greater involvement in health care was the establishment of the Task Force on Health Research (APA, 1976) by APA's Board of Scientific Affairs to survey the nature and extent of contributions by psychologists to basic and applied research on behavioral factors in physical illness and health maintenance. The Task Force surveyed and analyzed the research literature to this purpose. Suggestions were also made by this group for research into areas of neglect and recommended special training needs for the "health care" researcher.

As psychology got more involved in applying psychological principles to medical settings, attempts at conceptualization of the area of application and research began. Semantic confusion characterizes these efforts, and the final definition is probably not in. However, it is useful to review those efforts for the purpose of understanding the role of psychologists in this endeavor.

MEDICAL PSYCHOLOGY

Asken (1979) defines medical psychology as "the study of psychological factors related to any and all aspects of physical health, illness and its treatment at the individual, group, and systems level" (p. 67). Asken asserts that medical psychology can conceptualize problems from any desired orientation and represents no particular theoretical orientation and involves all areas of scholarly interest, including research, clinical intervention, application and teaching. The major distinction between medical psychology and traditional psychology is the nature of their relationship to physical illness and the nonpsychiatric physician. Asken suggests that the four major areas which comprise medical psychology are psychosomatics, somatopsychology, behavioral medicine, and health care studies.

Difficulties with this definition include the adoption of a formal definition of behavioral medicine at the Yale conference (Schwartz & Weiss, 1978a) to be "the interdisciplinary field concerned with the development and integration of behavioral and biomedical science knowledge and techniques relevant to health and illness and the application of this knowledge and these techniques to prevention, diagnosis, treatment, and rehabilitation" (Schwartz & Weiss, 1978b, p. 250). Thus Asken's definition, which subsumes behavioral medicine under medical psychology, is logically inconsistent with this definition. When defined as an interdisciplinary field, behavioral medicine consists of psychology, sociology, psychiatry, medicine (including most of its specialties), epidemiology, nursing, and nutrition. It further includes every discipline that is involved with health care at nearly every level (education, prevention, treatment).

Masur (1979) points out that the term behavioral medicine has been confusing because some consider the word "behavioral" to reflect a particular theoretical and/or technical orientation to treatment. Thus the techniques within behavioral medicine were thought to be relaxation training for muscle-contraction headaches, biofeedback training for epilepsy, and so on, that is, those techniques derived exclusively from behavior therapy. The term used in the context of behavioral medicine should, according to the Yale Conference definition, be conceptualized in a more generic sense, that is, behavioral sciences. Medical schools, for example, have used this term to include a variety of disciplines that contribute to our overall understanding of human behavior. If conceptualized this way, medical psychology joins the ranks of a multitude of disciplines within the interdisciplinary field of behavioral medicine.

Masur (1979) presents a conceptualization of behavioral medicine as a point of convergence for a variety of biomedical and behavioral disciplines. Behavioral disciplines are psychology, anthropology, epidemiology, sociology, and nutrition; the biomedical disciplines are nursing, physical therapy, dentistry, pharmacy, and medicine (especially clinical psychiatry). This conceptualization permits interface between psychology and any or all of the behavioral and biomedical disciplines. There exist many cross-links that represent both the knowledge base and techniques that have shared relevance at these interfaces.

Other terms have also been used to designate the area of interface between psychologists and other professionals involved in health and illness. Notably, "health care psychology" and "health psychology" have been used to designate this area. Some psychologists have attempted to avoid the use of "medical," proposing that any use of the term presupposes a tacit endorsement of the medical model of disease. They also contend that the term, when used to designate the field in psychology, has a primary clinical service orientation, which is too narrow. These are the arguments, for example, given by those who worked in areas of health screening, primary prevention, evaluation of compliance models, and so on, when the name was proposed for the new division of APA which was to be concerned with health issues as they relate to psychology. "Health care psychology" was similarly proposed instead of "medical psychology" because it would place an emphasis on health rather than disease. The term "care," however, seemed too restrictive for some since it ignored the role of education and prevention by stressing patient care. Thus "health psychology" was the agreed upon name in spite of the fear of being overinclusive by some.

DISTINCTIONS OF HEALTH PROFESSIONAL FROM MENTAL HEALTH PROFESSIONAL

Schofield (1969) argues that psychology is one of the health sciences and that certain patterns of training in the disciplines of psychology can appropriately prepare the psychologist to function as a health professional. The health impact of psychology has been too restrictively identified with clinical psychology, with psychiatry, and with mental illness, according to Schofield. He points to the majority of manpower distribution in clinical settings, distribution of research efforts to schizophrenia, psychotherapy, and neurosis, to the exclusion of the remaining 22 health-illness topics. He warns of the serious implications for the potential role of the psychologist as a health professional. The need is for the development of a new and broader image of the psychologist as a health professional who can contribute meaningfully to the evaluation and management of health problems beyond those entailing emotional or psychiatric components as usually conceived.

Health psychology is based on the fact that psychological factors are a primary concern in many health-related issues. Thus psychologists can make unique and specific contributions in the prevention and treatment of illness and promote health-seeking behaviors. While psychologists have provided valuable services in the area of psychiatric problems, health psychology stresses psychology's expansion into nonpsychiatric health problems. As the American Psychological Association's Task Force on Health Research (1976) noted, clinical psychologists may help achieve a comprehensiveness and integration of health care. But this will be reached only when the functional unity of the individual is recognized and there is a respect for the involvement of psychological factors in physical illness, injury, disability, and health in general.

Psychology as a health science and profession has two major influences. One is the progress of behavioral, medical, and public health sciences. The second is the sociopolitical forces in the American health care crisis. Reconceptualizations of the mind-body problems and physical health-mental health dichotomies have followed a history of research and the recent adoption of holistic medicine, "the new medical model" (Engel, 1977), and the new psychosomatic model (Lipowski, 1977). These influences have resulted in comprehensive ecological perspectives on health and illness as "biopsychosocial" phenomena.

The other factor involves the rapidly increasing costs of health care and the controversial movement toward national health insurance. Psychologists must become involved to insure their inclusion in the national health insurance (Wiggins, 1979) and the potential of psychology to deliver cost-effective health care (Cummings, 1977).

The thrust of efforts of today's psychology is to enter the arena of scientific and professional involvement represented by psychosomatic theory. The problem of assessing the relative contribution of psychological, biological, and social factors to the development, course, and outcome of physical and psychiatric disorders has regained a dominant position in both medicine and psychiatry after being dormant for almost two decades. The theoretical assumptions and tradition of addressing the mind-body problem in research and clinical practice is provided within psychosomatic medicine. Growing in breadth, complexity, and diversity, it is attempting to answer very old questions about human health and disease with the aid of modern investigative methods. Its concepts have been endorsed by the 27th World Health Assembly, held in 1974 (World Health Organization, 1974), when all nations were urged to support research on the role of psychosocial factors in health and disease. Thus a holistic and ecological approach to medical research, practice, and training was adopted. This group contended that these factors can precipitate and counteract physical and mental illness and are thus crucially important in the prevention and management of all disease. Psychology, as has recently been formally recognized by the APA Task Force on Health Research, has a prominent role to play. To provide a focus on the issues that are relevant to this endeavor and to provide some assessment of this interdisciplinary approach, the status of psychosomatic theory and research will be reviewed.

PSYCHOSOMATIC THEORY

Three interrelated facets jointly define the scope of psychosomatic theory:

1. It is a scientific discipline concerned with the study of the relationships of biological, psychological, and social determinants of health and disease.
2. It is a set of postulates and guidelines embodying a holistic approach to the practice of medicine.
3. It encompasses consultation-liaison psychiatry (Lipowski, 1977).

Masur's (1979) conceptualization would also add to the third facet other areas of the biomedical component, for example, clinical psychiatry, family medicine, neurology, and the behavioral component, such as clinical psychology, medical psychology, neuropsychology, rehabilitative psychology, as well as the other disciplines included in the behavioral medicine paradigm.

The definition of psychosomatic theory includes both the scientific and clinical aspects of the field. As a scientific discipline, psychosomatic medicine has focused on the reciprocal relationships between psychological and physiological variables. The correlation between specified conditions and changes in the person's social environment has been accomplished by employing research methods, explanatory concepts, and languages belonging to three distinct levels of abstraction— sociology, psychology, and physiology. The major scientific task has been to define the precise role of defined social and psychological factors in maintaining health and codetermining the development and course of disease. Another complementary task has involved the study of the effect that specified physiological variables have on psychological functioning in all of its principal aspects—information processing, motivation, emotions, and psychomotor behavior, both normal and abnormal. Thus, both antecedents and consequences of health and disease are the areas of concern.

Psychosomatic theory has always addressed issues of the nature of man and methods of medical practice as well. In health and disease, the prominence of neither mind nor body alone is important, but rather the person is the focus of study and treatment. People thus are conceived of as individual mind-body complexes ceaselessly interacting with the social and physical environment in which they are embedded. The psychosomatic conception of man, from this perspective, is integrative, holistic, and dynamic. The theory advocates a unified concept of health and disease, a distinct approach to prevention, diagnosis, and management of disease.

It is instructive to review those assertions that may have been attributed to psychosomatic medicine previously. It is not an affirmation of metaphysical dualism, nor an advocacy of psychological causation of physical illnesses, nor a study of the so-called psychosomatic disorders. The modern view embraces instead the doctrine of multicausality of all disease. It is consonant with this doctrine to view social and psychological factors as condeterminants of health and illness. Thus both have etiological and modifying significance in human morbidity. The relative contribution of these factors varies from disease to disease, from person to person, and from one episode of the same disease in the same person to another episode (Lipowski, 1977).

Lipowski (1977) pointed out that to distinguish a class of disease as "psychosomatic disorders" and to propound generalizations about "psychosomatic patients" is misleading and redundant. Concepts of single causes and of unilinear causal sequences—for example, from psyche to soma and vice versa—are simplistic and obsolete. The dynamic interaction of multiple factors occurring in varying constellations and time sequences, and modified by feedback effects, underlies all changes in health (Lipowski, 1977). The chief objectives of psychosomatic medicine today are to break down this complexity into testable hypotheses and validate them, to formulate integrated theories, and to develop effective preventive and therapeutic methods.

In essence, psychosomatic medicine is a body of empirical knowledge and practical precepts regarding the role of symbolic processes and their emotional correlates and behavioral consequences in health and disease.

Historical Perspective

In its present form, psychosomatic medicine is about 50 years old. Its roots are placed within the origins of Western medicine and thought in Greece in the fifth century B.C. Many similar themes in psychosomatic research and theory were formulated and recurrently addressed over the centuries. As early as 1747, Gaub, a professor of medicine, wrote that "the reason why a sound body becomes ill, or an ailing body recovers, very often lies in the mind. Contrariwise, the body can frequently both beget mental illness and heal its offspring" (cited in Rather, 1965, p. 71).

The groundwork for psychosomatic theory was laid in 1872 when Tuke compiled observations and anecdotes recorded in Western medical literature which addressed the influence of mind on the body in health and disease. Yet psychosomatic medicine was not recognized as a discipline for another 50 years. Empirical study of the mind-body problem was made possible by three independent developments. It was from Freud, Pavlov, and Cannon that new methods of research and explanatory concepts permitted exploration of the mind-body problem.

By the 1920s, psychosomatic medicine emerged from a background of philosophy and medical folklore. The concepts that began as a cluster of hunches, clinical anecdotes, and imaginative speculation became the subject of scientific investigation. The conceptual and research tools were finally available, and for the next 30 years, the field followed two major lines of investigation, psychodynamic and psychophysiological. The former was inspired by psychoanalytic theory and relied on psychoanalytic concepts and methods of making observations. Alexander (1950) was the most influential representative of this trend. He dominated the field until about 1955 with his specificity theory, which linked in a causal chain specific, unresolved, unconscious conflicts with specific somatic disorders.

Alexander (1950) is important for formulating many of the core assumptions of psychosomatic medicine. He postulated a decisive role of unconscious conflicts and related emotions in the development of such disorders as bronchial asthma, ulcerative colitis, thyroxicosis, essential hypertension, rheumatoid arthritis, neurodermatitis, and peptic ulcer, the seven "psychosomatic disorders." This approach stimulated much clinical research and raised hopes of effective therapy aimed at the resolution of pathogenic conflicts. His methodological approach had weaknesses. It causally linked variables of very different levels of abstraction, for example, conflict and peptic ulcer, without due regard to the intervening psychophysiological mechanisms. Validation of this hypothesis proved predictably difficult (Alexander, French & Pollock, 1968) and the efficacy of therapy did not materialize despite some successes (Kellner, 1975). The hypotheses were very popular, however, and were applied by uncritical supporters as simplistic "psychosomatic formulae" that were applied indiscriminately to all patients suffering from one of the psychosomatic disorders (Lipowski, 1977). By 1955, this approach was abandoned with widespread disenchantment with psychosomatic medicine as a whole. Popularity and credibility both dropped.

The second major direction in psychosomatic research and theory was concurrently developed by Wolff and his collaborators at Cornell University over a period of 30 years. This line of investigation was marked by careful scientific and experimental design, quantification of the studied variables, focus on conscious and thus more readily elicited psychological factors. Above all, Wolff was concerned with the mechanisms mediating between symbolic stimuli and processes and the peripheral physiological changes. Wolff developed a theory of psychological stress that was applied to a wide range of somatic diseases (Wolff, 1953). His psychophysiological studies employed epidemiological methods on the role of social and psychological factors in disease. Wolff's work has had the decisive influence on psychosomatic research since the mid-1960s (Lipowski, 1977).

Psychosomatic Theory Today

Difficulties of validating proposed primacy of unconscious psychological factors such as conflicts in the pathogenesis of various somatic disorders lessened the influence of psychoanalysis on psychosomatic medicine since the early 1960s. The specificity theory of Alexander still has a few adherents and attempts to validate its hypotheses continue (Alexander *et al.*, 1968). This theory has some value for clinical prediction and therapy of patients suffering from one of the seven "psychosomatic disorders" (Kellner, 1975), but it has not generated new research and clinical applications. Psychoanalytic concepts, such as conversion, somatization, physiological regression, repressed affects, and psychogenesis continue to be used by some to account for various somatic disorders. There is less of a tendency today to claim that these concepts can adequately explain the occurrence of any of the major diseases prevalent today. Their value appears to be in understanding certain somatic complaints not based on demonstrable pathology (Lipowski, 1968).

Some psychoanalytic concepts and methods of observation have been retained, however. They contribute knowledge of the unconscious significance of all information for the person, of the symbolic meaning of body parts and functions, and of unconscious motivation and conflicts. These factors influence a person's psychological responses to life events and situations, and susceptibility and psychological reactions to illness. Thus they codetermine the timing of onset, course, and outcome of disease. However, unconscious factors must be placed in context of other classes of relevant variables to achieve comprehensive knowledge.

Psychosomatic theory is influenced by a host of factors and theories. General systems and information theories, the doctrine of multicausality of somatic function and behavior, notions of psychophysiological response specificity and activation, the theory of conditioning and self-control of visceral functions, the hypotheses of loss as an antecedent of disease and the concepts of psychosocial stress, cognitive appraisal and meaning, individual susceptibility to disease, adaptation, coping, and feedback all influence current psychosomatic theory (Reiser, 1975; Lipowski, 1977, 1968). The most influential theoretical formulations have been generated by Wolff (1953), Grinker (1953), Engel (1960), and Lazarus (1960).

The first phase of psychosomatic medicine (between about 1925 and 1955) differs markedly from the present phase. Today there is relatively less emphasis on individual psychodynamics and more on psychophysiological responses to environmental stimuli. Theoretical perspectives now encompass the effects of social factors on health such as family interaction and disruption, conditions and relationships on the job, urbanization, poverty, migration, and rapidly changing value systems and life-styles (Lipowski, 1977). This biopsychosocial trend complements traditional psychodynamic and psychophysiological approaches. The social and ecological dimension has markedly expanded the previous two-dimensional psychosomatic theories that focused only on psychophysiological interactions (Lipowski, 1973). The current view is reflected by Dubos (1968): "The understanding and control of disease require that the body-mind complex be studied in its relation to external environment."

Current concern with conscious emotions and cognitive processes and their anatomical substrate and physiological concomitants represents another major shift in focus. Since these psychological variables are more easily elicited and quantified than the unconscious ones, they are more amenable to scientific study.

The current psychosomatic theories, in their growing complexity and holistic hypotheses, "reflect the scientific zeitgeist marked by acceptance of complexity, by attempts to study and relate multiple variables, and by striving for theories straddling interdisciplinary boundaries" (Lipowski, 1977, p. 286).

Dominant Theoretical Concepts and Formulations

The dominant concern of psychosomatic research is to answer several questions:

> Why does a person respond to particular social situations and specific life events with a given pattern of psychological and physiological changes?
>
> Which psychological variable may help predict when an individual will become ill and what illness he or she will develop?
>
> Through which pathways and mechanisms do symbolic stimuli bring about changes in susceptibility to somatic illness?
>
> Which kinds of social situations and events are most likely to predispose to and precipitate illness in a given person or group?
>
> Which behaviors, attitudes, and social conditions are most conducive to health and to adaptive coping with illness?
>
> What are the psychological characteristics of people who most readily become ill or complain of bodily symptoms, or both (Lipowski, 1977, p. 236)

Investigation of these questions can identify those psychosocial variables that increase susceptibility to illness as well as those that enhance resistance to and adaptive coping with disease. Social and psychological measures can then be developed that will help to prevent and ameliorate disease causing chronic disability and premature death. Evidence is beginning to suggest that this goal may be achieved by modifying specific behaviors, attitudes, and emotional responses and by improving social supports.

The general framework of current psychosomatic theory has two core assumptions. One assumption asserts that man's symbolic activity, subserved by the cerebral structures and functions, influences organismic processes at all other levels of organization down to the cellular level. Thus symbolic activity (conscious and unconscious perceptions, thoughts, memories, imagery, and fantasy) constitutes a set of factors affecting homeostasis, adaptation, and health. Environmental stimuli and bodily processes that directly affect the cerebral functions influence the symbolic activity. Social situations and events, significant sources of information, can affect the individual insofar as it is appraised, consciously or unconsciously, or both, and is endowed with subjective meaning. This meaning then activates emotions, which then, in turn, have physiological concomitants and cognitive and behavioral consequences, all of which can bring about changes in health (Lipowski, 1973). These propositions constitute the concept of psychosocial stress.

The second core assumption pertains to the role of enduring psychological and physiological tendencies to react to specific stimuli with individually specific patterns of cognitive, emotional, behavioral, and physiological responses. These tendencies, partly inborn and partly learned, are subject to modification and self-control (Shapiro & Surwit, 1974). Developmental factors and the kinds, timing, duration, and intensity of especially social stimuli during the early development of the organism and personality help shape future psychophysiological response patterns and individual susceptibility to disease (Ader, 1974).

Three sets of concepts and hypotheses reflect the preceding assumptions: psychosocial stress, psychophysiological response specificity, and individual susceptibility to disease.

Psychosocial Stress

Psychosocial stress implies that social situations and events as well as such psychological states as conflicts and frustrated strivings may disturb homeostasis and impose adaptive demands on the organism. This class of variables has been variously referred to as "stressors" (Hinkle, 1974; Mason, 1975a), "stressful life events" (Dohrenwend & Dohrenwend, 1974), or "life changes" (Rahe, 1975).

The three meanings of the term "stress" have produced ambiguity. For different investigators, stress refers to a state of the organism; the stressors; or an area of study including stressful stimuli, an organism's responses to them, and the totality of intervening variables (Wolff, 1953; Lazarus, 1960; Hinkle, 1974; Mason, 1975a). The relative specificity versus nonspecificity of physiological changes evoked by various stressors is also not clear (Mason, 1975a). The following definition is proposed by Lipowski (1977): "Psychosocial stress refers to external and internal stimuli that are perceived by and are meaningful to the person, activate emotions, and elicit physiological changes that threaten health and survival" (p. 237).

Because psychosocial stress is defined by subjective meaning, stress can include extremes of temperature, pathogenic microorganisms, and physical trauma (Lipowski, 1968; Wolff, 1953; Engel, 1960). Psychosocial stress can be beneficial as well as pathogenic. Its beneficial effect on health depends on the person's coping capacity, social support, and other factors. The key intervening variables in psychosocial stress are information, its cognitive appraisal, and subjective meaning and emotions (Lipowski, 1977).

Lipowski (1975c) distinguishes five categories of subjective meaning of information: threat, loss, gain or relief, challenge, and insignificance. Information that signifies threat, loss, or both for the person is likely to evoke dysphoric emotions of fear, anxiety, anger, grief, depression, guilt, and shame. These emotions play an important role in mediating the adverse effects of such information on the functions of the body and on illness behavior. Three defensive behavioral tendencies are possible to these emotions: fight, flight, or immobility (conservation-withdrawal) (Engel & Schmale, 1972). Subjective meaning of information has sociocultural, personality, and experimental determinants and influence what constitutes stress for the individual.

Emotions are the intervening variables between meaningful information and bodily changes elicited by it (Levi, 1975) and may also be activated by direct stimulation of the limbic-hypothalamic system (Lipowski, 1977). Physiological concomitants of emotions are well-known (cardiovascular, respiratory, glandular, musculoskeletal, and so forth) and may have one or more of the following effects: (1) be perceived and augment, reduce, or change the quality of the emotion; (2) predispose to, precipitate, make manifest, exacerbate, or ameliorate a pathological bodily process; (3) motivate behavior inimical or conducive to health; (4) set in motion ego mechanisms of defense and coping strategies aimed at relief of distress; and (5) be communicated as somatic symptoms and foster adoption of the sick role (Lipowski, 1975c).

Psychophysiology of emotions has been one focus of stress theory (Levi, 1975), with neuroendocrine mechanisms of key importance. The identification of social and psychological variables which constitute the most common forms of stress by virtue of the emotions they arouse is a major focus of research. The postulation proposed by this line of investigation is that the more disturbing an event or situation is for a person, the higher the probability that it will lead to bodily dysfunction and disease. The kind, intensity, and duration of the evoked emotions are the decisive variables.

Examples of common psychosocial stressors are bereavement (Clayton, 1973), loss of job (Kasl, Gore, & Cobb, 1975; Meissner, 1974), disturbed family interaction (Minuchin, Baker, & Rosman, 1975), specific work conditions (Mc-Lean, 1974), and sensory and information overloads (Lipowski, 1975f). The two major approaches to study psychosocial stress are qualitative and quantitative. Qualitative researchers have proposed that object loss is a common antecedent of illness (Engel, cited in Schmale, 1972; Lipowski, 1975c). Thus, actual, antici-pated, or fantasied loss of a valued person, possession, body part, or life-style is likely to lead to a psychological state called the "giving up—given up syndrome" and its associated emotions of helplessness or hopelessness. The quality or subjective meaning of a life change is postulated to be correlated with onset of illness. The quantitative approach, represented by Holmes and Masuda (1974) and Rahe (1975), asserts that the magnitude of recently accumulated life changes is predictive of near-future illness and its severity. These two approaches are viewed as mutually complementary rather than exclusive.

Hinkle (1974) has questioned the value of the concept of stress and semantic ambiguity has detracted from its usefulness. Investigation of the role of stress in health is further hampered by the difficulty in distinguishing between stress-induced illness and illness behavior (Dohrenwend & Dohrenwend, 1974). The concept of stress is however considered valuable for its integration of observations on the relationship of social factors, the individual's symbolic activity, and changes in health.

Psychophysiological Specificity

As currently revised, psychophysiological specifity refers to the probability that a person will respond to a given stimulus situation with a predictable set of psychological and physiological changes (Roessler & Engel, 1974). The prediction is based on the following three sets of variables:

1. The nature, intensity, and duration of the stimulus situation. Stereotypy occurs when the stimulus situation evokes similar responses in many individu-als.

2. Individual response specificity refers to the enduring psychological and physiological response characteristics of the person. Personality, genetic factors, developmental history, past exposure to illness, unconscious conflicts and modes of defending against them, behavior patterns, attitudes, and operant conditioning have all been proposed to account for individual psychophysiological response characteristics and for susceptibility to illness.
3. The current psychophysiological state of the person. The variables subsumed under this heading include current emotional state, fatigue, level and pattern of autonomic arousal, presence of physical illness, and state of consciousness.

The psychophysiological specificity concept epitomizes attempts to study the interactions of multiple variables influencing psychophysiological functioning in health and disease. The concept, broader than earlier proposals, is applicable to both normal and pathological responses and is also less ambiguous and more general than the concept of stress. Its strength is the freedom from value judgments of what is stressful but the individual unit of study constitutes a serious weakness.

Individual Susceptibility to Disease

The two classes of psychosomatic theory of etiology are the specificity and the generality theories. Both propose that social and psychological variables contribute to morbidity but the nature of the causal links and pathogenesis are different. Specific psychological variables have a predictable relationship to specific physiological variables, somatic disorders, or both according to specificity theory. These specific psychological characteristics such as particular emotions, unresolved unconscious conflicts over sexual, dependent, or hostile strivings, personality style, temperament, attitude, behavior pattern, and mode of communicating distress have been correlated with specific normal and abnormal physiological characteristics. Causal links have been claimed or implied between some of these psychological variables and specific disorders. Thus, the specificity theories postulate that specific psychosocial factors contribute to specific, or individual susceptibility to disease.

The generality theories postulate that a wide range of life events may increase the probability that a person will become ill. A state of general susceptibility to disease is thought to be the intervening variable (Thurlow, 1967). A positive correlation between the magnitude of life changes and the subject's near-future illness and its severity has been demonstrated in epidemiological studies (Dohrenwend & Dohrenwend, 1974). The generality theories also postulate lowered resistance of the host to all kinds of pathology (Cassel, 1976).

Rather than competing with one another, Lipowski (1977) views the generality and specificity theories as complementary. The specificity theories identify conditions in a person's life whose occurence increases the probability of imminent illness, whereas the generality theories allow a measure of prediction of which events are potentially hazardous for a given person or class of people sharing one or more psychological characteristics and which illness is more likely to follow exposure to such events. The combination of theories enhance ability to predict illness and to identify persons at risk. No causal relationships between life events or specific psychological characteristics and disease is possible, but the theories provide a basis for social and psychological preventive measures for individuals whom they help identify as vulnerable.

Current Trends in Psychosomatic Research

Because of the increased diversity of studies and methods of investigation characteristic of psychosomatic research today, many studies relevant to the area are not specifically labeled as "psychosomatic." Nevertheless they contribute to the development in this area. In today's conceptualization, any study which focuses on correlations among social, psychological, and physiological variables may be designated "psychosomatic." The broadened view of psychosomatic theory encompasses all studies concerned with these variables as they relate to issues of health and illness.

Lipowski (1977) categorizes five major groups of studies as characteristic of psychosomatic research in the 1970s, as follows:

1. Study of the role of specified social and psychological factors in the etiology of a wide range of human disease.
2. Study of mediating mechanisms (of neuroendocrine, neurophysiological, and immune processes) intervening between the central nervous system activity expressed in psychological terms and the normal and abnormal physiological functions of organs and tissues.
3. Study of psychosocial responses to physical illness and their effects on its course and outcome.
4. Study of the influence on specified somatic processes on psychological functioning.
5. Study of the effectiveness of behavior-modifying therapies on somatic disorders.

Most of psychosomatic research is multidisciplinary and multifactorial. The methodology encompasses three general approaches: psychophysiology (laboratory and experimental work using human and animal subjects); epidemiology; and clinical studies (Lipowski, 1977a).

Etiological Studies

Engel (1960) urges researchers to revise simplistic concepts of etiology to conceive of it in terms of the dynamic interaction of several sets of factors, including psychosocial ones, of different weight and temporal relationships that together enable a given disease to develop.

The major effort of etiological research is directed at the etiology of the chronic diseases responsible for the highest rates of premature mortality and the greatest burden in disability, suffering, and cost. Coronary and cerebrovascular diseases, respiratory disorders, cancer, diabetes, essential hypertension, rheumatoid arthritis, multiple sclerosis, and epilepsy have been of major concern (Lipowski, 1977). Since psychosocial factors are generally believed to have a direct bearing on their incidence, course, and outcome psychosomatic studies have focused on these and all major diseases (Cassel, 1976; World Health Organization, 1974).

Investigation of the precise role of social and psychological factors in the etiology of coronary heart disease (Jenkins, 1976a, 1976b; Eliot, 1974; Gentry & William, 1975) suggests that these factors do play a role in the genesis of the disease. These factors are especially potent in predisposing an individual to, and precipitating acute cardiac events (myocardial infarction, arrhythmias, angina pectoris, and congestive heart failure) (Lipowski, 1975e). It has been found that even behavior related to eating habits, smoking, exercise, and work may affect coronary heart disease by means of the so-called risk factors (Lipowski, 1975e). Attention has focused on the hypotheses that specific personality characteristics manifested by a recognizable behavior pattern and rewarded by affluent societies may have a direct effect (pathogenic) through chronic or repeated activation of specific neuroendocrine mechanisms (Friedman & Rosenman, 1974; Jenkins, 1976a, 1976b).

Essential hypertension is another condition that has been researched (Lipowski, 1975e). Results are not conclusive but it is believed that emotional and autonomic arousal induced by a variety of stressful stimuli in genetically predisposed people will provoke repeated pressor responses that may lead to chronic hypertension. Clinical studies have focused on repressed hostility as a predisposing factor to the disease (Pilowsky, Spalding, & Shaw, 1973) and on the effects of biofeedback (Goldman, Kleinman, & Snow, 1975). The findings to date support the hypothesis that certain social conditions and personality characteristics, although not singly decisive, combine to increase the probability of a person's developing hypertension.

Cancer is an example of an organic disease which has been investigated from the psychosomatic viewpoint. Psychological clinical studies have focused on two variables, personality and emotional characteristics, and emotional antecedents of cancer. Some cancer victims were found to be characterized by a marked tendency to repress experience or suppress expression of certain emotions, especially anger (Greer & Morris, 1975; Abse et al., 1974). A second group of studies (Schonfeld, 1975, 1966) attempting to relate the onset of cancer to recent object loss have produced contradictory results. Another line of investigation on immune mechanisms led to the proposition that events at man's symbolic level of organization and their emotional correlates may modify (enhance or inhibit) the body's immune defenses to cancer.

For example, in animal studies, stressed animals develop tumors more rapidly than nonstressed ones (Riley, 1975). Riley proposes an endocrine theory to account for increased individual susceptibility to cancer.

Etiology in general morbidity rather than specific diseases is another line of research. Epidemiological approaches are taken by Rabkin and Struening (1976), Holmes and Masuda (1974), and Rahe (1975). Hinkle (cited in Rabkin & Struening, 1974) proposes that exposure to social change may lead to a major change in health if the change is subjectively important in the presence of preexistent illness or susceptibility to it, and if there is a significant change in the subject's activities, habits, ingestants, exposure to pathogens, or in a physical character of his environment. When these variables occur in combination, a life event or situation can contribute to morbidity (Dohrenwend & Dohrenwend, 1974). Holmes and Masuda (1974) believe that the magnitude of life change is related to the time of disease onset and the seriousness of the resulting chronic illness. These life changes may contribute to causation of disease by lowering resistance to it. Exposure to life change may also lead to perception of physical symptoms and reports of near-future illness (Rahe, 1975). Several intervening variables (subject's past experience, psychological defenses, coping style, and degree of physiological activation) modify the impact of life change on health, as do social supports (Cassel, 1976; Rabkin & Struening, 1976; Cobb & Rose, 1976). There is evidence that onset of illness is more likely to occur after a person has experienced an event that made adaptive demands on him or her, especially those events signifying a loss for a person.

Lower socioeconomic classes generally have higher rates of morbidity, mortality, and disability (Syme & Berkman, 1976). Although there exists evidence that low status integration is a major form of social stress contributing to disease (Dodge & Martin, 1970), personality variables, enduring behavior patterns, chronic life situations and social conditions need further study to establish its etiological role.

Studies of Mediating Mechanisms

If causal links between social and psychological factors and physiological and pathological changes are to be established, identification of mediating physiological processes and pathways are needed. Research on neurophysiological (Kiely, 1974), neuroendocrine (Whybrow, 1974), and immune mediating mechanisms (Stein, Schiavi, & Camerino, 1976; Amkraut & Solomon, 1974) contribute knowledge to these links.

The most important work in this area recently has been by Mason (1975b). In his work on psychoendocrinology of emotions he has investigated concurrent assays of about 10 hormonal responses to a variety of psychosocial stimuli. Responses to a given situation are affected by the subjects' emotional state, psychological defenses, developmental history, and current psychosocial situation. Mason found that emotion-arousing stimulation produced variations in levels of cortisol, adrenaline, nonadrenaline, thyroxine, insulin, growth hormone, and testosterone. He concluded that psychological influences profoundly alter hormonal balance in the body on both a short and long-term basis and thus may affect all metabolic processes.

Another area of psychophysiological research involves laboratory analogues of "natural" stress and to the daily stresses, such as commuting (Patkai, 1974; Frankenhaeuser, 1975). Increases in catecholamine levels in the blood occur in response to both pleasant and unpleasant situations and during both understimulation and overstimulation. This line of research suggests that repeated and protracted increases in adrenaline and noradrenaline secretion occasioned by recurrent emotional arousal evoked by noise, crowding, appetitive stimuli provided by the media, driving in heavy traffic, and other common stimuli provided by the contemporary affluent environment may contribute to the high prevalence of cardiovascular disease (Pilowsky et al., 1973). Potentially injurious arousal is elicited by novel, discrepant, and unpredictable stimuli and information as well (Lipowski, 1975e, 1975f).

Experimentation in natural settings and situations have also been targets of this line of research. For example, outside of the laboratory, Taggart, Carruthers, and Somerville (1973) have shown that public speakers exhibited tachycardia, changes in ECG, and increased levels of plasma noradrenaline, trigycerides, and free fatty acids. The psychophysiological experimentation in the last two decades has advanced knowledge of the relationship between social stimuli, psychological responses, and the changes in a wide range of physiological functions and indices (Lipowski, 1977). These physiological changes provide links in the sequence of events leading from psychosocial factors to bodily disease.

Stuaies of Psychosocial Responses to Disease

The term somatopsychology has been applied to the study of the influence of psychosocial factors on the course and outcome of all kinds of physical illness (Lipowski, 1975d). The subjective meaning of illness-related information has been shown to be more important for the occurrence of maladaptive responses to disease than the severity of the disease (Lipowski, 1975c). Thus concepts such as coping, illness behavior, and the sick role have come under scrutiny (Lipowski, 1975c; Twaddle, 1972). The patient's response to illness is influenced by the patient's personality, family interactions, and the conscious and unconscious meaning for him or her of the diseased organ, dysfunction, and diagnostic label (Lipowski, 1975c). The meaning of illness affect the kind and intensity of the emotional response to personal illness are related to the meaning of the illness and affect its course and outcome. Anxiety generated by subjective evaluation of illness in cardiac patients may precipitate every major complication of heart disease (Gentry & William, 1975; Lipowski, 1975e; Pilowsky et al., 1973; Cay, Vetter, & Philip, 1972) can also contribute to psychogenic invalidism following myocardial infarction (Cay et al., 1973).

Lipowski, 1975d, for example, found that that psychiatric complications are common among the physically ill. Medical and psychiatric disorders coexist in 25 to 50% of the patients studied in every type of treatment setting. This high incidence of psychological concomitants of physical illness underscores the necessity for integrated medical and psychological health care and for continued growth of health care professionals concerned with psychological factors of illness and disease.

Psychological reactions to modern medical and surgical treatment and therapeutic environments are common (Lipowski, 1972; Aitken & Cay, 1975). All varieties of medical procedures (open-heart and coronary bypass surgery, chronic renal hemodialysis, and organ transplantation) have brought both benefits and psychiatric casualties (Howels, 1976; Abram, 1975). Research in thanatology further suggests psychological reactions in both patient and family in terminal illness (Lipowski, 1975a).

As in all areas involving psychological complications, attempts to develop preventative procedures and tactics have been attempted. However, psychosomatic etiological studies have had limited success (Hurst, Jenkins, & Rose, 1976) in this area. Current medical practice and training, however, reflect development of effective prevention and treatment of psychological complications of disease and disability developed by somatopsychological research (Lipowski, 1977).

Studies of Influence of Somatic Processes on Behavior

This area of research refers to the study of psychological aspects of cerebral function and dysfunction. Recent research on brain-behavior relationships has contributed to the understanding of psychosomatic processes (Kurczmar & Eccles, 1972). Recent studies of psychopathological manifestations of cerebral disorders has yielded a more precise understanding of these relationships (Lipowski, 1975b). Recently, a biopsychosocial perspective of behavior which argues that all verbal and nonverbal behaviors have physiological, endocrine, and neural components has shown implications for studies of emotion, anxiety, and all interventions, including verbal psychotherapies (Schwartz, 1978).

Studies of Behavior-Modifying Therapies

The application of treatments aimed at modifying behavior to somatic disorders has enjoyed rapid development in recent years. This development has depended on advancement in psychopharmacology and behavior modification. Studies on biofeedback (Hauri, 1975; Birk, 1973), behavioral modification (Price, 1974), and various relaxation techniques (Benson, Greenwood, & Klemchuk, 1975) have had a tremendous impact on the control of psychological concomitants of disease and illness. Therapeutic applications in medicine are commonplace today in medicine and treatment centers. These techniques reflect the belief that man has a measure of volitional control over visceral functions, which may be used to counteract potentially injurious physiological arousal elicited by the stresses of modern life. The somewhat older techniques used with psychiatric patients for years (psychotropic drugs (Solow, 1975), individual and group psychotherapies (Kinston & Wolff, 1975; Stein, 1971), and hypnosis (Frankel, 1975)) are variously applied to modify physiological functions and somatic disorders by means of effects on psychological functions and behavior.

IMPLICATIONS OF PSYCHOSOMATIC THEORY FOR PSYCHOLOGISTS

The psychosomatic aspects of health and illness presented above constitute one of the most vital areas of contemporary science, thought, and medicine (Lipowski, 1977). The relevance of psychosocial factors to health in times of rapid social change demanding adaptation is compelling (World Health Organization, 1974). It is important to note again that it is at the interface between the various disciplines concerned with man, and with health and disease, that the foremost intellectual challenge faces science today. Current psychosomatic theory is more diversified, scientifically rigorous, methodologically resourceful, and therapeutically relevant than ever before. Its hallmarks include a multifactorial approach to the study of the health and disease, formulation of testable hypotheses and their careful validation, and concern with the clinical applicability of research and development of integrative theories to harness its complexity. The implications of the current advances in the field of medicine, psychiatry, and the behavioral sciences are far reaching and continued growth is inevitable (Engel, 1974; Freyham, 1976). The scientific and clinical issues that this discipline has addressed have a bearing on man's survival and quality of life (Lipowski, 1977).

Many psychologists have in the past narrowly confined their involvement in health care service to "mental health." However, in recent years a growing number of them have begun to apply psychological principles which are often adapted from clinical psychology to physical illness as well. This is presently seen as a kind of revolution among clinicians and researchers (Masur, 1979) and has come to be termed "medical psychology" in the psychological community.

The term *medical psychology*, even though widely used and even accepted, is still objected to by many psychologists because of the tacit endorsement of the medical model of disease they believe it presupposes. However, psychologists must recognize that some of the most significant contributions made by medical psychologists have resulted from their unique psychological/behavioral paradigms which are different from a strictly medical approach. The point has been made that the psychologist is better equipped to deal with problems at the interface between psychology and health than the psychiatrist because the medical model orientation is theoretically or practically inappropriate (Masur, 1979).

Behavioral medicine, as it is currently defined (Schwartz & Weiss, 1978b), embraces the concepts of psychosomatic theory and research and application. It might be proposed, then, that behavioral medicine is a term that is a current adaptation to that endeavor previously termed "psychosomatic." Leigh and Reiser (1977) have, in fact, suggested that the modern approach to medicine be relabeled behavioral medicine. However, the fact that psychosomatic theory and research has been developed and embraced primarily by medicine should not predispose the psychologist to reject it. Such a short-sighted reaction would be tantamount to an unscientific reaction to legitimate scientific endeavor in areas relevant to the work of psychologists. Contrariwise, the psychologist should take the responsibility of building on those findings within the expertise of psychological/behavioral methodology and techniques. As an integral component of behavioral medicine, medical psychologists have an important role to play. Psychology as a discipline can and does interface with almost all of the other behavioral and biomedical disciplines. Researchers and clinicians of all disciplines must further define the cross-links that substantiate the integration of these various disciples.

It is instructive to note that psychologists have become involved in many of the research areas delineated by psychosomatic theory, although there is no formal acknowledgment of that fact. The literature suggests that there exists a belief among some psychologists that if new terms are used, the connection to psychosomatic medicine will be lost. Thus, the terms health and health care psychology are often used instead of the offensive word medical psychology, and the call of psychologists to contribute to knowledge about health and disease is presented as a new idea and endeavor which has no history. The point must be made that psychologists' involvement in health and health care, in disease and illness, indeed does have a history. In the enthusiasm to journey into new vistas, psychologists must not fail to recognize the roots of that journey.

To illustrate the point, comparisons may be made of the areas of involvement for psychologists in the psychological aspects of health and disease proposed by the APA Task Force on Health Research (1976) to those areas of psychosomatic research already outlined. This comparison shows that the Task Force highlighted most of the areas presented by Lipowski (1977) as legitimate areas for extended psychological involvement. Particularly stressed were those areas designated as the study of psychosocial factors in (1) etiology, (2) response to illness, (3) influence of somatic processes on psychological functioning, and (4) application of behavior-modifying therapies on somatic disorders. The areas the Task Force pointed out as most neglected involves psychologists' potential in effecting important improvements in health maintenance, illness prevention, and health care delivery, that is, the areas designated as psychosocial factors in etiology and psychosocial factors in the course and outcome of physical illness, and the larger area of systems analysis.

In reviewing the current patterns of psychological research on health, the Task Force was able to identify a low number of approximately 500 psychologists who have definite interests in health research. The Task Force used the PASAR system to identify literature cited in *Psychological Abstracts* on psychological aspects of (1) physical illness, (2) physical disability, or (3) health. They also included the role of the psychologist and of psychological research in the delivery of health services, excluding mental health services unless they were more generally a part of health services. During the years 1966–1973, the Task Force was able to identify only 350 relevant articles. Psychobiological aspects of health accounted for 66% of the abstracts. These abstracts included topics such as effects of stress, psychosomatics, social and environmental factors, and the effects of physical health and biological cycles on personality and behavior. Research related to health care delivery accounted for 18% of the abstracts which typically dealt with relatively specific aspects of treatment and rehabilitation rather than with larger issues or systems research. Studies of attitudes related to health and health care accounted for the remaining 16% of the abstracts. Based on this analysis and other work suggesting that psychologists publish mostly in traditional areas such as psychotherapy, mental retardation, and schizophrenia, the Task Force concludes that American psychologists have not sufficiently addressed the problems of health and illness either in applied or basic research activity, nor have they perceived the potentials for their work effecting important improvements in health maintenance, illness prevention, and health care delivery.

The Task Force acknowledges that "humanity's total functional health is threatened whenever either side of the interactive mind-body equation is neglected"

(1976, p. 271). They call for graduate education to instill in researchers an early awareness of the needs and opportunities to apply psychological principles and methods to the understanding and improvement of health behaviors. Furthermore, they outline a role for psychologists of virtually every specialty in the quest for factors determining health or illness at the molecular or molar levels. Thus, subtle physical responses to perception of threat is within the purview of the psychophysiologist; the behavioral predispositions (attitudes) to illness or health is within that of the personality researchers; the influence of group mores on susceptibility or resistance to health education and practices is within that of the social psychologist; the design of instruments to quantify important qualitative variables of health services is within that of the measurement expert; design of health care delivery systems is within that of the organizational psychologist; and the identification of variables which influence understanding, storing, and action upon health-related information is within that of the educational psychologist.

Most of all, the Task Force emphasizes that areas open to psychological investigations have a wide range, from health care practices and health care delivery systems to the management of acute and chronic illness and the psychology of medication and pain. They stress that psychologists should acknowledge that they are life scientists and consequently health scientists. There is need for psychologists to be aware of research by other psychologists and other disciplines. A further need suggested by the Task Force is to design innovative programs of graduate training to prepare psychologists to carry their expertise effectively into the general clinic, the hospital, the rehabilitation center, the community health center, and the group medical practice.

PSYCHOLOGY'S INTERFACE WITH PEDIATRICS

Pediatric psychology, as it has been researched and practiced to date, represents most of the areas of investigation and practice suggested above. As one of the earliest groups of psychologists to become formally concerned with the interface of psychology and health and illness, they have struggled with a definition of their specialty, the roles and role boundaries, their techniques, their substantive areas of involvement both in research and practice. Most of all, pediatric psychologists have exemplified the scientist-practitioner model of psychology, being productive in design of new delivery of services, program design, and research in those areas as well as other areas, including psychosocial factors in specific disease entities, health maintenance attitudes and practices, response to illness and therapeutic procedures, compliance behavior, and the sick role, as it applies to children.

The role of the pediatric psychologist in interface with pediatricians is yet evolving, but the strong activity both in practice and research during more than a decade has yielded a body of knowledge which describes the functions and potentials of this specialty. The specifics of that role as the pediatric psychologist develops an important place in the medical care of children is presented in the chapters that follow. It is clear at this point that although the roles are not mature, important advances have been accomplished and the potential development is enormous.

SUMMARY

This chapter reviews the emergence of pediatric psychology as the first identifiable group of professional psychologists to expand psychological/behavioral principles into nonpsychiatric health settings. The first definition of pediatric psychology embraced the notion that the interface between psychologist and nonpsychiatric childrens' medical settings was the area of concern for the pediatric psychologist. Note is made of the fact that early in the development of the specialty, the scope of involvement of the psychologist in pediatric settings was broad, covering such areas as developmental considerations, parent training in preventive measures, concern with the effects of physical illness and hospitalization on the physically ill child. From this early inception, the interdisciplinary model was also accepted.

As the general psychological community became more aware of the potentials for psychologists' contribution to health care and the understanding of health-related behaviors, conceptualizations of this integration of psychology and medicine were articulated. Within the concepts of *medical psychology, behavioral medicine, health psychology* and *health care psychology* were contained the many roles and concerns of the early pediatric psychologists. Indeed, pediatric psychology is a member discipline of the group now designated "medical psychology," which is itself a part of the larger interdisciplinary field designated today as "behavioral medicine." Distinctions between health professional and mental health professionals were made in the deliberations of various groups of psychologists from within and without APA. Mental health is considered a part of the health sciences, and indeed the life sciences, but is a very small part of the total possible endeavor of psychologists, that is, the part integrating psychology with another member of the behavioral medicine field, psychiatry. The possibilities of involvement of psychology is very much broadened in today's view, as the conceptualization of behavioral medicine with its cross-links to a myriad of other biomedical and behavioral disciplines is now being explored. While clinical psychologists are involved in this movement into interface with other health disciplines, it is by no means the only specialty of psychology which can and does play a role. Virtually every specialty area within psychology has been proposed to have potential in the total consideration of health care, health maintenance, and health care delivery.

The influences which have been designated as focusing psychology's attention to the potentials in this fertile area consist of the progress of behavioral, medical, and public health sciences, as well as the sociopolitical forces in the American health care crisis. Reconceptualizations of the mind-body problems and physical health—mental health dichotomies have resulted in a new medical model embracing a holistic view of the physically ill person and a new psychosomatic model. An ecological perspective on health and illness as "biopsychosocial" phenomena has thus emerged.

The thrust of efforts of today's psychology is to enter the arena of scientific and professional involvement represented by psychosomatic theory. Since the theoretical assumptions and tradition of addressing the mind-body problem in research and clinical practice is provided within psychosomatic medicine, that theory in its current status is herein presented. This presentation stresses that psychological, biological, and social factors must be considered as codeterminants of the development, course, and outcome of physical and psychiatric disorders. A historical perspective, dominant theoretical concepts and formulations of psychosomatic theory are also presented. The current status of research in several areas are also briefly reviewed, for example, etiological studies, studies of mediating mechanisms, of psychosocial response to physical illness, of influence of somatic processes on psychological functioning, and effectiveness of behavior-modifying therapies on somatic disorders.

Implications of psychosomatic theory for psychologists are then considered in light of the current view that psychosomatic aspects of health and illness are vital areas of contemporary science and thought, as well as of medicine. Psychology's potent role in the integration of psychology and medicine is stressed.

The recommendations of the APA Task Force on Health Research for psychologists' involvement in the health system in great part parallels the concerns and conceptualizations of psychosomatic theory and research. Those recommendations encompass psychological investigation ranging from health care practices and health care delivery systems to the management of acute and chronic illness and to the psychology of medication and pain.

Finally, pediatric psychology is discussed in terms of its development in research and clinical applications of psychology in interface with pediatrics as it relates to health and illness in children. Pediatric psychologists have exemplified the scientist-practitioner model of psychology. They have been productive both in design of new service delivery and research in many areas, including psychosocial factors in specific diseases, health maintenance, attitudes and practices, response to illness and therapeutic procedures, compliance behavior, and the sick role. The role of the pediatric psychologist in interface with pediatricians is still in the process of evolving, but strong activity in practice and research during more than a decade has yielded a body of knowledge which describes the functions and potentials of this specialty. The descriptions of developments advanced by these pioneering "medical psychologists" is the purpose of the succeeding chapters in this book. With documentation of what pediatric psychologists have accomplished to date, new applications in research and clinical practice and innovations in training are possible.

REFERENCES

Abram, H. S. Psychiatry and medical progress: Therapeutic considerations. *International Journal of Psychiatry and Medicine,* 1975, **6,** 203−211.

Abse, D. W., Wilkins, M. M., & Van de Castle, R. L. Personality and behavioral characteristics of lung cancer patients. *Journal of Psychosomatic Research,* 1974, **18,** 101−113.

Ader, R. The role of developmental factors in susceptibility to disease. *International Journal of Psychiatry and Medicine,* 1974, **5,** 367−376.

Aitken, C., Cay, E. L. Clinical psychosomatic research. *International Journal of Psychiatry and Medicine,* 1975, **6,** 29−41.

Alexander, F. *Psychosomatic medicine.* New York: Norton, 1950.

Alexander, F., French, T. M., & Pollock, G. H. (Eds.) *Psychosomatic specificity.* Chicago: University of Chicago Press, 1968.

Amkraut, H., & Solomon, G. F. From the symbolic stimulus to the pathophysiologic response: Immune mechanisms. *International Journal of Psychiatry and Medicine,* 1974, **5,** 541−563.

APA Task Force on Health Research. Contributions of psychology to health research: Patterns, problems, potentials. *American Psychologist,* 1976, **31,** 263−274.

Asken, M. J. Medical psychology: Toward definition, clarification and organization. *Professional Psychology,* 1979, **10,** 66−73.

Benson, H., Greenwood, M. M., & Klemchuk, H. The relaxation response: Psychophysiologic aspects and clinical applications. *International Journal of Psychiatry and Medicine,* 1975, **6,** 87−98.

Birk, L. (Ed.) *Biofeedback: Behavioral medicine.* New York: Grune & Stratton, 1973.

Cassel, J. The contribution of the social environment to host resistance. *American Journal of Epidemiology,* 1976, **104,** 107−123.

Cay, E. L., Vetter, N., & Philip, A. E. Psychological status during recovery from an acute heart attack. *Journal of Psychosomatic Research,* 1972, **16,** 425−435.

Cay, E. L., Vetter, N., & Philip, A. E. Return to work after a heart attack. *Journal of Psychosomatic Research,* 1973, **17,** 231−243.

Clayton, P. J. The clinical morbidity of the first year of bereavement: A review. *Comparative Psychiatry,* 1973, **14,** 151−157.

Cobb, S., & Rose, R. M. Hypertension, peptic ulcer and diabetes in air traffic controllers. *Journal of the American Medical Association,* 1973, **224,** 489−492.

Cummings, N. Prolonged (ideal) versus short-term (realistic) psychotherapy. *Professional Psychology,* 1977, **8,** 491−501.

Dodge, D. L., & Martin, W. T. *Social stress and chronic illness.* Notre Dame, IN: University of Notre Dame Press, 1970.

Dohrenwend, B. S., & Dohrenwend, B. P. (Eds.) *Stressful life events: Their nature and effects.* New York: Wiley, 1974.

Dubos, R. *Man, medicine and environment.* New York: American Library, 1968.

Eliot, R. S. (Ed.) *Stress and health.* Mount Kisco, NY: Futura, 1974.

Engel, G. L. A unified concept of health and disease. *Perspectives in Biological Medicine,* 1960, **3,** 459−485.

Engel, G. L. Memorial lecture: The psychosomatic approach to individual susceptibility to disease. *Gastroenterology,* 1974, **67,** 1080−1093.

Engel, G. L. The need for a new medical model: A challenge for biomedicine. *Science,* 1977, **196,** 129−136.

Engel, G. L., & Schmale, A. H. Conservation withdrawal: A primary regulatory process for organismic homeostasis. In *Physiology, emotion and psychosomatic illness.* Ciba Foundation Symposium 8 (new series). Amsterdam: Elsevier, 1972.

Frankel, F. H. Hypnosis as a treatment method in psychosomatic medicine. *International Journal of Psychiatry and Medicine,* 1975, **6,** 75–85.

Frankenhaeuser, M. Experimental approaches to the study of catecholamines and emotions. In L. Levi (Ed.), *Emotions—Their parameters and measurement,* New York: Raven Press, 1975.

Freyham, F. A. Is psychosomatic obsolete? A psychiatric reappraisal. *Comprehensive Psychiatry,* 1976, **17,** 381–386.

Friedman, M., & Roseman, R. H. *Type A behavior and your health.* New York: Knopf, 1974.

Gentry, W. D., & William, R. B. (Eds.) *Myocardial infarction and coronary care.* St. Louis: Mosby, 1975.

Goldman, H., Kleinman, K. M., & Snow, M. Y. Relationship between essential hypertension and cognitive functioning: Effects of biofeedback. *Psychophysiology,* 1975, **12,** 569–573.

Greer, S., & Morris, T. Psychological attributes of women who develop breast cancer: A controlled study. *Journal of Psychosomatic Research,* 1975, **19,** 147–153.

Grinker, R. R. *Psychosomatic research.* New York: Norton, 1953.

Hauri, P. P. Biofeedback and self-control of physiological functions: Clinical applications. *International Journal of Psychiatry and Medicine,* 1975, **6,** 255–265.

Hinkle, L. E. The concept of "stress" in the biological and social sciences. *International Journal of Psychiatry and Medicine,* 1974, **5,** 335–357.

Holmes, T. H., & Masuda, M. Life change and illness susceptibility. In B. S. Dohrenwend & B. P. Dohrenwend (Eds.), *Stressful life events: Their nature and effects.* New York: Wiley, 1974.

Howells, J. G. (Ed.) *Modern perspectives in the psychiatric aspects of surgery.* New York: Brunner/Mazel, 1976.

Jenkins, D. C. Psychologic and social risk factors for coronary disease. *New England Journal of Medicine,* 1976, **294,** 987–994. (a)

Jenkins, D. C. Recent evidence supporting psychologic and social risk factors for coronary disease. *New England Journal of Medicine,* 1976, **294,** 1033–1038. (b)

Kasl, S. V., Gore, S., & Cobb, S. The experience of losing a job: Reported changes in health, symptoms and illness behavior. *Psychosomatic Medicine,* 1975, **37,** 106–122.

Kellner, R. Psychotherapy in psychosomatic disorders. *Archives of General Psychiatry,* 1975, **32,** 1021–1028.

Kenny, T. J. Pediatric psychology: A reflective approach. *Pediatric Psychology,* 1975, **3,** 8.

Kiely, W. F. From the symbolic stimulus to the psychophysiological response: Neurophysiological mechanisms. *International Journal of Psychiatry and Medicine,* 1974, **5,** 517–529.

Kinston, M., & Wolff, H. Bodily communication and psycho-therapy: A psychosomatic approach. *International Journal of Psychiatry and Medicine,* 1975, **6,** 195–201.

Kurczmar, A. G., & Eccles, J. C. (Eds.) *Brain and human behavior.* New York: Springer-Verlag, 1972.

Lazarus, R. S. *Psychological stress and the coping process.* New York: McGraw-Hill, 1960.

Leigh, H., & Reiser, M. F. Major trends in psychosomatic medicine: The psychiatrists evolving role in medicine. *Annals of Internal Medicine,* 1977, **87,** 233−239.

Levi, L. (Ed.) *Emotions—Their parameters and measurement.* New York: Raven Press, 1975.

Lipowski, Z. J. Review of consultation psychiatry and psychosomatic medicine: Theoretical issues. *Psychosomatic Medicine,* 1968, **30,** 395−422.

Lipowski, Z. J. (Ed.) *Psychological aspects of physical disease.* Basel: S. Karger, 1972.

Lipowski, Z. J. Psychosomatic medicine in a changing society: Some current trends in theory and research. *Comprehensive Psychiatry,* 1973, **14,** 203−215.

Lipowski, Z. J. Consultation-liaison psychiatry: Past, present and future. In R. O. Pasnau (Ed.), *Consultation liaison psychiatry,* New York: Grune & Stratton, 1975. (a)

Lipowski, Z. J. Organic brain syndromes: Overview and classification. In D. F. Benson & D. Blumer (Eds.), *Psychiatric aspects of neurological disease,* 1975. (b)

Lipowski, Z. J. Physical illness, the patient and his environment: Psychosocial foundations of medicine. In S. Arieti & M. F. Reiser (Eds.), *American Handbook of Psychiatry,* 2nd ed., Vol. 4. New York: Basic Books, 1975 (c)

Lipowski, Z. J. Psychiatry of somatic diseases: Epidemiology, pathogenesis, classification. *Comprehensive Psychiatry,* 1975, **16,** 105−124. (d)

Lipowski, Z. J. Psychophysiological cardiovascular disorders. In A. M. Freedman, H. I. Kaplan, & B. J. Sadock (Eds.), *Comprehensive textbook of psychiatry,* 2nd ed., Vol. 2. Baltimore: Williams and Wilkins, 1975. (e)

Lipowski, Z. J. Sensory and information overload: Behavioral effects. *Comprehensive Psychiatry,* 1975, **16,** 199−211. (f)

Lipowski, Z. J. Psychosomatic medicine in the seventies: An overview. *American Journal of Psychiatry,* 1977, **134,** 233−244.

Lipowski, Z. J. (Ed.) *Psychosocial aspects of physical illness.* Basel: S. Karger, 1972.

Lipowski, Z. J., Lipsitt, D. R., & Whybrow, P. C. (Eds.). *Psychosomatic medicine: Current trends and clinical applications.* New York: Oxford University Press, 1977.

Mason, J. W. A historical view of the stress field. *Journal of Human Stress,* 1975, **11,** 6−12. (a)

Mason, J. W. Emotion as reflected in patterns of endocrine integration. In L. Levi (Ed.), *Emotions—Their parameters and measurement.* New York: Raven Press, 1975. (b)

Masur, F. T. An update on medical psychology and behavioral medicine. *Professional Psychology,* 1979, **10,** 259−264.

McLean, A. (Ed.) *Occupational stress.* Springfield, IL: Charles C. Thomas, 1974.

Meissner, W. W. Family process and psychosomatic disease. *International Journal of Psychiatry and Medicine,* 1974, **5,** 411−430.

Minuchin, S., Baker, L., & Rosman, B. L. A conceptual model of psychosomatic illness in children. *Archives of General Psychiatry,* 1975, **32,** 1031−1038.

Patkai, P. Laboratory studies of psychological stress. *International Journal of Psychiatry and Medicine,* 1974, **5,** 575−585.

Pilowsky, I., Spalding, D., & Shaw, J. Hypertension and personality. *Psychosomatic Medicine,* 1973, **35,** 50−56.

Price, K. P. The application of behavioral therapy to the treatment of psychosomatic disorders: Retrospect and prospect. *Psychotherapy: Theory, Research and Practice,* 1974, **2,** 138−155.

Rabkin, J. G., & Struening, E. L. Life events, stress, and illness. *Science,* 1976, **194,** 1013–1020.

Rahe, R. H. Epidemiological studies of life change and illness. *International Journal of Psychiatry and Medicine,* 1975, **6,** 133–146.

Rather, L. J. *Mind and body in eighteenth century medicine.* Berkeley: University of California Press, 1965.

Riley, V. Mouse mammary tumors: Alteration of incidence as apparent function of stress. *Science,* 1975, **189,** 465–567.

Reiser, M. F. Organic disorders and psychosomatic medicine. In S. Arieti (Ed.), *American handbook of psychiatry,* 2nd ed., Vol. 4. New York: Basic Books, 1975.

Roessler, R., & Engel, B. T. The current status of the concepts of physiological response specificity and activation. *International Journal of Psychiatry and Medicine,* 1974, **5,** 359–366.

Schmale, A. H. Giving up as a final common pathway to changes in health. In Z. J. Lipowski (Ed.), *Psychosocial aspects of physical illness.* Basel: S. Karger, 1972.

Schmale, A., & Iker, H. The psychological setting of uterine cervical cancer. *N.Y. Academy of Sciences,* 1966, **125,** 807-813.

Schofield, W. The role of psychology in the delivery of health services. *American Psychologist,* 1968, **24,** 565–584.

Schonfeld, J. Psychological and life experience differences between Israeli women with benign and cancerous breast lesions. *Journal of Psychosomatic Research,* 1975, **19,** 229–234.

Schwartz, G. E. Psychobiological foundations of psychotherapy and behavior change. In S. L. Garfield & A. E. Bergin, *Handbook of psychotherapy and behavior change: An empirical analysis,* 2nd ed. New York: Wiley, 1978.

Schwartz, G. E., & Weiss, S. M. Behavioral medicine revisited: An amended definition. *Journal of Behavioral Medicine,* 1978, **1,** 249–251. (b)

Schwartz, G. E., & Weiss, S. M. Yale conference on behavioral medicine: A proposed definition and statement of goals. *Journal of Behavioral Medicine,* 1978, **1,** 3–12. (a)

Shapiro, D., & Surwit, R. S. Operant conditioning: A new theoretical approach in psychosomatic medicine. *International Journal of Psychiatry and Medicine,* 1974, **5,** 377–387.

Solow, C. Psychotropic drugs in somatic disorders. *International Journal of Psychiatry and Medicine,* 1975, **6,** 267–282.

Stein, A. Group therapy with psychosomatically ill patients. In H. I. Kaplan & B. J. Sadock (Eds.), *Comprehensive group psychotherapy.* Baltimore: Williams & Wilkins, 1971.

Stein, M., Schiavi, R. C., & Camerino, M. Influence of brain and behavior on the immune system. *Science,* 1976, **191,** 435–440.

Syme, S. L. & Berkman, L. F. Social class, susceptibility and sickness. *American Journal of Epidemiology,* 1976, **104,** 1–8.

Taggert, P., Carruthers, M., & Somerville, W. Electrocardiogram, plasma catecholamines and lipids, and their modification by oxprenolol when speaking before an audience. *Lancet,* 1973, **3,** 341–346.

Thurlow, H. J. General susceptibility to illness: A selective review. *Canadian Medical Association Journal,* 1967, **97,** 1397–1404.

Twaddle, A. C. The concepts of the sick role and illness behavior. In Z. J. Lipowski (Ed.), *Psychosocial aspects of physical illness.* Basel: S. Karger, 1972.

Whybrow, P. C., & Silberfarb, P. M. Neuroendocrine mediating mechanisms from the symbolic stimulus to the physiological response. *International Journal of Psychiatry and Medicine,* 1974, **5,** 531–539.

Wiggins, J. G. The psychologist as a health professional in the health maintenance organization. In C. A. Kiesler, N. A. Cummings, & G. R. VandenBos (Eds.), *Psychology and national health insurance: A sourcebook.* Washington, DC: American Psychological Association, 1979.

Wolff, J. G. *Stress and disease.* Springfield, IL: Charles C. Thomas, 1953.

World Health Organization. *Technical discussion 6,* 27th World Health Assembly, Geneva, 1974.

Wright, L. The pediatric psychologist: A role model. *American Psychologist,* 1967, **22,** 323–325

CHAPTER 2

Psychological Effects of Physical Illness and Its Concomitants

Diane J. Willis
Charles H. Elliott
Susan M. Jay

OVERVIEW OF NORMAL GROWTH AND DEVELOPMENT IN CHILDREN

The psychological effects of illness on a child can be best understood within a developmental framework. As Travis (1976) stated, "What illness means to a child at the time it occurs, and the impression it leaves on his personality, are largely affected by his stage of development" (p. 57). Erik Erikson's theory of psychosocial development is particularly relevant in understanding and conceptualizing the psychological impact of physical illness in children. Erikson (1964) emphasized the importance of external social and environmental events in influencing personality development. He described eight stages, each of which involves a particular kind of encounter with the environment. Developmental "tasks" must be mastered at each stage in order to progress optimally to the next stage. Serious problems or disruptions at any one stage may prevent optimal growth and mastery of later developmental tasks. Physical illness may be conceptualized as an event which has definite implications at each stage of development, and which has the potential to prevent or increase the difficulty of optimal progression from one stage to the next.

Erikson's scheme is presented in order to clarify the psychological implications of physical illness at each stage of development. Aspects of other developmental theories will be incorporated in order to consolidate and integrate relevant aspects of a child's social, emotional, and cognitive development.

Basic Trust (Birth to 1½ Years)

Erikson (1964) maintains that the primary developmental task of infancy is the attainment of a sense of basic trust. During the first 1½ years of life the infant progresses from a helpless organism dominated by physiological needs to a toddler who is capable of independent social and motoric action and reciprocal interaction with significant others. During the early weeks of life, the infant's waking contacts with external reality are minimal and are confined to hunger arousal, feeding, and subsequent need reduction. Physiological processes are dominant; the infant exists in a world of undifferentiated sensation.

Around two months of age, the infant becomes aware that need satisfaction comes from outside the self. The infant begins to associate need satisfaction with visual, olfactory, and tactile contact with the mother. The infant enters what Mahler (1965) refers to as the symbiotic stage, which is the beginning of the social relationship between the mother and the child. The infant is no longer completely self-absorbed; instead the infant becomes increasingly invested in the mother and an emotional bond develops between mother and child which has been referred to by Bowlby as attachment (Bowlby, 1969). The mother becomes the focal point of the child's world and it is in this symbiotic relationship that the origins of basic trust reside. The mother is the infant's first social contact; the majority of the infant's experiences with the outside world are mediated through the mother. She feeds the infant when he/she is hungry, soothes the infant when he/she cries, and provides the infant with visual, tactile, auditory, and social stimulation. The quality and consistency of the mother's responsiveness and care of the infant during this time are critical in defining the infant's perception of the "goodness" or "badness," the dependability or lack of dependability, of the external world.

As the attachment between mother and child is strengthened, separation anxiety and stranger anxiety become prominent. Such anxiety indicates the infant's heightened capacity to distinguish the familiar from the strange, and to distinguish mother from others. The infant begins to smile differentially at the mother. The infant is also beginning to differentiate self from others. The infant begins to actively manipulate objects, to explore his body, the mother's body, and the external environment; the infant's curiosity and interest seem unlimited. Piaget and Inhelder (1969) emphasized the critical importance of the infant's active interaction with the environment during this period; they maintain that the origins of intelligence lie in the child's sensorimotor experience.

Through numerous experiences with the mother and with others, and through various experiments with objects, the infant develops the concept of object permanence. The infant learns that when an object disappears from view, it still exists even though he or she cannot see it. Likewise, the infant learns the mother will reappear after her departure. As Erikson (1964) stated, "The infant's first social achievement, then, is his willingness to let the mother out of sight without undue anxiety or rage, because she has become an inner certainty as well as an outer predictability" (p. 247). The development of object permanence means that the infant can maintain an image of mother which can sustain the absence of the mother and allay the infant's anxiety during her absence.

The implications of serious illness during the first 18 months of life are numerous. Physical illness and/or hospitalization may interrupt, delay, or inhibit the attachment process between mother and child. Due to the nature of the illness or to hospitalization procedures, the infant may be deprived of essential experiences with the mother such as being held, spoken to, rocked, cuddled, and soothed when distressed. According to Barowsky (1978), such deprivation impedes normal emotional and intellectual development. Severe or prolonged maternal deprivation may result in "failure-to-thrive" syndrome and/or to what Spitz (1965) referred to as "anaclitic depression." In such syndromes, the infant becomes listless, apathetic, and withdrawn, and social and intellectual development may be delayed.

The physically ill infant's first contacts with the external world may consist of isolation or painful and traumatic experiences over which the mother has little control. Such experiences may result in initial perceptions of the external world as painful, frightening, and unfulfilling, precipitating frustrated withdrawal by the infant and contributing to delays in the development of a sense of trust and assurance in relation to external reality.

Physical illness and/or hospitalization often result in numerous separations, thus making normal resolution of separation anxiety difficult. Poorly resolved separation anxiety may result in what Bowlby (1969) termed "anxious attachment" manifested by clinging, crying, and dysphoric behaviors as opposed to a confident, unproblematic attachment. If physical activity and exploration of objects and environment are severely inhibited by physical illness, intellectual delays may result. The development of object permanence may be delayed, thus compounding the anxiety of separation since the infant has no internal image of the mother to allay anxiety. The task of developing basic trust is made difficult when early experiences with the external world are traumatic and painful, when emotional attachment is tentative, and when intellect is too primitive for comprehension or organization of such circumstances.

Autonomy (1½ to 3 Years)

Just as the infant learned a sense of trust in others and in the environment in the first 18 months of life, the task of developing confidence in his or her own abilities and actions is mastered with the approach to the second year of life. Autonomy is the child's quest; increasing motoric abilities allow unlimited opportunities to test newly gained independence. The child cherishes the separateness of a new identity which is declared at every chance by saying "no," by being oppositional, and by being demanding and often unreasonable. The toddler values himself to the point of being omnipotent and egocentric. Egocentrism and omnipotence are evident in thinking which is highly intuitive, imaginative, and magical. For toddlers, causality is rooted not in logic but in magic, and they experiment, pretend, and fantasize without regard for logical cause-and-effect reality (Erikson, 1964; Piaget & Inhelder, 1969).

The acquisition of language allows a breakthrough in communication with others and increases the child's repertoire of self-enhancing and self-confirming skills. Language is useful in the development of internalized prohibitions since the child learns to substitute words for actions. As the toddler is constantly manipulating the environment, exploring new possibilities, and testing his or her own limits as an autonomous individual, parental discipline and limit-setting become necessary in curbing unmanageable behavior. The toddler needs to feel this new independence and individuality are accepted and appreciated but also needs to receive protection and security through external controls on her or his behavior. Through kind but firm parental discipline, the child gradually develops control of impulses and learns bowel and bladder control.

For the toddler, restricted physical activity and exploration due to physical illness may preclude sufficient opportunity to experiment with a newly gained autonomy. Bed-ridden children may become passive, apathetic, and overly dependent on others. They may exhibit regressive behavior such as baby talk, clinging, temper tantrums, and so on. Painful and intrusive medical procedures may contribute to feelings of helplessness and lack of control over the environment. The child may react to this lack of control by becoming extremely demanding and controlling of others, as if to disprove total helplessness.

Although the young child needs firm limits, parents may feel reluctant to discipline the sick child resulting in delayed development of impulse control. The undisciplined child may become manipulative, demanding, and disobedient, thus magnifying an already troublesome situation. Children at this age are likely to view illness and/or hospitalization as punishment. Children may react to such "punishment" with overly compulsive, eager-to-please behavior as if to repent for wrongdoing. Although separation anxiety is lessened at this age, it is still manifest, particularly in stressful situations, and when the mother is absent for longer than a routine, short separation.

Initiative (3 to 6 Years)

In the third stage of childhood, a new sense of initiative emerges. Whereas previously the child's self-will inspired acts of defiance and protested independence, initiative now becomes more goal-oriented and self-activated. The "I" replaces the "no" in the child's motivation toward action (Fraiberg, 1959). The child takes pleasure in conquest and attack and fantasizes about being powerful. At the same time the child becomes aware of genital differences and develops a sense of self as male or female. Identity at this age is merged with the feeling of completeness and integrity of one's physical body; how the child feels about his or her body will determine in large part how the child feels about himself or herself. Bodily integrity is a major issue and children at this age may develop fantasies and fears of bodily damage and mutilation. Such fears and fantasies are tremendously magnified when reality confirms them, as in the case of children who undergo surgical procedures and who suffer from disfigurement resulting from illness. The physically ill child may develop a sense of inadequacy due to the fact that his/her body is not functioning in an optimal manner.

The preschool child begins to exhibit a more intensive attachment and interest in the opposite-sexed parent and may fantasize replacing the same-sexed parent. However, the rivalry is gradually overcome by the child's identification with the same-sexed parent. Identification indicates that egocentrism is giving way to a more other-oriented social adaptation. The child's personal identity and self-concept crystallize during this stage on the basis of bodily perception, experiments in initiative and action, and resolution of competition and rivalry with the same-sexed parent. Since magical thinking and egocentrism dominate the preschool child's cognitive structure, confusion over causality of illness may develop. The child may view illness and/or hospitalization as punishment for oedipal fantasies. Disproportionate guilt, self-blame, and poor self-esteem may develop as a result of confused causality about illness and/or hospitalization.

Industry (6 to 12 Years)

When the child reaches school age, she or he enters the world of the classroom and becomes more involved with peers in the school and neighborhood. Consequently school and neighborhood become major socializing agents and the child's time spent at home with the parent is less influential, although still important. The child's exuberant imagination becomes tamed by imposed academic requirements. Skill acquisition becomes very important not only in school but in activitities, games, and sports. The child learns to win recognition by producing things and by being successful. Erikson (1964) maintains that if skill acquisition is not encouraged or reinforced, the child's sense of personal industry and mastery may give way to inferiority and inadequacy. The risk of inferiority and inadequacy is enhanced when illness prevents regular school attendance and thus the opportunities for skill acquisition may contribute to delay in social development and the physically ill child may become lonely and ostracized.

Whereas the preschool child's thinking was magical and fantasy-oriented, the school-aged child becomes more of a logical thinker, has a somewhat clearer understanding of illness, and is less likely to concoct magical and unrealistic explanations. However, the child's thinking is still very concrete and tends to be very literal. The child at this age tends to see things as black or white and is not able to grasp the subtleties of abstraction. Rules become important and are viewed in absolute, fixed terms.

Adolescence (12 to 18 Years)

As the child enters adolescence, thinking becomes less concrete and attains formal cognitive patterns that allow for abstractions and relativistic thinking. The adolescent begins generating theories, questioning values, and idealizing about the future. Cognitively, the adolescent can master comprehension of physical illness but emotional complications may result.

Erikson (1964) maintains that the major issue in adolescence involves resolving the crisis of personal identity. The adolescent is faced with multiple developmental tasks to be mastered in the establishment of her or his identity. Physically the body is maturing very rapidly; the body becomes a source of extreme self-consciousness. The adolescent must struggle with biological and sexual urges and must form a confident sexual identity through dating and social relationships with members of the opposite sex. As the child struggles for independence, parents still have to be relied upon. Adolescents must delineate occupational and educational goals and are faced with the decision of what to do with their lives. Erikson (1964) noted that the adolescent is forced to struggle with two major systems, both of which are in flux. Internal, cognitive, and physiological changes are occurring at the same time that the adolescent is dealing with the external pressures and stresses of dating, working, and trying to find a meaningful place within a peer group and within society. Adolescence is a time of turmoil, confusion, and ambivalence.

Physical illness seriously complicates and compounds the adolescent's struggle for identity and independence. Illness may cause changes in physical appearance which increase self-consciousness and threaten an already shaky sense of self-esteem. Questions of physical adequacy are compounded. Illness may force the adolescent into a dependent position which is deeply resented. The adolescent is likely to rebel against the lack of control and autonomy inherent in physical illness, which could lead to refusal to comply with the medical regime. The task of developing meaningful social relationships with opposite-sexed peers is made much more difficult and the adolescent may consequently withdraw from social participation thus delaying appropriate psychosexual development.

In summary, the implications of physical illness differ depending on the age and developmental status of the child. The problems resulting from illness during the first year of life are of a different nature from those resulting in the school-aged child. The child's emotional and cognitive development dictate the implications of previous illness. Parental responses to illnesses, past experiences, environmental circumstances, and the severity and longevity of illness all interact with developmental variables in determining the impact of illness on the child.

THE IMPACT OF PHYSICAL ILLNESS ON THE CHILD

The preceding discussion of developmental issues is relevant as one considers the range and scope of the impact of physical illness on the child. An important variable in determining the implications of physical illness is the chronicity versus brevity dimension (Dombro & Haas, 1970). The social and psychological consequences of physical illness upon children, if brief in duration, appear to be negligible. Davenport and Werry (1970) studied the behavior of 145 children in the United States and Canada who were undergoing tonsilectomies. When the children were compared to siblings and normal controls, no significant evidence of posthospitalization behavioral upsets was indicated. If the illness which precipitates hospitalization is serious and requires prolonged treatment, problems could be expected more readily. Often in serious illnesses and/or prolonged hospitalization, a child's normal development may be impeded since the focus becomes centered on the disease and its treatment, and normal family routine becomes disrupted.

The problems associated with chronic illness such as asthma, diabetes, advanced kidney disease, leukemia, hemophilia, chronic cardiac problems, juvenile rheumatoid arthritis, sickle cell anemia, spina bifida, spinal cord injuries, or muscular dystrophy, to name a few, are serious and can affect all aspects of the child's personal development as well as place considerable stress on the family (Dombro & Haas, 1970; Prugh, 1972; Prugh & Eckhardt, 1975; Steinhauer, Mushin, & Rae-Grant, 1974; Travis, 1976). The social and psychological problems presented by children who have chronic or serious health problems depend on the nature of the child's illness, the family's attitude toward the child, the child's ability to cope, and the child's developmental level. Prugh and Eckhardt (1975) noted common reactions manifested by children during acute illness or injury and subsequent hospitalization. Prugh and Eckhardt (1975) and Prugh (1972) reported that restlessness, irritability, malaise, listlessness, and disturbances in sleeping and eating may be viewed as direct behavioral effects of illness upon children. More serious behavioral reactions may also be observed in the hospitalized child and these include regression, depression, anxiety, misinterpretation of the illness or the reasons for certain medical procedures, conversion reactions, and mild learning problems once the child returns to school (Prugh & Eckhardt, 1975).

The personality patterns of children with a chronic illness fall along a continuum ranging from mild to severe psychopathology. Prugh and Eckhardt (1975) and Prugh (1972) reported that the personality patterns of chronically ill children range from "overdependent, overanxious, and passive, or withdrawn patterns—with strong secondary gains from illness—to overindependent, aggressive modes of behavior—with strong associated tendencies to deny illness, even to markedly unhealthy extremes" (Maddison & Raphael, 1971). The authors also reported that there are children who do develop realistic notions about their illness and subsequent capabilities and seem to accept their limitations. These children develop adequate compensatory mechanisms and adequate social outlets.

Examples of the problems encountered by children with certain medical disorders may illustrate how such disorders can affect their adjustment. Children and youth with juvenile rheumatoid arthritis (JRA) may tend to avoid contact with peers and have a poor self-image. Since there can be disfiguring aspects to JRA, children and youth with this medical problem often feel inferior, are especially sensitive to criticism, and exhibit frustration over their disability (Parker, 1979). Cleveland and Brewer (1970) report that these children also have difficulty expressing anger in an appropriate manner. Children and youth with progressive muscular dystrophy may tend to withdraw, lose interest in people and their environment, and retreat into themselves (Zitler & Allsop, 1976). Children with disorders of the respiratory system such as asthma often exhibit anxiety, insecurity, and dependency. Because the child may not understand how an asthmatic attack is precipitated the child may continually exhibit a high level of anxiety (Parker, 1979). Due to certain restrictions placed on the child by the family and physician, the child may feel he or she is being punished and depression may ensue.

To counteract the child or youth's negative reactions to physical and health-related problems, active intervention techniques involving medical/psychological personnel, the family, and the school must be established. For example, children need to gain self-confidence and need to feel that they have some control and freedom over their lives. Purcell, Weiss, and Hahn (1972) found that programs designed with an emphasis on physical activities with peers improved asthmatic children's physical fitness, sociability, self-assertion, and group activity skills. Furthermore, school absences decreased. Children with muscular dystrophy can feel more self-assured by performing necessary physical tasks for themselves such as feeding and dressing and making things with their hands (Parker, 1979). Children with JRA often need restrictions in physical areas but school personnel and parents can encourage the child to act in healthier ways and encourage classmates to include the child in certain activities. Parents must be encouraged against overprotecting and fostering dependency in the child.

Children and youth with chronic, long-term illnesses which require considerable medical support and frequent absences from school will inevitably have school-related and peer-related problems. Swanson and Willis (1979) emphasized the need for open communication between medical and school personnel. School personnel need to have knowledge concerning the child's medical problem so that appropriate services may be provided for the child. Medical personnel often lack knowledge about the services schools can and must provide children. An awareness and knowledge of Public Law 94-142 is essential. This law guarantees every child a free public education and includes free ancillary services to those exceptional children who need such services (speech therapy, occupational and physical therapy, psychological services, etc.). Medical services required to determine the need for special education are also included in this law if requested by the school personnel. Public Law 94-142 includes within its definition orthopedically impaired, other health impaired, multihandicapped, and other children with a variety of sensory or mental impairments.

Parker (1979) reports that most children and youth with chronic health-related problems can be served within the regular classroom. When the child must be hospitalized for varying lengths of time it becomes imperative that the classroom teacher and the hospital personnel maintain open communication and close cooperation. Homebound instruction may be provided for the child, or hospital-bound instruction can be offered, depending on the health of the child. Often the child who misses a great deal of school is hesitant about returning to the classroom. By working with the school counselor, teacher, and parents, the child can be eased back into the classroom without undue upset. Teachers can be helpful in preparing students for the return of one of their classmates.

In planning educational goals for children with disorders of the nervous system, Scherzer, Ilson, Mike, and Landoli (1972) reported that several factors must be analyzed: (1) degree of medical involvement, (2) level of intelligence, (3) social development, and (4) family stability. Scherzer et al. (1972) reported an 80% accuracy in predicting educational placement and development in regular schools by analyzing the aforementioned factors.

IMPACT OF PHYSICAL ILLNESS ON FAMILIES

Once a medical diagnosis has been made on a child the parents may respond in numerous ways, depending on the nature of the child's illness. Richmond (1958) cited an initial phase of denial and disbelief. The parents may be stunned and shocked by the medical diagnosis. Secondarily, parents feel a sense of fear and frustration particularly if the medical problem the child presents may be chronic or handicapping. During this period of time parents need considerable emotional support and medical information because they tend to feel responsible for or guilty about the child's problem (Freiberg, 1972; Prugh, Staub, Sands, Kirschbaum, & Lenihan, 1953). An example of how unrealistic parents can be in assuming responsibility for the child's illness is cited. When three-year-old Julie was diagnosed as having a seizure disorder, the mother, searching for her own cause for the seizure disorder, decided she had caused her daughter's medical problem because she bathed her in Phisohex. Parents of a child born with a cleft palate/lip condition have cited God's punishment of them for premarital sex or infidelity as the cause of their child's congenital defect. During the fear and frustration phase, parents may blame not only themselves but each other, the hospital, or the physician. It is critical that the physician discuss the child's medical problem with the parents. It has been demonstrated that the reasons for anxiety among parents during their child's hospitalization include lack of information about diagnosis and lack of information about procedures and treatment (Freiberg, 1972; Meadow, 1969). Freiberg found that lack of information was repeatedly discussed as the major reason for anxiety among mothers. All 25 of the mothers interviewed also reported that the hospitalization of one of their children upset the entire family (Freiberg, 1972). Parents, particularly mothers, need more information relative to their child's medical problem, treatment plan, and prognosis. In another study 114 out of 130 mothers interviewed indicated a strong need for more information on ways they could be involved to help their child (Meadow, 1969). These mothers were worried about their child, bored with their stay at the hospital, and earnestly desired to have a definitive role in caring for their child.

Once the parent is counseled through the phase of fear and frustration they are likely to enter a phase of intelligence, inquiry, and planning. They are less bewildered and are now able to actively carry out programs the child might require. Unfortunately, during hospitalization parents are given insufficient information on how they can participate in the care of their child. Eventually parents become adapted to the child's medical problem and the family routine may return to normal. Siblings, on the other hand, may feel guilty and anxious as though they somehow caused the illness. The siblings' reactions vary depending on their age, how close they felt to the ill child, and under what circumstances the illness occurred. Parents' behavior toward their ill child ranges from overprotectiveness, overindulgence, overpermissiveness, overly demanding, restrictive, to neglectful. Enabling parents to understand realistic limitations placed on the child as a result of the illness and encouraging the parents to treat the child as nearly normal as possible decreases chances of robbing the child of independence and positive self-esteem. Any time a child is seriously ill, however, it must be remembered that the family equilibrium is upset. Hospital personnel, including the physician, must not only meet the medical needs of the physically ill child but must consider the impact of the illness on the family and strive to offer services to all (Freiberg, 1972; Galdston & Hughes, 1972; Prugh, 1965). Extremely anxious parents, if not offered support and increased medical information, impart their anxiety to the child and may even interfere with the medical treatment. The goal becomes, as Prugh (1965) mentioned, gaining a therapeutic alliance between the parents and hospital personnel.

As parents traverse through the phases of denial, fear and frustration, intelligent inquiry, and planning they reach a point when they begin to adapt to the child's illness (Garrard & Richmond, 1963; Mattsson, 1972b). Prior to mature adaptation, parents usually suffer emotional disorganization but they soon reintegrate (Garrard & Richmond, 1963). Parents who are unable to mobilize psychological defenses and reintegrate to a realistic cognizance about their child's illness will need therapeutic intervention. The alert hospital worker (nurse, physician, psychologist, social worker, etc.) must constantly be "tuned in" to the needs and feelings of parents and attempt to intervene on their behalf.

The psychosocial adjustment of physically or chronically ill children is dependent, to a large degree, upon the reactions and attitudes of parents (Garrard & Richmond, 1963; Maddison & Raphael, 1971; Mattsson, 1972b). Mattsson (1972a) found that children who demonstrated poor adjustment to their illness had parents who were: (1) fearful and overprotective; (2) over solicitious and guilt ridden; or (3) embarrassed and ashamed of their child's illness or handicap. The parents who demonstrate good adaptation to their child's illness could offer encouragement and guidance to their child and treat the child realistically. These parents were able to master self-accusatory and guilt feelings (Mattsson, 1972a), as well as guard against being oversolicitous and overprotective. Mattsson (1972a) reported that children and youth who demonstrate good psychosocial adaptation to their illness are (1) functioning well at home and school, (2) realistic about accepting limitations imposed by their illness and did not seek secondary gain from their illness, (3) able to compensate for their limitations, (4) able to express negative emotions, (5) using to some degree the defense mechanism of denial. Mothers, rather than fathers, are prone to treat their ill child in a manner that is not conducive to good mental health. Maddison and Raphael (1971) find it crucial to provide the mothers of chronically ill children access to one person to whom they can form a relationship and to whom they can ventilate their anxieties, resentment, and guilt. The person can be a social worker, nurse, physician, or psychologist but availability of the person to the mother and continuity of care are important.

Travis (1976) artfully discussed the degree and manner of family burden different physical illnesses might create. She mentioned numerous factors that need to be considered when weighing the family burden, including:

1. Any sleep disturbances the child's physical illness might cause the parents, such as breathing problems in the asthmatic child or pain in the arthritic child.
2. Physical burdens the illness might create for the parents, such as dressing, lifting, feeding, giving physical therapy treatments, and so on, to the child with arthritis, spina bifida, spinal cord injury, muscular dystrophy.
3. Complicated special diets which must be prepared for children with diabetes, asthma, or advanced kidney disease, and which require extra time.
4. Extra housecleaning often necessary to prevent problems for the asthmatic child.
5. Added financial strain and the stress this places on families.

6. Housing adaptation that may be needed for the child whose illness requires a wheelchair, ramp, downstairs sleeping arrangement, hospital bed, and so on.

7. The unpredictable nature of the child's illness, which children have with kidney disease, heart problems, hemophilia, leukemia, sickle cell anemia or cystic fibrosis (Travis, 1976).

Travis (1976) reports that the family size, structure, and relationships are also important factors in that at least a two-parent family can share the emotional and physical load of caring for the ill child. If the couple is mutually supportive, the consultation and support offered them can be focused.

> The psychological effect upon siblings of the chronic illness of one child seems to depend on when, how long, and how much they are deprived of the things they want; the sick child's behavior and their retaliation with consequent guilt; and the strengths in the family, including parental attitudes toward them and the sick child. Some siblings develop a protective attitude toward the sick child, even when he is older than they are. Deprivation of affection and attention from the parents and deprivation of material wants because of the sick child's needs, create resentment that in some cases becomes very deep and destructive. (Travis, 1976, p. 56)

FACTORS MEDIATING THE IMPACT OF ILLNESS

As noted, the social, educational, and psychological effects of physical illness on children can be both pervasive and profound. Clearly, however, these effects are far from uniform and vary greatly depending on a multitude of mediating factors. These factors can be loosely grouped as (1) those that involve the psychosocial aspects of the child and (2) those that are more directly related to the illness itself.

With regard to the psychosocial factors, Shontz (1972) implicated a number of components which determine an adult's response to illness including fear of outcome, expense, fear of hospitalization, dislike for the physician, and missing out on activities. In our review of the literature on the impact of illness on children, we found the following list of additional psychosocial variables to be especially pertinent: the meaning of illness to a child, cognitive styles, typical coping behavior, and defense mechanisms. Considering the multivariate nature of these factors, it is hardly surprising that investigators have failed to demonstrate a consistent, predictable relationship between the severity of an illness and the response to it (Lloyd, 1977).

The literature to date suggests rather strongly that a child's response to an illness will be affected by the meaning the child has attached to concepts such as disease, injury, illness, and surgery. A consistent though not empirically validated finding is the observation that children frequently develop fantasies about their illnesses and the treatment for them. Clearly, the emotional impact of illness depends more on the child's perception of what is happening to him than what is actually happening (Howe, 1968). Interesting examples have been reported such as a 7-year-old male who had developed visual problems and mistakenly assumed he had been admitted to the hospital for removal of his eyes, and a 4-year-old female who assumed her insatiable appetite was caused by a little man in her stomach who ate her food (Petrillo & Sanger, 1972). In our own experience we have observed several children who believed they had come to the hospital to die because a sibling, friend, or other relative had died in a hospital before. We and others (e.g., Sheridan, 1975) also have often observed children who felt that they were personally responsible for their illness, even when this was clearly not the case. With a surprising frequency, children in the Diabetic Clinic at Oklahoma Children's Memorial Hospital have confided that they got their diabetes from eating too much sugar and more than a few cardiac patients have stated they developed problems from playing too hard. Along a similar vein, a number of accounts have reported that children often believe that their illness is a form of punishment for some misdeed or even bad thoughts (e.g., Korsch, 1961; Sheridan, 1975).

Observations have also been made concerning the substantial inaccuracies frequently seen in the meanings and attributions children attach to their treatment regimens. For example, Sheridan (1975) noted that many younger children believe that it is possible to bleed to death from blood tests. In addition, various procedures such as use of needles, surgery, intravenous solutions and dressing changes can be painful as well as bewildering to a child of limited cognitive abilities. As Sheridan (1975) noted, children often find it difficult to believe that all that pain is really for their own good.

The reason that children form such misattributions about their illnesses and treatments is not entirely clear. Nor are there adequate data concerning the percentage of children that form them at various ages. Some investigators have speculated that both the form and frequency of such misattributions is dependent on a given child's stage of psychosexual development (e.g., Gaddini, 1979). Actual data in support of this assumption is virtually nonexistent and represents an area where further study needs to be encouraged.

Several reports recently have focused on the child's level of cognitive development, in a Piagetian sense, as a key determinant of children's conception of illness (Carandang, Folkins, Hines, & Steward, 1979; Neuhauser, Amsterdam, Hines, & Steward, 1978; Simeonsson, Buckley, & Monson, 1979; Whitt, Dykstra, & Taylor, 1979). For example, Simeonsson *et al.* (1979) studied 60 hospitalized children in three age groups (5, 7, 9 years). Conception of illness causality were broken down into three stages as follows:

1. Responses scored as belonging to this stage were global, undifferentiated conceptions of illness. A typical response to "How do children get sick?" being "When you kiss old people."
2. Responses were characterized as concrete and overly specific such as responding to the same question with "Eating poison."
3. Responses demonstrated the abstract generalized principle as seen in the response "Sometimes you get sick by catching it from other people's germs."

The authors demonstrated a clear developmental progression in the types of causality conceptions in their sample of children. Thus stage 1 responses represented 39% of all responses of 5-year-olds and dropped to 10% of all responses for the 9-year-olds. Stage 2 responses accounted for 61% of 5-year-old responses, 74% of 7-year-olds, and 54% of 9-year-olds. Stage 3 responses apparently were rather infrequent, accounting for none of the 5-year-old responses and only 6% of the 7- and 9-year-old groups. In addition, the children's causality conception scores were found to correlate significantly with other measures of cognitive level in the areas of conservation, egocentrism, and physical causality.

Neuhauser et al. (1978) also found support for the notion of a developmental progression in children's concepts of healing. In this study, children in general had trouble conceptualizing the process of healing, but children in the stage of concrete operations gave much more accurate perceptions than those in the preoperational stage of development. Carandang et al. (1979) essentially replicated these findings with a sample of children aged 6¼ to 15. Additionally, the authors found that children who had a sibling afflicted with diabetes surprisingly had a lower level of conceptualization of illness than children without such a sibling, possibly due to the stress imposed on the whole family by having an ill child.

These investigations highlight the importance of first determining the child's perceptions of illness, healing, and their role as patient, and then presenting the child information that would be consonant with their current level of cognitive processing. Failure to do so could result in considerable added stress to a child.

Whitt et al. (1979) has presented a number of excellent illustrative examples of the application of both appropriate and inappropriate communication with ill children. As Whitt et al. (1979) accurately noted, the preoperational child has difficulty in appreciating the multiple meanings of words. Thus, some children could become centered on the notion of "death" when told that the doctor will inject some "dye." A number of metaphors more appropriate to the child's cognitive stage are presented by the authors, and it seems likely that following their approach would minimize misunderstanding and enhance the child's ability to call upon his own coping mechanisms. Much benefit could likely be derived by an increased effort to sensitize all members of the health care team to improving communication with children regarding their health and diseases.

Unfortunately, what we also need and do not have in this area are data. A few reports (e.g., Simeonsson et al., 1979; Neuhauser et al., 1978) have managed to demonstrate the logical assumption that increased understanding of illness and healing occurs roughly along the lines of predictable changes in cognitive development. Furthermore, Meichenbaum and Butler (1979) have recently described the process by which a person's emotional reactions are strongly influenced by the meaning system that the individual employs in response to a situation. However, we still do not have a clear understanding of the specific nature of children's meaning systems regarding illness and health. We also do not know the various effects of these meaning systems on children's overall coping in response to illness.

Cognitive styles are another set of variables which quite likely mediate the impact of illness on children in a way somewhat different from cognitive level. Included under this category are dimensions such as internal-external locus of control, repression-sensitization, minimization-vigilant focusing (Lipowski, 1970), and monitor-distractor (Miller, 1979).

As noted by Neuhauser *et al.* (1978), a child's general perceived locus of control may affect his or her perception of control over the healing process. Appropriately, the authors also noted the possibility that this very perception could affect the healing process itself. For example, if a child came to feel he or she had no control over the healing process it is possible that a general state of learned helplessness and depression, which are detrimental to healing, could develop. A model describing the development of such states has been presented by Seligman (1975) and has been updated recently (Abramson, Seligman, & Teasdale, 1978).

Neuhauser *et al.* (1978) administered a child's version of a locus of control scale (Nowicki & Strickland, 1973) and several measures of children's concepts of, and perceived control over, healing to a group of twelve 8- to 9-year-old children and twelve 4- to 5-year-old children. Children were also administered a Piagetian conservation task to verify their stage of cognitive development. Preoperational and concrete operational children did not differ significantly on the internal-external locus of control measure. However, the I-E scores did demonstrate a significant correlation with perceived control over healing from an illness. In other words, the more internally controlled children were on the I-E scale, the more control they perceived themselves to have over the healing process. Unfortunately, all the children studied were apparently well children and possible past experience with actual illness was not reported. In addition, this study did not allow for investigation into a possibly more interesting question: To what extent does one's perceived control over illness and healing affect the process of coping?

The effect could be substantial. For example, in the more general area of problem solving, Diener and Dweck (1978) found that differences in children's locus of control were predictive of substantial differences in specific thoughts and affects while working on a problem-solving task.

Some attempt to formulate a more specific "health locus of control" (Parcel & Meyer, 1978) has been made but no studies to date have systematically investigated the interaction of this specific variable with children's actual responses to illness. Yet, as Johnson (1979) recently implied, this type of relatively "specific" variable probably has a much greater chance of increasing our knowledge and predictive abilities than the more general personality assessment that has frequently proven fruitless in similar areas of investigation.

The next three cognitive styles—repression-sensitization, minimization-vigilant focusing, and monitor-distractor—all seem to be describing a similar construct. Thus, repressors, minimizers, and distractors are people who tend to use selective inattention, denial, avoidance of information, rationalization, and so on, when dealing with a stressful event. On the other hand, sensitizers, vigilant focusors, and monitors are people who actively seek information, pay attention to details of treatment, and so on. On the surface, it may seem as though the desirable part of the continuum for a child to be on would be the sensitizer, vigilant focusor, monitor end. In fact, a recent study by Burstein and Meichenbaum (1979) suggests that this assumption may be correct. In that study, a group of children who were to undergo surgery were assessed on various measures of anxiety and defensiveness. It was found that children who were low on defensiveness and who actively engaged in worry and play with stress-related toys prior to surgery reported less distress and anxiety following surgery than children who were high on defensiveness and who avoided playing with stress-related toys. Thus, in this case at least, it appears that the "work of worrying" was helpful to the sample of children who utilized it. However, the children were allowed simply to use their natural coping style with no attempts at independent manipulation. It may be that the children who utilized repression were already on their "last stand" in terms of coping. If pressed to use "constructive worry," the psychological trauma would possibly have been worse. This general idea has been expressed by Miller (1979), who stated that a subject's arousal level will probably be lower when his or her habitual coping style of monitoring versus distracting is matched by the opportunity to act accordingly. In other words, Miller suggests that monitors ideally should be given maximal information and distractors minimal information. Furthermore, Kiely (1972) suggested that this style should be confronted directly only when it leads the patient to avoid needed treatment. The danger of confronting the minimizer was underscored by observations of reactions that reportedly even included premature death following the induction of reality either by direct "spilling of the truth" by physicians or by phenothiazine medication (Kiely, 1972).

Overall, the data suggest that cognitive styles play a vital role in mediating the impact of illness. However, the nature of that role remains poorly understood. At this point, it would be impossible to even make recommendations for change based on knowledge of an individual child's responses to an illness and the child's cognitive style. Unquestionably, this area merits substantial investigation.

The assessment of other aspects of cognition would also appear to be an area that holds considerable promise for increasing our understanding of the impact of illness on children as well as providing suggestions for helping children reduce the impact. Kendall and Korgeski (1979) recently reviewed various approaches for a multidimensional assessment of cognition including the areas of imagery, beliefs, self-efficacy, specific self-statements, attributions, and cognitive style. In addition, Meichenbaum and Butler (1979) have noted the importance of understanding an individual's current concerns. For example, some children who are physically ill might be preoccupied with the concern of gaining attention and acceptance from professional or authority figures; other children might have concerns such as a fear of being overwhelmed by anxiety, a desire to maintain independence and autonomy, a fear of abandonment, a desire to maintain a particular body image, a fear of being evaluated or a desire to escape from a home situation. Current concerns such as these almost certainly would partially determine a child's response to illness. The determinants of these concerns include the level of psychosocial development à la Erikson, the aforementioned meaning attached to the illness situation, and, finally, the degree of emotional arousal that might be induced by the illness itself, pain, or the previously noted images, beliefs, and so on. As Meichenbaum and Butler (1979) noted, the relationship is bidirectional with cognitions influencing emotional responses, but with emotional states also influencing cognitions.

A technology for multilevel and multidimensional assessment of cognition is developing and has been reviewed by Kendall and Korgeski (1979). However, to date, only minimal application of these procedures has been made in the area of children's response to illness.

This lack of investigative effort is unfortunate given that such assessment may aid not only our understanding of the impact of illness on children but also our understanding of the factors involved with the patient's role in the treatment and/or healing processes. For example, compliance with medical regimens and instructions is an area that has received much attention in the literature because failure to comply is common and can often have disastrous effects. For example, diabetic children frequently break dietary rules, avoid testing their urine by writing up fake results, and sometimes even resist essential insulin injections; burn victims often actively resist dressing changes and often fail to consume a sufficient number of calories daily; and asthmatic children often fail to take prescribed medication and fail to avoid known allergens. Lack of knowledge of factual information about one's illness has often been cited as a possible explanation for these acts of non-compliance. However, a fairly extensive body of literature on this topic has yielded relatively little. Results have been conflicting but with an overall conclusion that knowledge per se is probably not a sufficient explanation for noncompliance (Tagliacozz & Ima, 1970). On the other hand, it is possible that knowledge combined with other cognitive variables such as a child's current concerns and perceived self-efficacy in being able to apply that knowledge might be highly predictive of noncompliance as well as suggest strategies for ameliorization.

Once again we see the value of applying recent advances in cognitive assessment to the area of children's responses to illness. This assessment will require a multidimensional approach. It will also be necessary to study not only children who cope poorly with illness but also those who cope well. By such comparisons perhaps it will be possible to determine the nature of the deficits in those children who cope poorly followed by the development of effective treatment strategies. The state of the art today was summarized by Johnson (1980) who noted that we still do not know under what circumstances to encourage or discourage confrontation with reality, the use of fantasy, the use of regression, and the use of other coping strategies.

ILLNESS-RELATED PHENOMENA

It should be clear that different children are affected by illness in various ways due to substantial differences in age, level of understanding, current concerns, defenses used, and so on. Differences in impact also occur due to wide variability in the diseases and treatments required for them. Illness and its treatment can result in a phenomenal range of stimuli impinging upon a child. This variability partly explains the difficulty in assessing the impact of illness. In fact, illness (and its treatment) is such an abstract concept that the only way to realistically deal with its impact is to break it into component parts such as pain, immobility, isolation, and disfigurement.

Illness itself, and perhaps its treatment even more, often results in substantial and prolonged pain. Diseases such as cancer, sickle cell anemia, and rheumatoid arthritis are well known for the considerable discomfort and pain they can produce. At least as excrutiating can be the iatrogenic pain produced in the treatment of these and various other disorders. Common pain-inducing procedures include dressing changes, debridement, and hydrotherapy for burn patients; bone-marrow aspirations, lumbar puncture, and venipuncture frequently inflicted on cancer patients; and various physical therapy procedures required for a variety of other dysfunctions. In addition, numerous procedures that induce much milder pain such as injections and intravenous lines are inflicted quite frequently in most hospitalizations.

Children's responses to these procedures vary, but anyone who has witnessed them will attest to the overwhelming impact such experiences can have in some cases. In spite of this impact, the study of pain in children has received relatively little attention in the literature. For example, Eland and Anderson (1977) conducted a thorough review of the medical literature from 1970 to 1975. Their search yielded 1380 articles of pain of which a scant 33 were devoted to children's pain. Thirty-two of these were articles on differential diagnosis and various diagnostic examinations with almost no data bearing on children's psychological response to pain or on means to improve coping. Unfortunately, at least for many, if not most children, medical treatments for their pain are woefully inadequate when the painful stimuli are as intense as those produced by many diseases and treatment procedures.

Understanding the individual differences in response to painful stimuli depends in part upon an understanding of the nature of pain itself. Although a thorough review of the various theories concerning pain mechanisms is beyond the scope of this chapter, a brief mention of a few points from these theories seems appropriate. The second author and colleagues have reviewed these theories in greater detail elsewhere (Elliott, Ozolins, & Ulissi, 1980). Recently, the theory of pain mechanisms receiving the most attention has been the gate control theory proposed by Melzack and Wall (1965). Further support and modifications of this theory are likely to occur from the very recent investigations in the biochemical study of specific brain peptides, labeled generically as endorphins (endogenous morphine). The original gate control theory proposed that a gating or regulating system located in the substantice gelatinosa of the spinal cord modulates the conduction of nerve impulses of both small and large fiber systems from peripheral nerves to spinal cord transmission cells (T-cells) which send impulses to the brain. The reticular formation, which receives fibers from the whole cortex, produces further inhibitory effects on T-cell transmission, which could account for the effects of cognitive processes, such as experience and attention, on the pain response. When T-cell output exceeds some critical level, presumably pain occurs.

Melzack (1973) further proposed three components of the pain experience: sensory-discriminative, affective-motivational, and cognitive-evaluative with various interconnected cortical sites postulated as responsible for the modulation of each component. The entire system is assumed to respond to both noxious and other kinds of stimuli, and when T-cell summation in the reticular system is below some critical level, brain areas subserving positive affect and approach tendencies are activated, and when summation exceeds this critical level, brain areas underlying negative drive and aversive affect are stimulated.

Gate control theory remains speculative and has justifiably been criticized on a number of points. However, to date, it is the only conceptualization of pain that provides an account both of various kinds of abnormal pain as well as a variety of motivational and cognitive variables known to interact with pain.

Motivational and cognitive influences have been dealt with by Fordyce, Fowler, Lehman and De Lateur (1968). Focusing on pain behavior, Fordyce suggested that pain behavior should be thought of in terms of respondant and operant pain. Respondant pain behavior is considered as the typical response to injury while operant pain behavior is thought to occur spontaneously and/or as an outgrowth from respondant pain. Respondant pain becomes operant pain as, over time, pain behavior almost inevitably comes under control of such social-interpersonal variables as attention and concern from significant others. Avoidance conditioning can also occur when pain behavior results in escape from other noxious situations which for children might be school, teasing from peers, or unpleasant chores. Fordyce's learning model provides an important elaboration of the role of motivational, cognitive, and interpersonal variables in the determination of response to pain. Unfortunately, the model does not provide an adequate means of separating the experiential-perceptual aspects of pain from pain behavior per se.

In addition, no conceptualization of pain to date has attempted to deal with its developmental aspects. Yet developmental issues would appear quite important for understanding children's response to and perception of pain. For example, it seems apparent that the motivational affective, cognitive-evaluative, and even sensory-discriminative components of pain discussed by Melzack almost certainly undergo maturational changes that would modulate the perception and expression of pain.

At this point, we are far from arriving at an adequate assessment of these developmental issues in regard to pain. What is clear, however, is that children can be profoundly affected by pain. A striking example of this effect can be seen in R. Seligman's (1974) observations that some children cope so poorly with burn pain that depressive withdrawal and sometimes death unnecessarily results. In addition, numerous authors (e.g., Beales, 1979) have commented on the potential for prolonged pain to disrupt normal psychological development. We have also observed numerous instances in which children's pain led them to actively avoid and/or resist needed treatment. Some children will even fail to report the presence of pain for fear of the pain induced by the injections to relieve it. Children in the burn unit at Oklahoma Children's Memorial Hospital have been observed at various times to beg, fight, defecate, urinate, run, and vomit as a means to avoid or stall their hydrotherapy treatments. It is also quite common to see children, because of the pain, utterly refuse any form of physical therapy even though they have been told that certain exercises will prevent disabling contractures later. Whether repeated and/or prolonged exposure to intense pain actually disrupts emotional and personality development is largely a matter of conjecture at this time. Complex longitudinal research will be needed to answer questions such as whether these children develop a future predisposition to developing depression, manipulativeness, hysteria, and so on. Regardless of these longitudinal questions, for reasons of humanitarianism as well as increasing cooperation with medical treatments, it will be important for us to increase our understanding of children's pain and way of dealing with it.

Some of the critical variables involved in children's dealing with pain have been raised previously in our section on the general psychosocial factors presumed to mediate the impact of illness on children. A brief note of the specific ways these variables affect the pain aspects of illness seems in order, however.

In particular, the literature has highlighted the role played by the meaning children attach to their painful experiences. During infancy the perception and comprehension of pain develop rapidly, although it is still unclear to what degree an infant perceives and remembers pain in the very first weeks of life (Gross & Gardner, 1980). One common myth is that newborn infants do not feel pain, but this assumption has been refuted by a variety of evidence. Szaz (1957) has suggested that pain is a stimulus that provides much of the means for a child to define and differentiate his body from other human objects. For the preschool child, temporal relationships are poorly understood, which diminishes the potential value to be derived from reassurance that the hurting will stop soon (Gildia & Quirk, 1977). The theme of punishment for misdeed and bad thoughts also appears common at this age. Beales (1979) has observed that younger children are most often concerned with and disturbed by insult to the surface of their bodies because they have little comprehension of their internal makeup, and thus little idea of the dangerous implications of pain originating from inside their bodies. Finally, due to the predominance of concrete and egocentric thinking at this age, it is difficult for these children to associate pain with an ultimate positive outcome (Gildia & Quirk, 1977). With school-age children (aged 10 and 11), Schultz (1971) found a virtually universal fear of bodily injury. Additionally, frequent concerns were found in the areas of losing control, fear over being treated like a baby, and inability to maintain favorite activities.

These observations provide us with helpful suggestions for dealing with children's pain in more effective ways. Unfortunately, very few of our data have been collected in a systematic, empirical fashion. We do not have anything that even remotely resembles norms of the ages at which children have particular beliefs about pain. Nor do we have adequate data regarding what ages particular current concerns of children are likely to influence their responses to pain. Research on these issues has been initiated with children in the burn unit at Oklahoma Children's Memorial Hospital and with a sample of normal school children. The research with the children on the burn unit involves a multidimensional assessment including behavioral observations, self-ratings of pain, a pain attitude scale, a structured interview, and a projective pain apperception test. The school children are being administered the pain attitude scale from grades kindergarten to 12. It is hoped that this type of broad-based assessment endeavor will elucidate the critical determinants of effective coping with pain and perhaps clarify the differences in these determinates at various age levels.

At this stage of our research, definitive conclusions cannot be made but several interesting trends have emerged from pilot work. For example, the good copers do not seem to be characterized by the absence of negative self-statements so much as they are by the presence of positive self statements that they use to counter the negative ones. Once the ways of dealing with the impact of pain are better understood, the development of more effective treatment strategies should follow quite readily.

Isolation and restriction are another set of factors that often impinge upon children during the treatment of their illnesses and diseases. A variety of degrees and types of isolation are often imposed upon children depending on the particular requirement of treatment. As Kornfield (1972) has noted, in many isolation rooms visiting is allowed only by gowned and masked staff and family, a practice that might even tend to reduce the overall number of visits. The visits that do occur certainly have the potential to be perceived as strange and unreal. Separation from family and the rest of the outside world could easily be intensified. As Kornfield (1972) noted, for a small number of patients, an acute psychotic reaction has been observed. A variety of other suggestions in the literature regarding the possible deleterious effects of isolation have been recently noted (Kellerman, Rigler, & Siegel, 1979). Once again, however, we are plagued by an overabundance of anecdotal reports rather than systematically collected data.

Standing in contrast to this trend, Holland and his colleagues reported (Holland, Harris, Plumb, Tuttolomondo, & Yates, 1970; Holland, Plumb, & Yates, 1977) the results of a systematic study of adult leukemic patients treated in a protected environmental unit with laminar airflow barrier isolation techniques. In these reports no acute psychiatric problems presumably associated with social isolation were observed. In addition, psychological stability as rated by nurses was maintained throughout. Kellerman, Rigler, and Siegel (1979) recently extended this study to the investigation of the effects of isolation in protected environments utilized in the treatment of children with advanced stage, solid, malignant tumors. A broad range of functions was assessed during the children's stay, which averaged 92.8 days. These areas included perceptual disturbance, sleep, intellectual functioning, physical discomfort, mood, activity patterns, social-communication, and sedation. In general, the study failed to reveal any short or long term debilitating effects from the prolonged isolation within the protected environmment. Great efforts were made, however, to provide the children with a comprehensive system of adjunctive care in the form of a play therapist, access to windows and clocks, regular family input, a school teacher, family counseling, and strong encouragement of daily activity schedules.

Clearly, isolation in the absence of such intensive adjunctive support could have a far more pervasive and negative impact. The types of isolation employed and the nature of supportive services available can vary widely with no way at present for determining the possible results. From a purely observational standpoint, we have seen children who were seemingly affected negatively by some of the partial isolation techniques at Oklahoma Children's Memorial Hospital. However, separating these effects from the concomitant effects of pain and other aspects of their disease is quite difficult. It would also seem logical to assume that at least some children, under certain conditions, would react negatively to isolation. This assumption has certainly not been ruled out by the Kellerman *et al.* report, especially when one considers that the total number of subjects in that report was only 14.

The encouraging aspect of the study by Kellerman *et al.* (1979) is that it at least seems possible to mitigate much of the potential effects of isolation. In the absence of more data, it would seem prudent to advise a special focus on the provision of psychosocial support systems whenever isolation is to be used with children.

Restrictions on mobility due to treatment consideration as well as disease process are another factor that many ill children must contend with. Once again, few data exist regarding the factors that potentiate effective coping as opposed to continued adjustment difficulties. Good observations of the effects of this restriction were made in the 1940s, but our understanding of the specific coping processes has not advanced much since. Bergman (1945) was one of the first to observe a rather unexpected but consistent contentment shown by children aged 2 to 16 who were severely immobilized for prolonged orthopedic treatment. A number of such children do indeed demonstrate an odd satisfaction and sometimes even pride while in an immobilzed state, but Bergman (1945) observed problems such as hyperactivity, rage, and temper tantrums manifested themselves during the phase of return to normal mobility. A few years later Burlingham (1953) and others made the same sort of observations. It almost appears as though the immobilization period represents a period of preparation and anticipation of recovery, possibly even a kind of atonement for some patients (Bergman, 1945). During actual gradual return of function, however, the effects of unrealistic expectations, frustrations, and a less clearly defined role manifest themselves. Patients no longer have the same salient cues to govern their behavior and are confronted with the frustrations of attempting and sometimes failing various tasks aimed toward improvement of function. Korsch (1961) has also noted that distortions in body image can occur during immobilization. The impact of this distortion might be particularly salient during the recovery phase. In addition, Korsch noted that the secondary gains during immobilization may be difficult to give up later.

Several authors have commented on the interaction between developmental level and the effects of immobilization (e.g., Porter, 1973; Williams, 1973). It was suggested in these accounts that movement restriction results in the disruption of normal tension and aggressive release channels. Presumably, this disruption could readily effect both cognitive development as well as psychological striving in areas such as orality, dependency, and various social modalities, depending upon the age at which restriction occurs (Williams, 1973). Additional variables that may affect an individual's reaction include past experience, type of restraints used, state of health, and attitude of those imposing the restriction (Porter, 1973; Williams, 1973).

Actual empirical research is almost nonexistent in this area as well. Almost all reports have been in nursing journals, with an almost total void in the psychology literature. Porter (1973) reported some preliminary data on a controlled study which suggested a trend for restricted hospitalized preschool children to have a greater incidence of enuresis than a control group of hospitalized children with no unusual restrictions on movement. An obvious need remains for broadening the parameters of investigation in this area to include variables such as degree of restriction, age, coping styles, and personality.

An indication that restriction may not need to be severe to have significant effects was suggested by Baekeland (1970) in a study on the effects of simple exercise deprivation. In this study, a group of college students was asked to refrain from their usual exercise routines but otherwise to continue a normal life style. Even this relatively minimal restriction resulted in a change in sleep patterns, increased reports of sexual tension, and a stated increase in the need to be with others.

One final aspect of disease and injury that must be dealt with by many children involves the disfigurement that often results from skin disorders, burns and various other disorders requiring deforming surgeries. In some ways, this aspect of illness, disease, and/or injury can be one of the most difficult to cope with. This particular difficulty is all the more understandable if one reflects on the high value placed on good looks and appearance by our culture (Addison, 1978). Most unfairly, the disfigured can often face wide ranging bias and discrimination. Frequently, conclusions are even reached concerning intelligence and general capabilities based solely on anomalies in appearance. Bernstein (1976) has commented that most children he has studied who were disfigured by facial burns find the experience and adjustment to it crushing and totally engulfing. He further noted that shame and self-consciousness constitute a long-term difficulty for such children, with depression and apathy frequently being the characteristic affect. Being stared at was one of the most common and difficult adjustment problems reported in interviews of hundreds of children (Bernstein, 1976). Some have suggested that a grieving process similar to that encountered with any loss is an almost universal response, but that the process is made more difficult by the lack of support that is available for other types of loss (West & Shuck, 1978).

One indication of the enormity of impact and difficulty in coping can be found in responses of patients following the initial, acute phases of their illness or injury. For example, Addison (1978) observed that following mutilating facial surgery, many patients state that had they really known the outcome they would have elected to forgo their surgery, even if the long-term outcome might have been fatal. We have also observed many adolescents with facial burns who, following discharge, refuse to wear a facial mask designed to reduce long-term scarring. Upon interviewing these patients, generally we have found that the failure to wear the mask is not based on lack of knowledge about the long-term consequences but rather on a fear of ridicule or of appearing more different than they already are. The previously noted social discrimination has been highlighted in a number of cases in which our patients were literally taken to the police station because store managers and bank tellers assumed that the mask was indicative of an intent to commit robbery. The traumatizing effect of such an experience has been profound in some of these cases.

Still, the extent of impact that disfigurement induces will depend once again on a variety of factors such as age, sex, value and meaning of the afflicted bodily part, premorbid body image, developmental level, and coping syles (Bernstein, 1976;

Woods, 1975). As Seligman (1974) noted, there is also a tremendous need for study of the long-term adjustment to disfigurement. Unfortunately, to date, no such studies have been conducted. Nor has there been any systematic study of possible correlations between responses during acute treatment and responses during later reconstruction. Finally, there has been an almost total disregard of the process involved with patients who cope unexpectedly well. As Bernstein (1976) noted, some patients seem to adjust far better than one would predict on the basis of the disfigurement and/or the person's premorbid adjustment. These "good responders" could teach us a great deal about ways to help "poor responders" and perhaps should be studied with at least the same intensity as the latter.

EFFECTS OF HOSPITALIZATION ON THE DEVELOPING CHILD

The Child's Reaction to Hospitalization

Factors mediating the impact of illness, as well as other illness-related factors such as chronicity, immobility, isolation, separation, disfigurement, and pain, all influence a child's reaction to hospitalization. Upon entering the hospital, the child's initial reactions may include crying, clinging, fearfulness, withdrawal, aggressiveness, destructiveness, poor eating and sleeping, anger, uncooperativeness in the treatment process, bodily concerns, and general regressive behavior (Barowsky, 1978; Belmont, 1970; Demaio, 1978; Duffy, 1972; Mason, 1965; Tekely & Dittemore, 1978). Additionally, the stress of hospitalization may result in physiological changes such as elevated pulse rate, blood pressure, and temperature (Skipper & Leonard, 1968).

In years past, hospitalization, like institutionalization, had deleterious effects on the child's cognitive, physical, and social well-being (Spitz, 1945). While drastic improvements in medical technology and hospital facilities have been made, hospitalization remains a stressful and anxiety-provoking experience for children and can produce emotional and behavioral problems that persist long after discharge. As stated in previous sections, the reactions to hospitalization that the child presents depend on a number of variables, such as potential separation from parents and home, the child's adaptive and coping capacity, the fantasies that the child elaborates about the experience, entering a strange, new environment, the parents' attitudes, medical procedures that may be painful and unexpected, observing the fate of other patients, forced dependency and restriction on mobility, the developmental stage of the child, and the nature of the illness (Becker, 1972; Belmont, 1970; Langford, 1961; Nagera, 1978; Wright, Schaefer, & Solomons, 1979).

Belmont (1970) reported that the age of children at the time of hospitalization is extremely important in the child's understanding the meaning of the hospital experience. First and foremost we must understand how normal children think and feel at various stages in their development and, secondarily, we must understand the effects of hospitalization on children and families. As reported earlier, Erikson's theory of psychosocial development and Piaget's theories lend themselves well as a framework within which we can understand children and the reactions that they may manifest.

Anxiety responses relevant to hospitalization and illness must also be considered. The level of anxiety contributes to a myriad of behaviors that may disrupt the course of healing in the hospital. As noted previously, children can totally ignore prescribed plans such as specialized diets, exercises, and bed rest simply because they want to deny their illness (Belmont, 1970). Other children may ward off their anxiety by aggressive misbehavior and overactivity. By creating a diversion they do not have to think of their illness. Yet another group of children may handle their anxiety by being overly submissive and compliant, or by regressing to earlier stages of development (Belmont, 1970; Tekely & Dittemore, 1978). A few children may be so fearful that literally they do not want to move or initiate any activity (Belmont, 1979). They become perfect patients with the probable conscious or unconscious notion that if they comply and obey, they will not die and they will go home. Children tend to show the greatest amount of stress and anxiety to procedures involving needles (shots, drawing blood, bone marrow taps, etc.), but the degree of heart rate acceleration demonstrated by the child can be reduced by "scheduling" the procedures involving needles (Burling & Collip, 1969). Preparing the child psychologically does reduce the level of stress in the child.

Besides understanding normal childhood development and a child's anxiety responses to hospitalization, we must have some notion of, and sensitivity to, children's fantasies regarding hospitalization. Most children between the ages of 3 and 8 to 10 years will likely distort the hospital experience to some degree. The more serious the illness and the more medical procedures that must be scheduled, the more complicated the situation, especially when no prehospital counseling is scheduled for the child and family. A few children with chronic illnesses such as leukemia may be subjected to bone marrow taps from early infancy and may assume that this is a normal procedure for all children. For example, Tommy had been seen twice a month since early infancy, and by age 7 he finally asked what age his older brother reached before the hospital personnel stopped doing bone marrow taps on him. Two other case examples will illustrate the impact of fantasy on a child's behavior and adjustment. Joe was 9 years of age and each time he entered the hospital he became extremely depressed and unresponsive. Exploration of his feelings revealed that he associated hospitalization and separation from his parents with dying. Hospitals and death were equated. Jimmy, by age 6 years, had had numerous surgeries on his testes. At home and school he presented serious behavior problems. In an initial play therapy session with Jimmy, the misperceptions or distortions surrounding his surgery were revealed. The therapist, using a medical/ surgical kit and two large anatomically correct dolls, introduced Jimmy to the play materials. Jimmy proceeded to "try to make the boy into a girl" by operating on the boys penis.

Postoperatively or posthospitalization, it is not uncommon for children to manifest emotional reactions once they are home. Parents frequently report the following symptoms in their children; (1) enuresis or encopresis; (2) sleep disturbances; (3) fears of death; (4) anxiety reactions; (5) depression; (6) eating problems; (7) behavior problems and anger; and (8) regression (Duffy, 1972; Kenny, 1975).

Shore and Goldston (1978, pp. 21–23) discuss seven areas dealing with the impact of hospitalization:

1. The recognition over the last three decades that behavior, such as attachment, is a significant area of study and can be subjected to vigorous and careful investigation. In essence, infants and small children adapt better when the mother or significant adult remains in the hospital with them.

2. The realization that psychic pain can have an effect as profound as, or even greater than physical pain, especially in children.

3. The effect of hospitalization must be reviewed within a developmental framework.

4. The child must be viewed within the context of his family.

5. "Anticipatory guidance" techniques to help a child master the potentially traumatic experience of hospitalization.

6. An interdisciplinary approach toward dealing with the hospitalization of children.

7. Hospital settings must be responsive to new knowledge about health care.

In this day of advanced knowledge, many medical procedures can be scheduled on an outpatient basis or hospitalization can be of very brief duration, thus reducing the stress to children (Shore & Goldston, 1978). In any event, we must recognize that children and families do react to hospitalization. We must understand the child's concept of hospitalization, and that the child's reaction to painful medical procedures is rarely rational or unemotional (Duffy, 1972). In one study it was found that those children hospitalized for a brief period of time did not demonstrate psychological reactions to the hospitalization two weeks after discharge (Davenport & Werry, 1970). Children hospitalized for two weeks or longer demonstrated psychological reactions after discharge from the hospital (Vernon et al., 1966). When a child remains hospitalized for longer periods of time the child begins to focus on his or her disease and ties to the school and home become strained (Dombro & Haas, 1970). And the younger the child (5 or 6 years of age and under) the more vulnerable the child is to harmful psychological effects as a result of the hospital experience because the child cannot conceptualize adequately, communicate readily, and has less social experience than older children (Duffy, 1972).

Preparing the Child for Hospitalization

As many as 70% of the nonchronic care hospitals for children throughout the United States are offering new and innovative programs to prepare parents and children for hospital procedures prior to the child's admission (Peterson & Ridley-Johnson,

1980). Unfortunately, most parents do not take advantage of the prehospital preparation. Hospital personnel may use booklets, films, tours, orientations, plant play therapy, or demonstrations to explain hospital procedures to parents and children (Azarnoff, 1976; Johnson, 1974; Jolly, 1975; Melamed *et al.*, 1976; Pomarico *et al.*, 1979; Rae & Stieber, 1976; Scahill, 1967). Johnson (1974) describes a program within a children's hospital that combines a puppet show with a tour of the hospital followed by a discussion period. The topics of fear, pain, anesthesia, and the recovery room are discussed by the puppets, and slides are shown of such equipment as intravenous tubes and traction (Johnson, 1974). Melamed *et al.* (1976) found that film modeling could be used successfully to reduce anxiety in children preparing for hospitalization and surgery. In this study children observed a film of a young boy entering the hospital for the first time to have a hernia operation. The boy in the film is shown at various stages from admission to discharge. Additionally, the boy narrates some of the scenes and describes his fears and feelings. Measures taken on the children who observed the film demonstrated a reduction in anxiety on a number of psychological behavioral and self-reported measures (Melamed *et al.*, 1976).

Many pediatric hospitals offer preadmission parties or tours of the hospital to orient the children and families. These "parties" may include tours of the induction room, recovery room, hospital play room, x-ray, physical therapy, and hospital rooms. The express purpose of preadmission tours is often threefold: (1) reduce the child's and parents' fears of hospitalization; (2) increase the hospital personnel's awareness of the emotional needs of children; and (3) sensitize the medical personnel to the fact that hospitalization can be stressful to the child and parents (Eckhardt & Prugh, 1978; Jolly, 1975, 1977; Pomarico *et al.*, 1979; Scahill, 1967).

Preparing children for painful medical and surgical procedures is extremely difficult, particularly if the children are between the ages of 8 to 10 months and 3 to 4 years. Eckhardt and Prugh (1978) noted that this age group is susceptible to separation anxiety, and they do not have sufficient cognitive development to understand why painful procedures are necessary. Nevertheless, simple and brief explanations are necessary for the 3- to 4-year-old children. It is rare for the medical personnel to assess the adaptive capacity of children when painful procedures or surgery is necessary. Often the medical procedure must be carried out regardless of the adaptive capacity or emotional state of the child. However, the emotional state of the child can be stabilized by carefully explaining procedures to parents, encouraging parents to be calm and supportive of the medical personnel, and not only establishing live-in facilities for parents but actively encouraging one of them to remain in the hospital with the child throughout the duration of the young child's hospitalization. The child can often be given a sedative in the hospital bed with one or both parents present, and it is advisable to have the parents present in the recovery room when the child awakens. Later, as the infant or child recovers from the medical procedures, play experiences utilizing doctor kits and other hospital equipment can be extremely useful in helping the child work out his or her anxieties or distortions of fantasy surrounding the medical procedure.

There are many ways of preparing children and adolescents for hospitalization.

Other methods include anatomical displays and discussions, as well as bibliotherapy. Booklets do and can be of therapeutic value before and after surgery in several ways:

1. The nurse can establish rapport with the child by reading to the child.
2. Books with pictures and simple discussion of another child's hospitalization can decrease the child's sense of aloneness, can instruct the child, and may answer questions he or she may not know how to ask.
3. Books can help entertain the bedfast child and may assist in the child's recovery.
4. Books can help the child's mental and emotional growth (Murphy, 1972).

Positive Aspects of Hospitalization

A child entering the hospital for the first time can find the experience traumatic or relatively constructive depending on a number of factors. The child's age, the nature of the child's illness, the care or sensitivity of the hospital personnel, the hospital procedures, and the support of significant adults all play varying roles. The emotional climate offered by the hospital and hospital personnel can be constructive for many children by (1) serving as a refuge from emotional strains, (2) promoting emotional education, (3) encouraging normal patterns of growth and development, (4) altering the parent-child relationship, (5) teaching and providing good nutrition, (6) enhancing a sense of mastery and fostering adaptive behavior (Adams, 1976; Azarnoff, 1976; Billington, 1972; Farrell & Biernan, 1977; Hartley & Goldenson, 1963; Morgenstern, 1968; Shore, Geiser & Wolman, 1965).

Serving as a Refuge from Emotional Strains and Promoting Emotional Education

Seriously abused, neglected, or emotionally deprived children often thrive on the emotional care and attention they receive while in the hospital. Infants admitted to the hospital for nonorganic failure-to-thrive begin to gain weight and thrive from the cuddling and regular feeding given them by the nursing personnel. Children from unbearable home situations may find the hospital to be a safe haven where the hospital routine, the regular nutritious meals, and personal attention offer a relief from the chaotic home environment. Children from low-income, multiproblem families, who experience the adverse effects of poverty, can also find hospitalization a positive experience (Guerin, 1977). Guerin (1977) reports that highly structured hospitals with good facilities and equipment, coupled with hospital personnel attuned to the emotional and physical well-being of children, can offer at least temporary respite for poor children.

Encouraging Normal Patterns of Growth and Development

In a psychologically sophisticated hospital the staff are more sensitive to the cognitive, behavioral, and psychosocial problems children present and efforts can be made to intervene in a positive way on behalf of the child. Another way in which the hospital can be constructive is its focus on health care in all its aspects. For example, a child of poverty may feel sick for prolonged periods and only during hospitalization may the full impact of the child's illness be diagnosed. The child may have otitis media, anemia, speech problems, a developmental lag, or any number of other problems. All of these areas of concern may well be addressed in the hospital attuned to the well-being of the whole child (Guerin, 1977). By assessing the child's patterns of growth and development, intervention within the home and school can occur. Frequently children at risk can be seen in follow-up clinics that provide parenting instructions and instructions for good health care.

Altering the Parent-Child Relationship and Teaching and Providing Good Nutrition

The hospitalization can be constructive in that the staff has the opportunity to observe mother-child interactions. As stated, at-risk parenting, poor mothering, or maladaptive interactions between parent(s) and child can be monitored and followed closely. Occasionally, the staff may detain the child in the hospital until the home situation becomes more stabilized. Often parents need services that social workers or case workers can help provide. These services may alleviate economical and/or other stress the family may be experiencing. For example, the family may need welfare services, food stamps, housing aid, a job, or a myriad of other services. By stabilizing the economical and/or housing situation of parents, less strain might result in the parent-child relationship. Occasionally day care services for the child can be provided. This removes the child from the home and gives the parent time alone. One other way in which parent-child relationships might be altered in the hospital setting is by modeling effects of providing the parents opportunities for identification. The parents may learn to relate to their child in a different manner by modeling the nurses, psychologists, or other hospital personnel's behavior.

Within the hospital and follow-up clinics, the staff can also interview parents about the child's food preferences and eating habits, and through this information can help the parent learn more about nutrition (Farrell & Biernan, 1977). Hospitalized children unaccustomed to balanced and regular meals often thrive, depending on the nature and severity of their illness, within the hospital setting. The family, including the patient, are a captive group for teaching and learning about nutrition (Farrell & Biernan, 1977).

Enhancing a Sense of Mastery and Fostering Adaptive Behavior

Play programs mentioned in the next section offer the best opportunities for enhancing the child's sense of mastery and fostering adaptive behavior (Adams, 1976). Additionally, based on Erikson's theory of psychosocial development, Calkin (1979) developed scales to assess how well small children might be adapting to the hospital experience. The scales assess such behaviors as toileting, eating, resting and sleeping, separation, independence, and dependence on adults (Calkin, 1979).

Play Experiences

A normal and natural part of a child's life is play. Through play the child has the opportunity to experience pleasure, develop intellectually, and resolve conflicts. It is easier now to convince hospital personnel that a play program for both inpatients and outpatients can be extremely beneficial. The importance of a hospital's facilities and space for play programs cannot be overlooked. When children enter the hospital they are entering an oftentimes strange and frightening environment. They are subjected to necessary but painful shots, needle pricks to draw blood for a laboratory workup, examination by the physician, and other intrusions. It can be a time of severe stress for many children. A play program introduces a semblance of normality and the child has an opportunity to interact with other hospitalized children. The child's sense of isolation can be drastically reduced. Of greater importance, play enables children to act out their fears and fantasies, to express their feelings and thus ventilate and reduce the anxieties and tensions that can so often thwart recovery (Adams, 1976; Billington, 1972; Hartley & Goldenson, 1963). Children undergoing surgery or prolonged treatment for serious illnesses, such as leukemia, benefit from play that affords them the opportunity to reenact and master the anxieties they feel and the fantasies they have conjured up about their hospital experience. The psychologist, recreational therapist, or child life worker can assist the child during play by enabling the child to explore and understand his or her feelings about illnesses and hospitalization. The child can then be helped to modify his or her defenses and develop more adaptive behavior (Adams, 1976).

Play programs are also beneficial in reducing the amount of staff time spent controlling or consoling children. The programs can also be used to increase a child's cooperation with medical treatment (Adams, 1976; Billington, 1972).

Hartley and Goldenson (1963) discussed the close relation between recreation and recovery. In Air Force studies the length of hospital stay for patients with major or relatively minor illnesses was drastically cut for those patients actively engaged in recreational and occupational therapy programs. Children who are bedfast for prolonged periods of time need play activities not only to help speed recovery but to stimulate them cognitively and to enhance their emotional and social development. Hospital recreation and Talk Time programs are both beneficial in speeding recovery by allowing the child or adolescent to express feelings and emotions (Sheridan, 1975; White, 1972).

In summary, play activities and play programs are viewed as essential in any hospital that admits children. Play activities can relieve a child's anxieties and fears, enable the child to cope and adapt to the hospital experience, and in general create a more cooperative patient whose recovery is likely faster with, than without, a play program. Those planning to implement a play program will want to read the play program described by Adams (1976), Hartley and Goldenson (1963), and Wolinsky and Koehler (1973). Toys unsafe for use in a hospital must also be considered, and features of such toys include those that can be swallowed, have ropes or loops, come apart easily, explode, burn, cut, or have sharp or rough edges (Frank & Drobish, 1975).

Parental Participation

Parents must be considered an integral part of the child's total hospitalization. Parents are the major support and security system of the child and they must be encouraged to stay with their child during hospitalization (Hardgrove & Rutledge, 1975). This is particularly important for the child 6 years of age and younger.

When it is not possible for parents to remain with their young child there are numerous ways in which the hospital staff and nursing personnel can maintain the hospitalized child's home ties. These include maintaining rituals such as rocking or cuddling the child prior to bedtime, leaving the child with a familiar toy or doll, and enabling the parents to call or write (Chadwick, Pflederer, & Ray, 1978). It is often helpful to teach parents ways in which they can be aware of their child's needs (Hardgrove & Rutledge, 1975). Irwin and Lloyd-Still (1974) utilized groups to mobilize parental strengths during their child's hospitalization. As a result of the weekly parent meetings, the parents were able to minimize their child's emotional reactions to hospitalization, and the hospital personnel became more responsive to parents and children entering the hopsital. The end result of parental participation and education in their child's hospitalization is that the child is happier and feels more secure, and the mother's fears and distress can be reduced significantly (Riley, Syme, Hall, & Patrick, 1965; Robinson, 1968).

SPECIAL PROBLEMS OF THE ADOLESCENT PATIENT

Adolescence is a period of development that has received a special focus in the literature on the impact of illness. The reason for this heightened attention can be readily understood by simply interviewing the medical staff in any children's hospital that has a significant adolescent population. For example, the nursing staff of the burn unit at Oklahoma Children's Memorial Hospital will quite readily discuss horror stories of their numerous adolescent problem patients for as long as anyone would care to listen. Furthermore, one of the medical residents assigned to the adolescent medicine service once told us, only partly tongue-in-cheek, that they really should have a psychologist there attending faculty, and they could then call in a medical consultant on the few occasions that it might seem necessary. For that matter, almost every service at one time or another has commented on the special difficulties presented by the adolescent.

We have already noted some of the special concerns that characterize normal adolescent behavior and will briefly note how these and other concerns may affect the impact of illness on adolescents. Issues of particular concern that have received wide attention include independence and autonomy, heightened awareness of body image, increased status needs, concerns about sexuality, and overall development of role function (e.g., Hofmann, Becker, & Gabriel, 1976; Kimball & Campbell, 1979; Oremland & Oremland, 1973; Schowalter & Loard, 1973). Quite obviously this last concern is in a state of constant change from early to late adolescence, with mid-adolescence (approximately ages 14 to 17) often being singled out as the period of greatest difficulty with respect to adjusting to illness. Enforced dependency, barriers to emancipation, and threats to body-image integrity often induced by hospitalization and illness, may be especially difficult to handle during this time (Hofmann et al., 1976). Examinations or invasive medical procedures may cause adolescents to feel as though their bodies have failed them. Wright et al. (1979) reported that the adolescent's self-esteem may be damaged by physical disability or disfigurement. Adolescents who suffer facial injuries through accidents or burns and adolescents who suffer injuries resulting in paralysis may have tremendous adjustment problems.

A sex difference was suggested by Weinberg (1970), who found that physical illness during adolescence leads to suicidal intent depending upon a somewhat different set of concerns for males and females. Thus, adolescent males were more likely to consider suicide if illness was perceived as a threat to masculine identity, and females were most likely to respond similarly if illness was perceived as a cause of rejection. For these reasons, Oremland and Oremland (1973), among others, have suggested that the impact of illness is greater during adolescence than any other period of development. Not surprisingly, this assumption has not been researched with any degree of thoroughness at this point.

In contrast to this trend, two extensive attempts to evaluate the effects of illness in adolescence were recently reported (Kellerman, Zeltzer, Ellenberg, Dash, & Rigler, 1980; Zeltzer, Kellerman, Ellenberg, Dash, and Rigler, 1980). In these reports, approximately 350 healthy adolescents were compared with 168 adolescents who were affected with various chronic or serious diseases on a variety of self-esteem, trait anxiety, health locus of control, and impact of illness. Although matching procedures and other methodological procedures were less than ideal, several interesting findings emerged. First, no difference between ill and healthy groups was found on measures of either trait anxiety or self-esteem. In terms of health locus of control, some, but not all, of the illness groups demonstrated a reduction in their own sense of control over health. Interestingly, this reduction of perceived control seemed to match reality in that the greatest reduction occurred in illness groups which are not especially responsive to the patient's actions. Prognosis, as rated by physicians, revealed an interesting relationship to anxiety. Those with a "stable" rating were found to have less anxiety than those with prognosis ratings of "uncertain," "deterioration," or "improvement." This finding would suggest that "change" per se, whether it represents deterioration or improvement, is a significant stressor for adolescents who are already attempting to cope with chronic disease and the numerous changes inherent with some normal development.

In terms of the impact of illness (e.g., leukemia or colds), healthy and ill adolescents surprisingly did not differ substantially in terms of their overall scores on a self-report illness impact questionnaire. Specific illness groups did differ somewhat, however, in terms of the particular area of report impact.

In discussing the meaning of these findings, the authors noted, at least for chronically ill outpatients, the disruption of psychological functioning brought on by illness appears to be amazingly small. They also note that this lack of impact may be at least partly due to a denial process which they see as possibly quite adaptive (Kellerman *et al.*, 1980).

The conclusion that denial is adaptive in these cases may be quite valid when applied to everyday functioning. We feel that the assumption is highly questionable when applied to intermittent disease and treatment-related problems. However, Verwoerdt (1972), Kagen (1976), Lloyd (1977), as well as numerous observations of our own, have all suggested that at least under certain circumstances and at certain points during treatment the overuse of denial can have very deleterious results. For example, as previously noted, we have seen patients blithely ignore needed dietary restrictions, forgo required surgery, fail to take necessary medication, and fail to wear Jobst suits needed to reduce scarring. Obviously, denial is not the only relevant variable in these cases, but it does seem to play a large role in many of them. Unquestionably, the relationship is complex. Denial may indeed by very helpful to adolescents (and others) at certain critical points and perhaps even during typical day-to-day life. However, it is plausible that this strategy can have a profoundly negative effect as well. The crucial task, therefore, will be to determine which patients, at which ages, at which points in time, under what conditions, can be best served by encouraging or discouraging this strategy.

SUMMARY

Our review of the psychological effects of physical illness and its concomitants suggests these effects can be both pervasive and profound, but a wide variety of mediating factors influence an individual child's specific reactions. We have noted Erikson's theory of psychosocial development and Piaget's theory of cognitive development are useful general frameworks for understanding some of these reactions. In addition, the emerging technology of cognitive assessment offers substantial promise for the eventual development of a refined analysis of the more specific role played by cognitive structures and process. For example, children's illness-related images and fantasies frequently appear to play a substantial role in determining the child's response to illness. An increased understanding of the frequency, causes, and precise function of such fantasies could be quite helpful in improving children's ability to cope with illness.

The child's reactions to hospitalization itself were also discussed. A variety of procedures for minimizing the negative effects were reviewed, and the potential for maximizing constructive aspects of hospitalization was also noted. Finally, particular problems common to the ill or hospitalized adolescent were presented.

Overall, research efforts in this area have tended to be limited in scope and deficient in the quality of methodological procedures. In part, these deficiencies are due to the difficulties inherent in conducting research in hospital settings. However, it should be clear from our review that the need for further investigations is substantial and that the ''pay off'' for such efforts is likely to be great.

REFERENCES

Abramson, L. Y., Seligman, M. E. P., & Teasdale, J. D. Learned helplessness in humans: Critique and reformulation. *Journal of Abnormal Psychology*, 1978, **87**, 49–74.

Adams, M. A. A hospital play program: Helping children with serious illness. *American Journal of Orthopsychiatry*, 1976, **46**, 416–424.

Addison, C. Social implication of sudden facial disfigurement. *Social Work Today*, 1978, **9**, 19–20.

Azarnoff, P. The care of children in hospitals: An overview. *Journal of Pediatric Psychology*, 1976, **1**, 5–6.

Baekeland, F. Exercise deprivation. *Archives of General Psychiatry*, 1970, **22**, 365–369.

Barowsky, E. I. Young children's perceptions and reactions to hospitalization. In E. Gellert (Ed.), *Psychosocial aspects of pediatric care*. New York: Grune & Stratton, 1978, pp. 37–49.

Beales, J. G. Pain in children with cancer. In J. J. Bonica & V. Ventafridda (Eds.), *Advances in pain research and therapy*, Vol. 2. New York: Raven Press, 1979, pp. 89–98.

Becker, R. D. Therapeutic approaches to psychopathological reactions to hospitalization. *International Journal of Child Psychotherapy*, 1972, **1**, 65–97.

Belmont, H. D. Hospitalization and its effects upon the total child. *Clinical Pediatrics*, 1970, **9**, 472–483.

Bergman, T. Observation of children's reactions to motor restraint. *Nervous Child*, 1945, **4**, 318–334.

Bernstein, N. R. Disfigurement and personality development. In *Emotional care of the facially burned and disfigured*. Boston: Little, Brown, 1976, pp. 41–46.

Billington, G. F. Play program reduces children's anxiety, speeds recoveries. *Modern Hospital*, 1972, **118**, 90–92.

Bowlby, J. Attachment and loss. In *Attachment*, Vol. 1. New York: Basic Books, 1969.

Burling, K.A., & Collip, P. J. Emotional responses of hospitalized children: Results of a pulse-monitor study. *Clinical Pediatrics*, 1969, **8**, 64–646.

Burlingham, D. T. Notes on problems of motor restraint during illness. In R. Lowenstein (Ed.), *Drives, affects, and behavior*. New York: International University Press, 1953, pp. 169–175.

Burstein, S., & Meichenbaum, D. Work of worrying in children undergoing surgery. *Journal of Abnormal Child Psychology*, 1979, **7**, 121–132.

Calkin, J. D. Are hospitalized toddlers adapting to the experience as well as we think? *American Journal of Nursing*, 1979, **4**, 18–23.

Carandang, M. S. A., Folkins, C. H., Hines, P. A., & Steward, M. S. The role of cognitive level and sibling illness in children's conceptualizations of illness. *American Journal of Orthopsychiatry*, 1979, **49**, 474–481.

Chadwick, B. J., Pflederer, D., & Ray, M. A. Maintaining the hospitalized child's home ties. *American Journal of Nursing*, 1978, **78**, 1361–1366.

Cleveland, S. E., & Brewer, E. J. Psychosocial aspects of juvenile rheumatoid arthritis. In E. J. Brewer (Ed.), *Juvenile rheumatoid arthritis*. Philadelphia: Saunders, 1970, pp. 116–131.

Davenport, H. T., & Werry, J. S. The effects of general anesthesia, surgery and hospitalization upon the behavior of children. *American Journal of Orthopsychiatry,* 1970, **40,** 806−824.

Demaio, D. J. Body image concerns of a six year old boy. *Maternal Child Nursing Journal,* 1978, **7,** 175−184.

Diener, C., & Dweck, C. An analysis of learned helplessness: Continuous changes in performance, strategy, and achievement cognitions following failure. *Journal of Personality and Social Psychology,* 1978, **36,** 461−462.

Dombro, R. H., & Haas, B. S. The chronically ill child and his family in the hospital. In M. Debuskey (Ed.), *The chronically ill child and his family.* Springfield, IL: Charles C. Thomas, 1970, pp. 163−180.

Duffy, J. C. Psychiatry: emotional reactions of children to hospitalization. *Minnesota Medicine,* 1972, **55,** 1168−1170.

Eckhardt, L. O., & Prugh, D. Preparing children psychologically for painful medical and surgical procedures. In E. Gellert (Ed.), *Psychosocial aspects of pediatric case.* New York: Grune & Stratton, 1978, pp. 75−81.

Eland, J. M., & Anderson, J. E. The experience of pain in children. In A. K. Joacox (Ed.), *Pain· A sourcebook for nurses and other health professionals.* Boston: Little Brown, 1977, pp. 453−473.

Elliott, C., Ozolins, M., & Ulissi, S. M. A review of children's responses to painful medical procedures. *Oklahoma Health Sciences Manuscript,* 1980.

Erikson, E. *Childhood, youth and society.* New York: Norton, 1964.

Farrell, Sister Ellen, & Biernan, B. S. A positive approach to nutrition for hospitalized children. *Maternal Child Nursing,* 1977, **2,** 113−117.

Fordyce, W. E., Fowler, R. S., Lehmann, J. F., & De Lateur, B. J. Some implications of chronic pain. *Journal of Chronic Disease,* 1968, **21,** 179−180.

Fraiberg, S. M. *The magic years.* New York: Scribner, 1959.

Frank, D. J., and Drobish, N. L. Toy safety in hospitals or beware of parents bearing gifts. *Clinical Pediatrics,* 1975, **14,** 400−402.

Freiberg, K. H. How parents react when their child is hospitalized. *American Journal of Nursing,* 1972, **72,** 1270−1272.

Gaddini, R. The relationship of reactions to illness to developmental stages. *Bibliotheca Psychiatrica,* 1979, **159,** 96−196.

Galdston, R., & Hughes, M. C. Pediatric hospitalization as crisis intervention. *American Journal of Psychiatry,* 1972, **129,** 721−725.

Garrard, S. D., & Richmond, J. B. Psychological aspects of the management of chronic diseases and handicapping conditions in childhood. In H. E. Lief, V. F. Lief, & N. R. Lief (Eds.), *The psychological basis of medical practice.* New York: Harper & Row, 1963.

Gildia, J. H., & Quirk, T. R. Assessing the pain experience in children. *Nursing Clinics of North America,* 1977, **12,** 631−637.

Gross, S. C., and Gardner, G. G. Child pain: Treatment approaches. In *Pain meaning and management.* New York: Spectrum, 1980, pp. 127−142.

Guerin, L. S. Hospitalization as a positive experience for poverty children. *Clinical Pediatrics,* 1977, **16,** 509−513.

Hardgrove, C., & Rutledge, A. Parenting during hospitalization. *American Journal of Nursing,* 1975, **75,** 836–838.

Hartley, R. E., & Goldenson, R. M. *The complete book of children's play.* New York: Crowell, 1963.

Hofmann, A. D., & Becker, R. D. Psychotherapeutic approaches to the physically ill adolescent. *International Journal of Child Psychotherapy,* 1973, **2,** 492–510.

Hofmann, A. D., Becker, R. D., & Gabriel, H. P. *The hospitalized adolescent.* London: Free Press, Collier-Macmillan, 1976.

Holland, J., Harris, S., Plumb, M. Tuttolomondo, A., & Yates, J. Psychological aspects of physical barrier isolation. Observation of acute leukemia patients in germ-free units. *Proceedings of the International Congress on Hematology,* 1970.

Holland, J., Plumb, M., & Yates, J. Psychological response of patients with acute leukemia to germ-free environments. *Cancer,* 1977, **40,** 871–879.

Howe, J. Children's ideas about injury. *ANA Regional Clinical Conferences.* New York: Appelton-Century-Crofts, 1968.

Irwin, S., & Lloyd-Still, D. The use of groups to mobilize parental strengths during hospitalization of children. *Child Welfare,* 1974, **53,** 305–312.

Johnson, B. H. Before hospitalization: A preparation program for the child and his family. *Children Today,* 1974, **3,** 18–26.

Johnson, M. Mental health interventions with medically ill children: A review of the literature 1970–1977. *Journal of Pediatric Psychology,* 1979, **4,** 147–164.

Johnson, S. B. Psychosocial factors in juvenile diabetes: A review. *Journal of Behavioral Medicine,* 1980, **3,** 95–113.

Jolly, J. The grand tour. *Journal of the Association for Care of Children in Hospitals,* 1975, **3,** 2–13.

Jolly, J. D. How to be in the hospital without being frightened. *Nursing Times,* 1977, **73,** 1887–1888.

Kagen, B. Use of denial in adolescent with bone cancer. *Health and Social Work,* 1976, **1,** 71–87.

Kellerman, I., Rigler, D., & Siegel, S. Psychological response of children to isolation in a protected environment. *Journal of Behavioral Medicine,* 1979, **2,** 263–276.

Kellerman, J., Zeltzer, L., Ellenberg, L., Dash, J., & Rigler, D. Psychological effects of illness in adolescence. I. Anxiety, self-esteem, and perception of control. Adolescent medicine. *Journal of Pediatrics,* 1980, **97,** 126–131.

Kendall, P. C., & Korgeski, G. P. Assessment and cognitive-behavioral interventions. *Cognitive Therapy and Research,* 1979, **3,** 1–21.

Kenny, J. The hospitalized child. *Pediatric Clinics of North America,* 1975, **22,** 583–593.

Kiely, W. F. Coping with severe illness. *Advances in Psychosomatic Medicine,* 1972, **3,** 105.

Kimball, A. J., & Campbell, M. M. Psychological aspects of adolescent patient health care. *Clinical Pediatrics,* 1979, **18,** 15–24.

Kornfield, D. S. The hospital environment: Its impact on the patient. *Advances in Psychosomatic Medicine,* 1972, **8,** 255–270.

Korsch, B. M. Psychologic reactions to physical illness in children. 107th Annual Session of the Medical Association of Georgia, Atlanta, 1961, **50,** 519–523.

Langford, W. S. The child in the pediatric hospital: Adaptation to illness and hospitalization. *American Journal of Orthopsychiatry,* 1961, **31**, 667–683.

Lipowski, Z. J. Physical illness, the individual, and the coping process. *Psychiatric Medicine,* 1970, **1,** 91–102.

Lloyd, G. G. Psychological reactions to physical illness. *British Journal of Hospital Medicine,* 1977, **18**, 352–358.

Mahler, M. Mother-child interaction during separation-individuation. *Psychoanalytic Quarterly,* 1965, **34,** 483–498.

Maddison, B., & Raphael, B. Social and psychological consequences of chronic disease in childhood. *Medical Journal of Australia,* 1971, **2**, 2165–2170.

Mason, E. A. The hospitalized child—his emotional needs. *New England Journal of Medicine,* 1965, **272**, 406–414.

Mattsson, A. Long-term physical illness in childhood: A challenge to psychosocial adaptation. *Pediatrics,* 1972, **50**, 801–805. (a)

Mattsson, A. The chronically ill child: A challenge to family adaptation. *MCV Quarterly,* 1972, **8,** 171–175. (b)

Meadow, S. R. The captive mother. *Archives on Diseases in Childhood,* 1969, **44,** 362–367.

Meichenbaum, D., & Butler, L. Cognitive ethology: Assessing the streams of cognitive and emotion. In K. Blankstein, P. Pliner, & J. Polivy (Eds.), *Advances in the study of communication and effect: Assessment and modification of emotional behavior.* New York: Plenum Press, 1979, pp. 1–54.

Melamed, B. G., Meyer, R., Gee, C., & Soule, L. The influence of time and type of preparation on children's adjustment to hospitalization. *Journal of Pediatric Psychology,* 1976, **1,** 31–37.

Melzack, R. *The puzzle of pain.* New York: Basic Books, 1973.

Melzack, R. & Wall, P. D. Pain mechanisms: A theory. *Science,* 1965, **150,** 971–979.

Miller, S. M. Coping with impending stress: Psychophysiological and cognitive correlates of choice. *Psychophysiology,* 1979, **16,** 572–581.

Morgenstern, F. S. Facilities for children's play in hospitals. *Developmental Medical Child Neurology,* 1968, **10,** 111–114.

Murphy, C. The therapeutic value of children's literature. *Nursing Forum,* 1972, **11,** 141–164.

Nagera, H. Children's reactions to hospitalization and illness. *Child Psychiatry and Human Development,* 1978, **9,** 3–19.

Neuhauser, C., Amsterdam, B., Hines, P., & Steward, M. Children's concepts of healing: Cognitive development and locus of control factors. *American Journal of Orthopsychiatry,* 1978, **48,** 334–341.

Nowicki, S., & Strickland, B. R. A locus of control scale for children. *Journal of Consulting and Clinical Psychology,* 1973, **40,** 2–8.

Oremland, E. K., & Oremland, J. D. *The effects of hospitalization on children,* Vol. 2. Springfield, IL: Charles C. Thomas, 1973.

Parcel, G. S., & Meyer, M. P. Development of an instrument to measure children's health locus of control. *Health Monographs, 1978,* **6,** 149–159.

Parker, H. J. Children and youth with physical and health disabilities. In B. Swanson & D. J.

Willis (Eds.), *Understanding exceptional children and youth*. Chicago: Rand McNally, 1979, pp. 377–407.

Peterson, L., & Ridley-Johnson, R. Pediatric hospital response to survey on prehospital preparation for children. *Journal of Pediatric Psychology*, 1980, **5**, 1–7.

Petrillo, M., & Sanger, S. *Emotional care of hospitalized children*. Philadelphia: Lippincott, 1972.

Piaget, J., & Inhelder, B. *The psychology of the child*. New York: Basic Books, 1969.

Pomarico, C., Marsch, K., & Doubrava, P. Hospital orientation for children. *AORN*, 1979, **29**, 864–870.

Porter, L. S. On the importance of activity. *Maternal-Child Nursing Journal*, 1973, **2**, 85–91.

Prugh, D. Emotional aspects of the hospitalization of children. In M. Shore (Ed.), *Red is the color of hurting*. Washington, DC: U.S. Government Printing Office, 1965, pp. 19–34.

Prugh, D. G. Children's reactions to illness, hospitalization and surgery. In A. M. Freidman & H. I. Kaplan (Eds.), *The child*. New York: Atheneum, 1972, pp. 181–194.

Prugh, D., & Eckhardt, L. O. Children's reactions to illness, hospitalization and surgery. In A. M. Friedman, H. I. Kaplan, & B. J. Sodock (Eds.), *Comprehensive textbook of psychiatry*. Baltimore: Williams & Wilkins, 1975.

Prugh, D., Staub, E. M., Sands, H. H., Kirschbaum, R. M., & Lenihan, E. A. A study of the emotional reactions of children and families to hospitalization. *American Journal of Orthopsychiatry*, 1953, **23**, 70–106.

Purcell, K., Weiss, J. H., & Hahn, W. W. Certain psychosomatic disorders. In B. B. Wolman (Ed.), *Manual of child psychopathology*. New York: McGraw-Hill, 1972, pp. 706–740.

Rae, W. A., & Stieber, D. A. Plant play therapy: Growth through growth. *Journal of Pediatric Psychology*, 1976, **1**, 18–20.

Richmond, J. B. The pediatric patient in illness. In M. H. Hollender (Ed.), *The psychology of medical practice*. Philadelphia: Saunders, 1958.

Riley, I. D., Syme, J., Hall, M. S., & Patrick, M. J. Mother and child in hospital—Ten years experience. *British Medical Journal*, 1965, **2**, 990–992.

Robinson, D. Mothers' fear, their children's well-being in hospital and the study of illness behavior. *British Journal of Medicine*, 1968, **22**, 228–233.

Scahill, M. Preparing children for procedures and operations. *Nursing Outlook*, 1967, **5**, 35–38.

Scherzer, A. L., Ilson, J. B., Mike, V., & Landoli, M. Educational and social development among intensively treated young patients having cerebral palsy. *Archives of Physical Medicine and Rehabilitation*, 1972, **54**, 478–484.

Schowalter, J. E. Psychological reactions to physical illness and hospitalization in adolescence. *Academy of Child Psychology*, 1977, **16**, 500–516.

Schowalter, J. E., & Loard, R. D. On the writings of adolescents in a general hospital ward. *Psychoanalytic Study of the Child*, 1973, **27**, 181–200.

Schultz, N. How children perceive pain. *Nursing Outlook*, 1971, **19**, 670.

Seligman, M. E. P. *Helplessness: On depression, development, and death*. San Francisco: Freeman, 1975.

Seligman, R. Psychiatric classification system for burned children. *American Journal of Psychiatry,* 1974, **131**, 41–46.

Sheridan, M. Talk time for hospitalized children. *Social Work,* 1975, **20**, 40–44.

Shontz, F. C. The personal meanings of illness. *Advances in Psychosomatic Medicine,* 1972, **8**, 63–85.

Shore, M. F., Geiser, R. L., & Wolman, H. M. Constructive uses of a hospital experience. *Children,* 1965, **12**, 3–8.

Shore, M., & Goldston, S. E. Mental health aspects of pediatric care. In P. Magrab (Ed.), *Psychological management of pediatric problems.* Baltimore: University Park Press, 1978, pp. 15–31.

Simeonsson, R. J., Buckley, L., & Monson, L. Conceptions of illness causality in hospitalized children. *Journal of Pediatric Psychology,* 1979, **4**, 77–84.

Skipper, J. K., & Leonard, R. C. Children, stress and hospitalization: A field experiment. *Journal of Health and Social Behavior,* 1968, **9**, 275–287.

Spitz, R. *The first year of life.* New York: International Universities Press, 1965.

Spitz, R. A. *Hospitalization: An inquiry into the genesis of psychiatric conditions in early childhood.* New York: International University Press, 1945, pp. 53–74.

Steinhauer, P. D., Mushin, D. N., & Rae-Grant, Q. Psychological aspects of chronic illness. *Pediatric Clinics of North America,* 1974, **21**, 825–840.

Swanson, B. M., & Willis, D. J. *Understanding exceptional children and youth.* Chicago: Rand McNally, 1979.

Szaz, T. S. *Pain and pleasure.* New York: Basic Books, 1957.

Tagliacozz, D. M., & Ima K. Knowledge of illness as a predictor of patient behavior. *Journal of Chronic Diseases,* 1970, **22**, 765–775.

Tekely, K., & Dittemore, I. Regressive behavior in a hospitalized preschool child. *Maternal Child Nursing Journal,* 1978, **7**, 185–190.

Travis, G. *Chronic illness in children.* Stanford, CA: Stanford University Press, 1976.

Vernon, D. T. A., Schulman, J. L., & Foley, J. M. Changes in children's behavior after hospitalization. *American Journal of Diseases of Children,* 1966, **3**, 581–593.

Verwoerdt, A. Psychopathological responses to the stress of physical illness. *Advances in Psychosomatic Medicine,* 1972, **8**, 119–141.

Weinberg, S. Suicidal intent in adolescence: A hypothesis about the role of physical illness. *Journal of Pediatrics,* 1970, **77**, 579–586.

West, D. A., & Shuck, J. M. Emotional problems of the severely burned patient. *Surgical Clinics in North America,* 1978, **58**, 1189–1204.

White, P. Hospital recreation helps adolescent patients. *Canadian Nurse,* 1972, **68**, 34–35.

Whitt, K., Dykstra, W., & Taylor, C. A. Children's conceptions of illness and cognitive development. *Clinical Pediatrics,* 1979, **18**, 327–334.

Williams, T. K. Infants' reactions to restraint of mobility: A review of literature. *Maternal-Child Nursing Journal,* 1973, **2**, 229–235.

Wolinsky, G. F., & Koehler, N. A cooperative program in materials development for very young hospitalized children. *Rehabilitation Literature,* 1973, **34**, 34–41.

Woods, T. L. Comments on the dynamics and treatment of disfigured children. *Clinical Social Work Journal,* 1975, **3**, 16–23.

Wright, L., Schaefer, A., & Solomons, G. *Encyclopedia of pediatric psychology*. Baltimore: University Park Press, 1979.

Zeltzer, L., Kellerman, J., Ellenberg, L., Dash, J., & Rigler, D. Psychologic effects of illness in adolescence. II. Impact of illness in adolescents-crucial issues and coping styles. *Journal of Pediatrics*, 1980, **97,** 132−138.

Ziter, F. A., & Allsop, K. G. The diagnoses and management of childhood muscular dystrophy. *Clinical Pediatrics*, 1976, **15,** 540−548.

CHAPTER 3

Assessment Techniques in Pediatric Psychology

Phyllis R. Magrab
Ellen Lehr

Psychological assessment in pediatric settings is part of a larger process of health care that aims at the optimum development and the quality of life of children and their families. The cognitive, emotional, and social dimensions of individual differences may be significantly altered by pediatric conditions. The contribution of pediatric psychological assessment to the process of health care is targeted toward an understanding of the interaction of psychological and physical well-being.

Because the population of children served by pediatric psychologists encompasses a spectrum of etiologically defined conditions and psychological problems, the need for specific appropriate assessment approaches is critical. The pediatric psychologist may be involved in assessing children with developmental problems, chronic and terminal illness, and behavioral or habit disorders. The assessment of children with developmental problems, including mental retardation, neurological deficits, moderate to severe learning disabilities, sensory impairment, and congenital malformations often focuses on the interaction of cognitive factors with social and emotional development. Deficits in language, motor, social, and cognitive skills place these children at risk for normal learning and educational gains. With children experiencing chronic or terminal illnesses such as pulmonary disorders, renal disease, cardiac disease, epilepsy, diabetes, muscular dystrophy, or cancer, the relationship of the disease process to psychological development and adjustment is a key assessment question. In addition, coping with the stress of a disease on normal developmental tasks and on family life is a complex psychological process. For the array of behavioral and habit disorders including feeding problems, enuresis, and encopresis, highly specific assessment questions and strategies emerge. The pediatric psychologist is compelled to develop complex assessment skills to address the various assessment issues for the broad pediatric population.

The role of assessment in the practice of pediatric psychology is both diverse and highly specialized. Essentially, psychological assessment in pediatric settings assists in determining the level of intellectual, emotional, behavioral, and/or social functioning of children with specific conditions or problems to be utilized for treatment and intervention planning. Developing a psychological profile of a child directly relates to determining appropriate intervention strategies both in terms of initial decisions and ongoing reevaluation. Frequently, in pediatric practice, assessment of baseline functioning is necessary to monitor development and to ascertain the effects of medical, behavioral, or educational treatments. Through repeated psychological assessments and follow-up, patient change-over-time can be documented both in relation to specific interventions and in relation to the condition itself. From a program development perspective, pediatric psychological assessments can contribute to an understanding of the types of intervention approaches that are most effective for particular problems. Although intervention planning represents the most significant arena for pediatric psychological assessment, there continues to be a need for more accurate descriptions of the psychological components of such conditions as genetic diseases and neurologically based disorders.

In developing an approach to assessing children and families, pediatric psychologists have come to rely on a variety of techniques and instruments that encompass the multiple dimensions of psychological functioning: developmental measures, intelligence tests, social/emotional and personality techniques, behavior scales, neuropsychological procedures, and interview and family techniques. Measures of developmental status that describe the progression of behaviors in functional categories such as language, motor, adaptive, cognitive, and social/ emotional skills are useful to obtain an overall picture of the developmental status of young children. These developmental measures range in depth from brief screening tools to complex assessment techniques. Measures of intelligence include well-known standardized individual intelligence tests as well as more recently developed instruments for special populations of children. Assessing the neuropsychological, emotional, and social components of pediatric conditions requires a blending of personality, behavioral, and adaptive measures and techniques as well as interview strategies. The family must be part of the assessment process and there are specific assessment techniques useful to pediatric psychologists for this purpose.

COGNITIVE ASSESSMENT

For the psychologist, assessing cognition is a complex undertaking. The process of thinking that permits us to manipulate and to interact with our environment is multifaceted and difficult to measure. Various psychologists have developed instruments that assist in understanding the cognitive functioning of children, but these measures do not derive from a single philosophical point of view. Many of these tests are intellectual measures that focus on the reasoning process, the adaptation of the child to the environment, and/or the child's patterns of verbal and performance behaviors. Cognitive assessment procedures vary substantially depending on the nature of the condition and the age of the child. The use of these measures with pediatric conditions has become increasingly important in pediatric care.

Infant Assessment

Major issues in infant cognitive assessment have been raised by psychologists who have advanced the state of the art of infant testing that serves as a prelude to any pediatric psychologist's attempt to utilize infant measurement techniques (Kopp, 1979; Ramey & Smith, 1976; Vietze & St. Claire, 1976). First of all, standardized infant measures clearly sample only a small segment of the developmental characteristics of the young child. Important areas of early development that impinge on cognition are excluded from typical infant assessment techniques such as measurement of play, attention, problemsolving strategies, and nonverbal communication (Johnson & Kopp, 1980). Second, psychologists need to document more than the infant's status on measures of progressive behaviors by assessing, in addition, the infant's process of learning at the time (Ramey & Smith, 1976). Related to this, in understanding the learning process of the infant it is important to look beyond the infant to the interactive process between the infant and parent or primary caretaker. Furthermore, Kopp (1979) asserts that infant tests lack a conceptual rationale and that the gap between what is measured and what should be measured in the face of new knowledge about infant learning and development is wide. Continually, questions are raised by reseachers about the reliablity and validity of the range of infant assessment instruments (Kopp, 1979; Vietze & St. Claire, 1976). For infants with major handicaps, tests fail to be adapted to their special needs and have not been appropriately normed. Given these constraints related to infant measures, pediatric psychologists must be cautious in the use of infant measures and supplement them with direct observation of learning style and play while applying a developmental conceptual framework to the overall assessment process.

Evaluation of the Newborn

The earliest evaluation of infant functioning that is at least partially related to cognitive potential is conducted at the moment of birth by the attending physician. The Apgar screening technique (Apgar, 1953) involves rating the newborn 60 seconds and 1, 5, or 10 minutes after birth for heart rate, respiratory effort, reflex irritability, muscle tone, and color. Often the physician will follow up on the Apgar screening with a neurological examination to determine gestational age and neurological status (Dubowitz, Dubowitz, & Goldberg, 1970; Prechtl & Beintema, 1964). The psychological assessment of infants by a pediatric psychologist should interface with these medical evaluations.

Increasingly, the behavioral repertoire of the newborn infant has come to be understood and valued in terms of predicting future developmental status. Two major assessment techniques are available to the pediatric psychologist that are designed exclusively for newborns: the Brazelton Neonatal Behavioral Assessment Scale (Brazelton, 1973) and the Graham-Rosenblith Neonatal Behavioral Examination (Rosenblith, 1961). The Brazelton Neonatal Behavioral Assessment Scale is the most widely used of the neonatal scales. Typically, it is administered during the first two or three days of life. The test consists of both behavioral and neurological items. Twenty-seven behavioral items scored on a 9-point scale assess habituation, motor activity, motor control, stimulus responsivity, and organization; 21 neurological items are scored on a 3-point scale to assess elicited reflexes. Obtaining optimum responses and administering items during appropriate levels of arousal is the key to an adequate assessment. Brazelton points out the need for repeat assessment to assure confidence in results. Although there is no formal standardization sample for the scale, researchers have provided their own normative data. Horowitz and Brazelton (1973) reported a high interrater reliability range.

The Brazelton scale has been used to document obstetrical medication effects (Aleksandrowicz & Aleksandrowicz, 1974; Standley, Soule, Copans, & Duchowny, 1974), maternal narcotic addiction effects (Kron, Finnegan, Kaplan, Litt, & Phoenix, 1975; Soule, Standley, Copans, & Davis, 1974; Strauss, Lessen-Firestone, Starr, & Ostrea, 1975), cross-cultural differences in neonates (Brazelton, Robey, & Collier, 1969; Brazelton & Tryphonopoulou, 1973; Freedman & Freedman, 1969), prematurity effects (Scarr-Salapatek & Williams, 1973; Sostek, Quinn, & Davitt, 1979), and the effects of high-risk conditions (DiVitto & Goldberg, 1979). Recent studies have begun to compare Brazelton scores with other tasks such as with later visual discrimination during infancy (McCluskey & Horowitz, 1975) and with auditory conditioning (Franz, Self, & Franz, 1976).

The Graham-Rosenblith Neonatal Behavioral Examination is a revision of the Graham Scale (Rosenblith, 1961) that was designed to differentiate between brain-injured and normal newborns. On the Graham-Rosenblith scale, a total maturation score is derived from two subscales: motor and tactile-adaptive. Each subscale has a maximum of 9 point yielding a maximum total maturational score of 18. The sensory scales include visual responsiveness and auditory responsiveness. Ratings of muscle tone and irritability are also obtained. No standardization data are completed. Interobserver reliability is reported by Brown, Bakeman, Snyder, Frederickson, Morgan, and Hepler (1975) with a range of .83−1.00; interexaminer reliabilities are reported ranging from .42 for the vision scale to .91 for the maturation scale (Bench & Parker, 1970; Rosenblith, 1975).

The Graham-Rosenblith was used as part of the collaborative Perinatal Project which included 1500 infants. Comparison data with later measures at 8 months and 4 years of age suggested that the test is useful in prediction of future cognitive status for infants below 37 weeks gestational age (Rosenblith, 1974a). Thus, it is particularly relevant for the study of high-risk infants. Rosenblith (1974b) also reported the predictive capability of this test for the incidence of Sudden Infant Death Syndrome (SIDS).

Cognitive Evaluation of the Infant

The field of infant assessment had its beginning with Arnold Gessell, and a revised version of his work continues in use today (*the Gessell and Amatruda's Differential Diagnosis;* Knobloch & Pasamanick, 1974). On these scales, behavior is divided into five areas: gross motor, fine motor, adaptive, language, and personal/social, to be examined at the key ages of 4, 16, 28, and 40 weeks, and 12, 18, 24, and 36 months. The Gessell Developmental Schedules have been extensively standardized and test-retest reliability is high (Knobloch & Pasamanick, 1974). The scale has been widely used in infant research and particularly in longitudinal studies (Fish, Shapiro, Halpern, & Wile, 1965) because it was designed to be used repeatedly over a number of years. Parmalee, Kopp, and Sigman (1976) pointed out that one of the most important strengths of this developmental measure is its capability for examination of intrainfant variability in motor, adaptive, language and personal/social behaviors.

The Cattell Infant Intelligence Scale (1940) was developed specifically as a downward extension of the Stanford-Binet Intelligence Scale and this continues to be one of its chief distinguishing features for clinicians. The scale extends from 2 to 36 months. Items are grouped by age level at intervals of one month during the first year, two months during the second year, and three months during the first half of the third year.

Cattell initially standardized the scale on 274 children participating in a longitudinal study at the Harvard School of Public Health. Test-retest reliability reports have ranged from .01 to .96 (Cavanaugh, Cohen, Dunphy, Ringwall, & Goldberg, 1957; Gallagher, 1953). Cattell indicated that the predictive validity with the Stanford-Binet at 3 years is adequate after 12 months of age. Other studies have indicated poor validity up to 24 months (Escalona & Moriarty, 1961).

The Griffiths Mental Development Scale (Griffiths, 1954) has an age range from 1 to 24 months. The scale is divided into five parts: personal/social, locomotor, hearing and speech, eye and hand coordination, and performance, similar to the Gessell Developmental Schedule. It offers similar advantages because of this. Initial standardization was on 604 British infants. Currently, no observer reliability data are available. Griffiths initially reported a .87 coefficient of stability on a sample of 60 children. Hindly (1960) and Roberts and Sedgley (1965) reported correlation of 6- and 8-month Griffiths Scores with IQ on the Stanford-Binet at 5 years. Data are not available on the predictive power of performance on the Griffiths scale during the first few months of life. Griffiths, in developing the scale, made clear that the role of the scale was to measure current functioning and not to predict future status.

The Bayley Scales of Infant Development (Bayley, 1969) are the most carefully developed and best standardized of all the infant scales. The Bayley Scales include a mental scale, a motor scale, and a behavioral scale. The age range for the Bayley Scales is 1 month to 2½ years and items are arranged in chronological order. The Bayley Scales have been standardized on 1262 infants stratified according to sex, race, and education of head of household. Test-retest reliability, interexaminer reliability, and split-half reliabilities that are reported by Bayley are satisfactory. The Bayley Scales scores do not appear to be influenced by repeated use of the instrument (Haskin, Ramey, Stedman, Blacher-Dixon, Pierce, 1978), which make it useful for many clinical follow-along situations.

The Bayley Scales have been correlated with measures of infant cognitive performance (Gottfried & Brody, 1975; King & Seegmiller, 1973, Matheny, 1975), with observations of mother-infant interaction (Lee-Painter & Lewis, 1974), and with hereditary or physiological influences (Nichols & Broman, 1974; Wilson,

1974). The comparative predictive strength of SES and infant Bayley scores was examined by Ireton, Thwing, and Grave (1970) and Willerman, Broman, and Fiedler (1970) who found SES to be a better predictor of high 4-year-old IQs, but Bayley scores, a better predictor of low 4-year-old IQs. Ramey, Campbell, and Nicholson (1973) reported high correlation of Bayley mental and motor scores with 3-year-old IQs in a group that had similar environmental day care over a 3-year period.

Two assessment procedures based on Piagetian theory have recently been developed: the Einstein Scales of Sensorimotor Intelligence (Corman & Escalona, 1969) and the Uzgiris-Hunt Ordinal Scales of Psychological Development (Uzgiris & Hunt, 1975). The Einstein Scales were constructed as part of a comprehensive study aimed at measuring early cognitive development. The three scales—comprehension, object permanence, and spatial relations—are designed for infants between the ages of 1 and 24 months. The scale defines four Piagetian stages and four substages. Little research has been done as yet using this scale.

The Uzgiris-Hunt Ordinal Scale of Psychological Development is similar to the Einstein scale but is divided into six scales: visual pursuit and permanence of objects, outcome-initiated action, development of imitation, development of operational causality, construction of object relations in space, and development of schemes for relating to objects. Limited data on the relationship between the Uzgiris-Hunt scale and other infant measures currently exists (King & Seegmiller, 1975; Uzgiris, 1976; Wachs, 1975).

Assessment Considerations with Special Populations of Infants

Developmental and psychological assessment of infants has two primary objectives. For conditions that are known to be related to cognitive impairments, assessment can be utilized to evaluate the extent of impairment and to monitor intervention or treatment procedures. In those conditions that do not directly affect cognitive development but have an impact on a child's general functioning, assessment has a preventative focus in attempting to identify problem areas as they arise.

For the group of infants who are at continued risk of cognitive deficits from birth, there have been numerous attempts to develop strategies for identification at the earliest possible moment. Some of these infants, because of the nature of their conditions, are easily recognized as at risk from birth—for others there is potential for more variable outcomes.

In some of the pediatric conditions that occur during infancy, lowered cognitive functioning is probably an effect of the disease process itself. Most prominent of these are the conditions that directly compromise the central nervous system either through infections (encephalitis, meningitis), congenital defects (hydrocephalus, phenylketonuria), nutrition (iron deficiency, lead poisoning), or trauma (head injuries). In other pediatric conditions the treatment may have an impact on cognitive development, either enhancing intellectual potential or possibly interfering with normal growth. Since cognitive and social/emotional development are closely integrated during this period of life, the interactional limitations experienced by these infants may have an adverse effect on their intellectual development as well. With high risk infants, multiple cumulative assessments are considered more predictive than any single infant assessment or variable. Sigman and Parmalee (1979) attempted to improve assessment of risk factors through multiple evaluation of infants and environmental characteristics. Prenatal, natal, and neonatal events and neonatal performance interact in an additive manner. Diagnostic measures utilized by Sigman and Parmalee (1979) included an obstetrical complication scale, postnatal complication scale, newborn neurological examination, visual attention rates, sleep polygraph, caregiver-infant interaction measure, developmental scale, cognitive scale, motor scale, novelty scale, and a pediatric complications scale. They found that early measures of neurological and behavioral states accounted for only a small part of outcome variance. Significant for pediatric psychological assessment, they pointed out in their results, is the importance of taking into consideration the ongoing transactions between child and environment in newborn and infant assessment.

Infants with respiratory distress represent a risk group that has been identified with clearly demonstrated variable outcomes. Some studies show early delays in development with normalization by the preschool years. (Ambrus, Weintraub, Niswander, Fischer, Fleishman, Bross, & Ambrus, 1970; Fisch, Bilek, Miller, & Engel, 1975). However, greater deficits are reported for those infants who have required ventilatory support (Harrod, L'Heureaux, Wagensteen, & Hunt, 1974; Johnson, Malachowski, Grobstein, Dailey, & Sunshine, 1974). For this group, Field, Hallock, Ting, Dempsey, Dabiri, and Shuman (1978) proposed a cumulative risk index to address the problem of predicting continued risk to cognitive development.

The preterm infant and low-birth-weight infant are at greater risk for cognitive delays or deficits and damage to the central nervous system than are other infants (Francis-Williams & Davies, 1974; Lubchenco, Bard, Goldman, Coyer, McIntyre, & Smith, 1974). The assessment of the premature infant poses an especially difficult problem for pediatric psychologists. Allowances must be made for prematurity since biological maturity continues to influence cognitive development for at least the first two years of life. Scoring of infant tests should be based on biological age as opposed to chronological age when attempting to document the infant's developmental status (Hunt & Rhodes, 1977).

Early assessment and frequent follow-up are useful in detecting possible neurological complications of medical conditions in infancy (Fishman & Palkes, 1974; Phatak & Phatak, 1973). Infant assessment can be especially useful in determining the early neurological effects of such conditions as meningitis, encephalitis, and sickle cell disease (Flick & Duncan, 1973). The risk of neurological involvement in meningitis and encephalitis, has been found to be particularly handicapping when onset occurs during the first two years of life (Boll, 1973; Finley et al., 1967; Ford, 1944; Vernon, 1967). In the case of iron deficiency (Oski & Honig, 1978), lead poisoning (Chisholm, 1973; Wright & Fulwiler, 1972), and malnutrition (Guthrie, Masangkay, & Guthrie, 1976; Klein, Freeman & Yarbrough, 1971), infant assessment can be useful not only in evaluating developmental delays but also in measuring improvement after effective treatment.

Assessing the cognitive status of multiply handicapped or sensory impaired infants presents special problems for the pediatric psychologist since most infant tests have not been standardized for this population. Some psychologists argue that administering infant tests according to standardized requirements gives a more accurate picture of the infant in relation to others; but most psychologists agree that adaptation of these tests to accommodate the specific handicaps of the infant offers a better understanding of the infant's skills and learning potential. Criticos (in press), in an extensive discussion of the applicability and adaptibility of infant tests for the multiply and sensory impaired infant, suggests that the Bayley Infant Scales have more cognitive items than most other infant scales and leave the most room for adaptation. Accounting for the handicap of the infant should be encouraged through item omissions, substitution, and alternative scoring. Visually handicapped infants require kinesthetic and physical guidance to compensate for visual clues. In selecting a test, the psychologist should keep in mind that the Griffiths Scales are less visually oriented than the Bayley Scales, and the Gesell Scale is a blend of auditory and visual items (Criticos, in press). For the auditorily impaired infant, language items are more difficult to adapt and greater examiner judgment is required.

Infants with chronic medical conditions during the first two years of life constitute a high-risk population for possible cognitive deficits and delays. For medically involved infants the loss of stimulation through prolonged hospitalization, restricted physical activity (either related to illness or treatment), and delayed or interrupted parent/child attachment may adversely effect cognitive development. Since many of these infants have either less experience in sensorimotor areas or have defects that prohibit learning or interacting through this mode, the heavy reliance on sensorimotor areas of the infant assessment scales may especially penalize the performance (Feldt, Ervert, Stickler, & Weidman, 1969; Lewis & McGurk, 1972). The positive influence of the mother's presence during testing should be kept in mind. When infants are tested in a hospital setting without benefit of their mothers present, spuriously low assessments may result (Haskin, Ramey, Craig, Stedman, Blacher-Dixon, & Pierce, 1978).

Many of the components of illness during the first two years of life interfere with optimal performance during assessment. Behaviorally, chronically ill infants may exhibit irritability, lessened interest in their surroundings, and decreased attentiveness (Oski & Honig, 1978). They may associate the presence of strange adults with painful medical treatments. Chronically ill infants also fatigue easily with correspondingly lowered performance on many of the timed sensorimotor tasks common on infant scales (Feldt et al., 1969).

Research on cognitive assessment of chronically ill infants is not extensive. Probably the most thoroughly studied group has been those infants diagnosed with congenital heart disease. According to Posey (1974), congenital heart disease is the leading cause of illness and death in infancy, even though improved treatment has increased the number of children who survive beyond the first year. The delayed motor milestones of these infants, especially those who are cyanotic, lowers their performance on infant scales such as the Bayley and Cattell (Feldt et al, 1969).

However, on follow-up assessments using verbally oriented scales such as the Stanford-Binet, there is no difference between cyanotic and normal children (Linde *et al.*, 1967). Surgical correction of congenital heart defects either is associated with a maintenance of prior average functioning or an increase of postoperative IQ (Landtman, Valanne, Pentti, & Aukee, 1960; Stevenson, Stone, Dillard, & Morgan, 1974; Whitman, Drotar, Lamberti, VanHeeckeren, Borkat, Ankeny, & Liebman, 1973).

It should be kept in mind that infant assessment can also be utilized with at-risk infants to document age-level or better functioning, not only to evaluate possible delays or deficits. Reassurance that an at-risk infant is developing at a level commensurate with developmental norms can encourage continued stimulation, promote infant-parent interaction, and lessen the overprotection that can interfere with developmental progress both cognitively and emotionally.

Preschool and School Age Cognitive Assessment

In assessing cognition and intelligence in young children and school-age children, pediatric psychologists must keep in mind that it is erroneous to view an intellectual assessment as a measure of an innate, fixed capacity. Intelligence tests are limited in the types of behaviors and problem-solving approaches they sample, and they do not measure the same aspects of intelligence at all ages. There are a variety of factors that affect cognitive testing, including familial, personality, socioeconomic, and cultural variables. These must be understood to adequately interpret and utilize assessment results. The bias in intelligence tests and their use with minority groups has been consistently challenged. A psychologist must exercise extensive caution in the use and interpretation of intellectual testing results with minority populations (Oakland, 1977). An equally important bias is the test item selection in standardized tests vis-à-vis children with specific handicaps, that is., audiovisual or motor deficits.

Sattler (1974) lists some important limitations of intelligence tests which should be a cautionary prelude for the clinician. These limitations include unreliability of test results for long-range prediction and the limited information gathered about the cognitive domain and processes that underlie test responses. The best use of intellectual assessments is to determine current levels of functioning for prescriptive and planning purposes, in conjunction with observation reports from parents and teachers.

Preschool Cognitive Assessment Measures

The Stanford-Binet Intelligence Scale (Terman & Merrill, 1973), the Merrill-Palmer Scale of Mental Tests (Stutsman, 1948), the Wechsler Preschool and Primary Scale of Intelligence (Wechsler, 1967), and the McCarthy Scale of Children's Abilities (McCarthy, 1972) are the four most frequently used tests with preschool children.

The Stanford-Binet Intelligence Scale, covering a chronological age range from 2 through 18 years, consists of a mixture of verbal and nonverbal subtests at each age level. It is important to note that the Stanford-Binet does not assess the same psychological processes at all age levels. From 2 to 5 years of age, the test largely measures such functions as visual-motor capacities, nonverbal reasoning, social intelligence, and language functions. These four areas comprise 85% of the items in the 2 to 5 year age range, whereas cognitive functions, such as memory and conceptual reasoning, are emphasized in the school-age years. The current edition of the Stanford-Binet (1972) was developed by renorming the 1960 edition without a corresponding revision of the test content. This procedure has been criticized by Salvia, Ysseldyke, and Lee (1975) because it jeopardizes the age placement characteristics of the test. Currently, the Stanford-Binet is in the process of a complete revision.

The McCarthy Scale of Children's Abilities (McCarthy, 1972), a relatively new test for ages 2½ to 8½, consists of 18 subtests that are grouped into six scales: verbal, perceptual-performance, quantitative, general cognitive, memory, and motor. A general cognitive index (GCI) can be attained; however, it may not be directly comparable to IQ scores derived from conventional tests (Gerken, Hancock & Wade, 1978; Phillips, Pasewark, & Tindall, 1978). Nagle (1979) in reviewing the reliability and validity studies of McCarthy, and Kaufman and Kaufman (1977), pointed to the importance of this new test because of the child-oriented nature of the tasks and its excellent reliability and standardization. It is increasingly being used in clinical settings because of the extensive profile it yields of a young child's abilities. The test's major limitations are the length of time required for assessment and the question of its validity for use with exceptional children (Salvia & Ysseldyke, 1978).

The Wechsler Preschool and Primary Scale of Intelligence (WPPSI) (Wechsler 1967), for ages 4 to 6½, includes 11 subtests and yields a language, performance, and full-scale IQ. The WPPSI can be easily adapted for use with special populations because the subtests are divided into these three areas.

The Merrill-Palmer Scale of Mental Tests (1948) is predominantly a performance test, although there are some verbal items covering ages 18 to 71 months. It is especially useful with hearing-impaired preschoolers and children with language delays because of its emphasis on perceptual-motor items. However, the available norms and technical aspects of the test are less adequate than more recently developed tests.

School Age Cognitive Assessment Measures

Among the individual intelligence tests used with developmentally disabled children, the Wechsler Intelligence Scale for Children-Revised (WISC-R) (Wechsler, 1974) is the most widely used test for school age children 6 to 16 years, 11 months. The test is designed so that it provides a full-scale IQ score as well as separate verbal and performance IQ scores. The test is composed of six verbal subtests and six performance subtests that correspond to different areas of functioning. The verbal area measures such functions as long-range memory or information, immediate auditory memory, language comprehension, and arithmetic reasoning; the performance area measures visual organization and sequencing, visual attention to detail, spatial relations, eye-hand coordination, and visual memory. The WISC-R is most useful in beginning to pinpoint the specific strengths and weaknesses of the child with an intellectual handicap. Nothing whether there is a discrepancy between the child's verbal and performance (nonverbal) IQ is a first step in delineating specific problems. Kaufman (1979a, 1979b) has developed a comprehensive summary of research with the WISC-R and its implications for assessing children with exceptional needs.

The Stanford-Binet Intelligence Scale, mentioned in the preschool section, is another important test at the school-age level. Because of its age span, it measures lower levels of intellectual functioning and is an important measure for the severely retarded school-age child. One must keep in mind, though, that at the school-age years, the Stanford-Binet is an extremely verbally oriented test and measures primarily conceptual and abstract reasoning processes. In this age range it does not include many nonverbal or performance items. Thus, the Stanford-Binet will not give a good reflection of the range of skills of school-age developmentally disabled children. Scores on the Stanford-Binet correlate most highly with verbal IQs of the WISC-R.

The Wechsler Adult Intelligence Scale (WAIS) (1955) for ages 16 years and older is similar to the WISC-R in structure. It is important for pediatric psychologists to be aware of the discrepancy between WISC-R scores and WAIS scores at the 16 to 17-year-old level, with the WAIS measuring consistently higher than the WISC-R at these ages (Sattler, 1974).

Special Cognitive Assessment Measures

There are a number of special tests that, because of their unique construction, can be used to assess intelligence in children with sensory and physical handicaps.

For use with the hearing-impaired child, the most adequate standardized scale is the Hiskey-Nebraska Test of Learning Aptitude (Hiskey, 1966), which was standardized on both deaf and hearing children, ages 3 to 16 years. Pantomime and practice exercises are used to instruct the child in the 12 subtests that cover visual memory, fine motor, spatial relation, pictoral analogy, and visual association tasks. The response requirements for all the subtests is nonverbal, utilizing a pointing or motor response.

For the visually impaired child, adaptations have been made of both the Stanford-Binet Intelligence Scale (Livingston, 1959) and the Wechsler Intelligence Scale for Children—Revised. The Interim Hayes-Binet (Hayes, 1949) was developed by utilizing and adapting all items that could be administered without vision from the Stanford-Binet, resulting in a test suitable for visually impaired children with mental ages of 7 years and older. The WISC-R adaptation consists essentially of the verbal subtests with a few substitutions for inappropriate items. The Blind Learning Aptitude Test (BLAT; Newland, 1969) offers an alternative approach for assessing the learning potential of school-aged visually impaired children (ages 6 to 20 years). Utilizing a bas-relief format similar to braille, it measures skills involved in discrimination, generalization, sequencing, analogies, and matrix completion tasks. The BLAT is well standardized on blind children and correlates with performance in both the Hayes-Binet and the WISC-R verbal scale as well as with measured educational achievement. It is particularly difficult to measure the intellectual functioning of visually impaired infants and preschoolers because of the heavy reliance of tests on measurement of verbal abilities. Usually assessments during these developmental periods are primarily done on an informal basis.

The Columbia Mental Maturity Scale (Burgemeister, Blum, & Lorge, 1972) serves as an important complement in testing the cognitive functioning of children 3½ years, 6 months to 9 years, 11 months of age, particularly those who have difficulty responding verbally since it does not require language for administration. The test consists of 92 plates, each with three to five pictures or drawings. The child must select from the alternatives the one drawing which "does not belong" with the others. The types of discriminations to be made involve differences and similarities among such variables as form, color, number, size, and function or use of the depicted alternatives. The Columbia is both appropriately standardized and technically adequate; however, it samples a relatively narrow range of intellectual behavior.

The Leiter International Performance Scale (Leiter, 1966) for ages 2 to 18 years requires little language or physical manipulation for completion. It covers a wide range of functions including visual discrimination, spatial relation, analogies, and series. Response mechanisms can be adapted without violating standardization procedures. The test is primarily untimed, which enhances its utility with motorically involved children, and it does not require a verbal response, which recommends it for language-involved children. However, the psychometric aspects of the Leiter are inadequate in terms of standardization and results should be used with caution (Ratcliffe & Ratcliffe, 1979; Salvia & Ysseldyke, 1978).

Neuropsychological Assessment

Many causes of cognitive limitations, sensory handicaps, and chronic medical conditions are also associated with neurological impairments of various kinds (Golden, 1978; Reitan & Davison, 1974; Wright, Schaefer, & Solomons, 1979; Pless & Pinkerton, 1975). Pediatric psychologists should be aware of the possibility of neurological involvement and assess the degree to which it impinges on psychological and developmental functioning. In practice, neuropsychological assessment is closely integrated with neurological evaluation and intervention, and represents a close working relationship between medicine and psychology (Lezak, 1976).

In general, the issues involved in the neuropsychological functioning of children are more complex than in adults. Age of onset and process of development (especially of the brain itself) complicate interpretation of neurological impairment and its implications for behavior (Boll, 1978). Research involving children with known neurological deficits, while recognizing the heterogeneity of this population, has found that early onset is related to more significant impairment than later onset (Boll, 1973; Dikman, Matthews, & Harley, 1975) and that generalized deficits are more commonly reported than specific deficits (Boll, 1978; Golden, 1978).

The basic objective of neuropsychological assessment is to identify cognitive strategies rather than content, that is, how a child learns, rather than what he or she knows (Lezak, 1976). Many tests are available that measure or purport to measure some aspect of neuropsychological functioning in children. However, no single test has demonstrated validity in identification of individual children, even though they have been effective in differentiating brain-damaged from normal children on a group basis (Golden, 1978; Graham & Berman, 1961; Herbert, 1964). Herbert (1964) and Davison (1974) review the available neuropsychological techniques utilized in evaluation of children and guidelines for test selection.

Thorough neuropsychological evaluation, because of the large amount of time required for administration and interpretation, is usually recommended only when central nervous system involvement is clearly suspected, or to delineate the impact of prior neurological insult.

The Halstead-Reitan Tests for Children are the best known neuropsychological techniques. There are two versions of the Halstead-Reitan Battery for Children which consist of adaptations of the adult forms of the tests and several tests developed especially for use with children. The Halstead Neuropsychological Battery for Children (Reitan, 1969) was developed for children from 9 to 14 years and the Reitan-Indiana Children's Battery (Reitan, 1969) was developed for use with children below 9 years of age. The test battery covers a broad range of abilities from fine motor and sensoriperceptual skills to cognitive and intellectual abilities. Usually, the WISC or WISC-R, an aphasia screening test, and measures of academic achievement are used in conjunction with the Halstead-Reitan tests. Normative data are available (Hughes, 1976; Klonoff & Low, 1974; Spreen & Gaddes, 1969); however, the adequacy of norms has been questioned and further work in this and other methodological areas is needed (Herbert, 1964; McFie, 1975).

Sensitivity of the individual tests of the Halstead-Reitan battery varies according to the age of the child being tested (Reitan, 1974). In addition, Boll (1974) found that the overall WISC-R subtest and full-scale scores, and many of the individual subtest scores, were as effective as the Halstead-Reitan tests in identifying neurological deficits. In spite of the test limitations and the complex nature of the field, neuropsychological assessment batteries have been able to differentiate children with epilepsy (Boll & Berent, 1977), head injuries (Klonoff & Paris, 1974), and minimal brain dysfunction (Reitan & Boll, 1973) from normal controls.

Considerations with Special Populations

Many of the assessment issues remain the same for school-age children as for infants but as the child increases with age the environmental impact increasingly compounds its effect. The most important role of assessment of intelligence during the school years is to assist in the planning of the most optimum learning environment for the child.

In assessing children with genetically determined conditions, it is important for the pediatric psychologist to be acquainted with the intellectual expectations of these children and the developmental patterns for the acquisition of cognitive skills. For example, children with Down syndrome show a wide range of intellectual functioning (Dicks-Mireaux, 1972), a positive correlation with their parent's and sibling's intellectual level (Frazer & Sadovnick, 1976) and a possible sex difference in the form of increased intelligence in females (Clements, Bates, & Hafer, 1976). Children with phenylketonuria (PKU), when placed on a proper diet early in life, will usually have normal intellectual functioning, but it has recently been shown that under some circumstances, mental development is impeded when the diet is discontinued (Brown & Warner, 1976; Koff, Kammerer, Boyle, & Pueschel, 1979; Smith, Lobascher, Stevenson, Wolff, Schmidt, Grubel-Kaiser, & Bickel, 1978).

In assessing school-age children who evidence sensory impairment, either visual or auditory, a number of considerations must be kept in mind. Not only the product of learning but also the process should be assessed. Because sensory impairments dramatically impinge on the learning process, it is essential that the pediatric psychologist make detailed and accurate observations about the child's learning style. How the child organizes the resources available for task performance will be a critical component in intellecutal development and functioning. The value of assessment for classroom planning and individualized programming for the child is dependent on the examiner's ability to develop an appropriate test battery that is adapted to the particular limitations of each individual child.

For the visually handicapped child, several special tests have already been mentioned, including the Interim Hayes-Binet and the Blind Learning Aptitude Test. Ellis (1978), Bauman and Kropf (1979), and Swallow (1977) review less well-known tests available for use with visually impaired children. Adapting existing tests for use with these children has been attempted for several traditional intelligence tests. This has involved both stimulus and response modification of test items. Spungrin and Swallow (1975) discuss an approach to scoring and modifying the WISC-R (Kaufman & Kaufman, 1977) and discuss adapting the McCarthy Scales for the visually impaired, and Criticos (in press) describes the use of parts of the Merrill Palmer Scale for haptic principles of size and shape.

For the hearing-impaired child, the impact of the handicap on the normal acquisition of language is enormous, as evidenced in substantially impoverished vocabularies. In testing the hearing-impaired child, Sullivan and Vernon (1979) point out several features the examiners must be alert to that will significantly influence test results: poor attending, impulsive responses, and lack of understanding of instruction. The examiner should ensure that the child wears a hearing aid during testing to maximize performance. Vernon (1976) points out that test scores for young hearing-impaired children are extremely unreliable. For all ages of hearing-impaired children, it is important to have supporting data, but this is especially true with young children.

In selecting tests for assessing the intelligence of children with a hearing deficit, verbal tests are not appropriate nor are nonverbal tests with verbal direction. In a recent review, Sullivan and Vernon (1979) recommend the Hiskey-Nebraska Test of Learning Aptitude (ages 3 to 17), the Smith-Johnson Non-Verbal Performance Scale (ages 2 to 4), Raven's Progressive Matrices (9 and up), and the WISC-R performance scale as the most appropriate measures for evaluation of hearing-impaired children.

One of the most difficult assessments of intelligence for the pediatric psychologist is the deaf and blind child. Adequate measures of intelligence do not exist and test adaptations usually fail because of the multiple sensory involvement and the inability to rely on a remaining intact sensory system. The only existing scale available, designed for low functioning, deaf and blind children, ages 0 to 9 years, is the Callier Azusa Scale (Stillman, 1975) which measures motor development, perceptual abilities, daily living skills, cognition, communication and language, and socialization. It has been suggested that for the psychologist to be truly able to evaluate these children, a knowledge of both sign language and braille should be obtained (Vernon, Blair, & Lotz, 1979).

Professionals involved with psychological assessment of chronically ill children have a vital role in the identification of potential and present cognitive deficits that are not likely to be apparent during routine medical examinations (Magrab, 1978; Pless & Pinkerton, 1975; Wright *et al.*, 1979). Application of assessment procedures to chronically ill children must reflect the change in perspective from a terminal all-pervasive perception of disease to a focus on survival and long-term coping with medical conditions. Since children with chronic illnesses are more frequently surviving into adulthood and are able to lead less restricted lives, the adequacy of their educational experiences and vocational preparation become areas of increasing concern (Travis, 1976). More definitive knowledge and understanding of the cognitive effects of specific medical conditions in terms of age at onset, type of treatment, severity of the condition, and particular impact of the disease process are necessary for comprehensive evaluation and planning for these children.

Chronic and terminal illnesses that are most commonly identified and dealt with during the school years include pulmonary disorders, especially asthma (2% of the population under 18); epilepsy (1%); cardiac conditions (0.5%); orthopedic illnesses (0.5%); and diabetes (0.1%) (Mattson, 1972). Other less frequently occurring diseases that pose particularly difficult and complex assessment and management concerns are cystic fibrosis, renal diseases (especially those requiring dialysis and possible transplantation), leukemias, and tumors (Magrab, 1978).

Clinicians involved in the cognitive assessment of chronically ill children should be aware of the possible sources of intellectual interference. In some children, cognitive delays and deficits may precede the onset of chronic illness, especially since particular congenital and chromosomal anomalies may be associated with a greater incidence of chronic disease. An example of this is the higher incidence of leukemia reported in Down syndrome children and their siblings (Kucera, 1971). Cognitive impairment may be directly associated with the disease process itself. These effects often are related to the potential CNS impact of many chronic diseases such as the possible effect of uremia (Massry & Sellers, 1976; Merkel, Ing, Ahmadian, Lewy, Ambruster, Oyama, Sulieman, Belman, & King, 1974; Wright *et al.*, 1978), CNS infiltrations in leukemia (Berry, 1974; Thatcher, 168), and possible effects of prolonged seizures (Dikman, Matthews, & Harley, 1975; Nelson & Ellenberg, 1976; Tarter, 1972; Whitehouse, 1971). Even though medical advances in treatment have in general improved longevity and reduced activity limitations, many treatments have the potential for interfering with cognitive processes to a greater or less degree. The possible concomitants for cognitive development of such treatments as cranial radiation (Eiser, 1978, 1979; Peylan-Ramu, Poplack, Pizzo, Adornato, & DiChiro, 1978), some of the chemotherapy agents used in cancer treatment (Allen, 1978; Meadows, & Evans, 1976), and medications that control seizures (Dodrill, 1975; Stores, 1975) are currently under examination.

Chronically ill children are often perceived to be less intelligent than their healthy peers, and subsequently less is often expected of them in terms of learning and achievement. Korsh, Cobb, and Ashe (1961) found that pediatricians frequently underestimated the intelligence of physically ill children. Parents are reported to have either lowered expectations for their children with cardiac illness, even when the disease is well controlled and interferes to a minimal degree in most daily activities, or unrealistically high expectations when compared with healthy siblings (Cleveland, Reitman, & Brewer, 1965; Kennell, Soroker, Thomas, & Wasman, 1969; Linde, Rasof, Dunn, & Rabb, 1966; McArney, Pless, Satterwhite, & Friedman, 1974). Therefore, intellectual assessment and follow-up of chronically ill children may provide a more accurate measurement of cognitive strengths and weaknesses than is possible through informal means, such as observation and parent report.

Probably the most important use of cognitive assessment during the school-age years pertains directly to appropriate educational placement and programming. When chronic illness has been identified at an early age, as is common in conditions such as hemophilia, leukemia, and muscular dystrophy, it is important to assess functioning prior to school entrance, especially if neurological involvement is suspected or confirmed (Wright, et al., 1979). Base-line functioning in the early school years can also be helpful in identifying later academic underachievement. Since underachievement is often cited in the studies of chronically ill children, even beyond the impact of school absences (Dorner & Elton, 1973; Green & Hartlage, 1971; Katz, 1970; Lawler, Nakielny, & Wright, 1966; Olch, 1971a; Rutter, Tizard, & Whitmore, 1970), the possible effects of learning disabilities and social/emotional factors, such as low self-esteem and motivation, need to be seriously considered (Pless & Pinkerton, 1975).

In addition, in terms of medical management, cognitive assessment can suggest the intellectual and developmental level at which to gauge explanations of disease and treatment procedures in order to obtain optimal understanding on the part of the child (Magrab, 1978; Wright et al., 1979). In those diseases where daily management is essential, such as diet control in diabetes and dialysis, it is possible to determine the level of cooperation and understanding that can be expected from a child (Garner & Thompson, 1974).

Although it is especially important to obtain an accurate and optimal performance from chronically ill children during cognitive assessment, several factors may interfere. The negative effect of illness and injury on test performance has been recognized for many years (Wallin, 1940). Scheduling of evaluation sessions requires a great deal of flexibility since the physical well-being experienced in an ongoing medical condition can rarely be predicted in advance. Testing sessions may need to be shortened or rescheduled because of fatigue, illness, or treatment (Sattler, 1974). Although conducting evaluations while a child is a hospital inpatient may be convenient, the situational effect of hospitalization may be a confounding one for reliable assessment. In order for the results of any one or a series of evaluations to be most useful with this population, the conditions of the session and behavioral observations of the child must be carefully documented. This is especially crucial when assessment findings are utilized in the analysis of disease progression and treatment effects.

The assumption often has been made that there would be intellectual differences between children with chronic illnesses when compared with their physically healthy peers. However, this bias has not been upheld in many of the chronic medical conditions that are prevalent during the childhood years. In spite of methodological difficulties, including small sample size, the question of appropriate comparison groups, and the need for additional data, recent research has tentatively found at least average intellectual functioning in children with hemophilia, juvenile arthritis, cystic fibrosis, diabetes, ulcerative colitis, sickle cell anemia, and rheumatic heart disease (Ack, Miller, & Weil, 1961; Allain, 1975; Cleveland, Reitman, & Brewer, 1965; Chodorkoff & Whitten, 1963; Fishler & Fogel, 1973; Gayton & Friedman, 1973; Levitt & Taran, 1963). However, in almost all of these conditions, academic achievement was significantly lowered even though intellectual functioning was adequate. The effect of asthma and renal disease on cognitive functioning has not been studied in even a preliminary manner, as far as could be determined. Those medical conditions which have been associated with cognitive impairment are usually related to CNS involvement of disease, treatment, or both. Seizure disorders, encephalitis, brain damage as a result of trauma, lead poisoning, multiple sclerosis, meningitis, and Rocky Mountain spotted fever all appear to have potential impact on cognitive functioning (Goldstein & Shelly, 1974; Levin & Eisenberg, 1979; Pueschel, Kopito, & Schwachman, 1972; Rie, Hilty, & Cranblitt, 1973; Tarter, 1972; Wright, 1972; Wright & Jimmerson, 1971). The direct effect and prediction of the impact of specific chronic illness on cognitive functioning is often unclear in the individual case; however, the age of the child at onset often appears to be related to intellectual impairment. In those conditions with potential cognitive effects, onset before 3 to 6 years of age is more often associated with lowered intelligence than is later onset (Sattler, 1974).

Wright's studies of the cognitive impact of meningitis, Rocky Mountain spotted fever, and lead poisoning (Wright, 1972; Wright & Fulwiler, 1972; Wright and Jimmerson, 1971) are excellent examples of the well controlled research necessary in elucidating the cognitive sequelae of chronic illness. Subjects were matched for age, sex, race, family income, and history of hospitalization, and compared on intellectual functioning (WISC-R) and perceptual-motor functioning. Wright and Jimmerson's (1971) findings of specific learning disabilities in postmeningial children who clinically appeared to have recovered from the disease with no permanent damage highlights the importance of careful psychological assessment of children with even short-term medical conditions.

PSYCHOSOCIAL ASSESSMENT

Assessing the social and emotional status of children with pediatric conditions implies an understanding of personality dynamics, behavioral patterns, and environmental characteristics. The goals of psychosocial assessment of these children include:

1. Identification of the interrelationship between the pediatric condition and psychosocial development.
2. Identification of children and families who are at risk emotionally and socially.
3. Differentiation of the characteristics that contribute to more adequate coping.
4. Suggestion of intervention approaches that can enhance emotional and social development.
5. Identification and referral for special treatment of children within this group who are also emotionally disturbed.

Psychosocial Assessment Techniques

There is a wide range of techniques utilized to evaluate the psychosocial functioning of children and adolescents with pediatric conditions. The techniques that are briefly discussed here include adaptive behavior measures, projective measures, standardized personality inventories, self-concept scales, behavior rating scales, family measures, interviews, and measures that have been designed to evaluate components of specific medical conditions. Observation techniques will not be discussed; however, the reader is referred to recent comprehensive reviews on this subject (Ciminero, Calhoun, & Adams, 1977; Cone & Hawkins, 1977; Haynes, 1978; Mash & Terdal, 1976).

Adaptive Behavior Measures

Adaptive behavior is an important aspect of social development that should be assessed by pediatric psychologists for children with pediatric conditions since it represents a tangible component of life adjustment, particularly for children with multiple handicaps, sensory deficits, and mental retardation. Adaptive behavior is defined as "the effectiveness or degree with which the individual meets the standards of personal independence and social responsibility expected of his age or cultural group" (Grossman, 1973). The adaptive behavior skills of children often stand in contrast to their academic and intellectual attainments; thus, these skills represent an important dimension in determining the overall coping of the child.

One of the most frequently used measures of social competence is the Adaptive Behavior Scale (Nihira, Foster, Shellhaas, & Leland, 1974). It measures a broad domain including independent functioning, economic activity, self-direction, responsibility, socialization, and rebellious behavior that relates to emotional and conduct disorders. The scale was developed to be used with mentally retarded, developmentally disabled, and emotionally disturbed children and adults. The informant must be someone familiar with the child on a day-to-day basis. Another measure of social competence, the Vineland Social Maturity Scale (Doll, 1965) assesses self-help, self-direction, communication, locomotion, and socialization from birth to 25 years of age. A social quotient can be obtained. Similar to the Vineland, but developed especially for trainable mentally retarded children, the Cain-Levine Social Competency Scale (Cain, Levine, & Elzey, 1963) also utilizes an interview format in assessing independence skills through the 5- to 14-year range. Coulter and Morrow (1978) thoroughly review the relative merits of various scales as well as the concept of adaptive behavior itself.

With sensory impaired and multiply handicapped children, each of these tools has significant limitations in both the array of items and the normative data. For the visually impaired or blind child the Social Maturity Scale for Blind Preschool Children (Maxfield & Buchholtz, 1961), which is an adaptation of the Vineland, is a viable alternative. With deaf-blind children, the Collier-Azusa Scale includes daily living and socialization items. Clearly, though, in-depth interviewing of parent and child and direct observation of these children will provide the best assessment of social competence and development. The use of adaptive behavior scales with mentally retarded and handicapped children can augment the psychologist's understanding of how the child is managing in daily life situations, but they should be incorporated into a broader view of the adaptation of the entire family.

Projective Techniques

Despite the criticism that projective measures have received regarding questionable validity and low reliability, their use in assessing emotional and social functioning is widespread (Klopfer & Taulbee, 1976; Zubin, Eron, & Schumer, 1965). In actuality, this probably reflects the application of projectives in clinical settings (Reynolds & Sundberg, 1976). Not only have traditional projective techniques been utilized with chronically ill and handicapped children, but experimental techniques designed especially for these populations have been developed recently. However, most of the traditional projective techniques are not appropriate for assessing sensory handicapped children because of stimulus and response characteristics of the measures.

There are two interrelated approaches for the use of projectives in the evaluation of chronically ill and handicapped children. Projective techniques have been utilized to compare the social-emotional effects of specific handicaps and illnesses and to assess the adjustment of individual children with pediatric conditions. Wright et al. (1979) recommend periodic projective assessment at 6- to 12-month intervals for those children and adolescents with high-impact and potentially terminal conditions such as leukemia, cystic fibrosis, and hemophilia. In these diseases and other chronic conditions, projective techniques can be helpful in identifying fantasies about the medical conditions and revealing unspoken concerns particularly in reticent or uncommunicative children.

The most commonly used projectives with this population are the Draw-A-Person, Children's Apperception Test (CAT), the Thematic Apperception Test (TAT), and the Rorschach.

Human figure drawings have been used as an estimate of intellectual development (Harris, 1965; Koppitz, 1968) and as a screening measure for emotional functioning (Koppitz, 1968). Drawings are most often used in conjunction with other measures, and their validity, especially for emotional assessment, is contested (Buros, 1974; Roback, 1968; Swenson, 1968). They have been utilized to study body image and anxiety of impaired children with equivocal results (Fox, Davidson, Lighthall, Waite, & Sarason, 1958; Khan, Herndon, & Ahmadian, 1971; Reite, Davis, Solomons, & Ott, 1972; Schoenfeld, 1964; Wysocki & Whitney, 1965). It is difficult to quantify specific aspects of drawings to accurately reflect the visual impact of drawings; however, the communicative potential of drawings, especially with young or depressed chronically ill children, is an area for further study. Because they are easy to administer and children usually enjoy them, drawings will probably continue to be used as screening procedures. Drawings also can provide a great deal of flexibility in attempting to understand the impact of various medical procedures and treatments. Having children draw themselves in the hospital, draw the inside of their bodies or themselves on dialysis has been helpful in identifying the psychological effects of pediatric conditions (Gellert, 1962; Magrab & Papadopoulou, 1978).

Storytelling measures such as the CAT and TAT (Bellack, 1975) require the child to make up a story about each of a series of pictures showing people in various situations. It is assumed that the stories will reveal the feelings, needs, motives, and personality characteristics of the storyteller. Attempts to quantify story characteristics have been made but often are complex and time consuming. A recent developmental norming of TAT scores, assessing both language ability and personality adjustment by Neman, Neman, and Sells (1973), deserves special mention. As part of the Health Examination Survey, they have developed scoring procedures and norms for 6 to 17 year olds based on a large national probability sample of children and adolescents in the United States. Storytelling measures that have been constructed to stimulate illness and hospital concerns include the Waechter Hospital Pictures (Waechter, 1971) and the Pain Apperception Test (Petrovich, 1957, 1958). Several of the pictures in the CAT-Supplement (Bellack, 1975) can also be used with young chronically ill and handicapped children, for example, the doctor and the crutches scene.

The Rorschach (Rorschach, 1921), with its 10 symmetrical ink blots, has been a widely used projective technique with chronially ill and handicapped children and adolescents (Goggin, Lansky, & Hassanein, 1976; Olch, 1971; Weiss, Quinlan, O'Neil, & O'Neil, 1978). One of the most valid scoring systems that could be useful in understanding the handicapped and chronically ill is Friedman's measure of developmental level (Friedman & Orgel, 1964). Although primarily used to assess cognitive functioning, it has had wider application, for example, the level of emotional disturbance and social participation can be assessed, and it reflects a broader measure of overall developmental level (Goldfried, Strickler, & Weiner, 1971). Exner (1974, 1978), in devising a comprehensive scoring system for the Rorschach and in his considerable contribution to Rorschach reseach, may have initiated a renaissance for the technique. Levitt and Truumaa's (1972) compilation of normative data for children and adolescents may also aid in research and clinical efforts in this area.

Standardized Personality Inventories

Standardized personality scales have long been criticized for their minimal usefulness in the assessment of chronically ill and handicapped children either because of social desirability response factors or their failure in identifying chronically ill and handicapped populations from normal controls (Purcell, Weiss, & Hahn, 1972; Seidersfeld, 1948). However, the latter criticism may be more a function of the population utilized than limitations of the assessment techniques themselves, as was discussed earlier.

Research utilizing the Minnesota Multiphasic Personality Inventory (MMPI) (Hathaway & McKinley, 1967) has often been as inconclusive as the research in social/emotional aspects of handicapping and medcal conditions in general. For example, studies of young asthmatic patient's MMPI profiles vary in findings from no differences, compared with normal controls, to findings of high anxiety, fearfulness, and a greater degree of psychopathology (Block, Jenning, Harvey, & Simpson, 1964; Fitzelle, 1959; Smith, 1962; Willams & McNichol, 1969). The MMPI may have clinical relevance in helping to assess depression, possible self-destructive tendencies, and the personality resources of parents with affected children (Murawski, Chagan, Balodimos, & Ryan, 1970; Wright *et al.*, 1979). However, interpretation of psychopathology should be made cautiously when utilizing the MMPI with medical and handicapped populations. Many items may reflect actual experiences related to a medical condition rather than the somatic complaints of the psychiatric population for which the MMPI was developed.

Although the MMPI in particular has been used in studies with older adolescents and adults with chronic diseases, objective and personality techniques have not been utilized often in research or routine evaluation of handicapped or chronically ill children. The series of tests developed by the Institute for Personality and Ability Testing (IPAT) are the most suitable instruments currently available for use with pediatric populations. The series includes the Early School Personality Question-naire (ages 6 to 8 years), the Children's Personality Questionnaire (ages 8 to 12 years), the Junior-Senior High School Personality Questionnaire (adolescents), and the Sixteen Personality Factors Questionnaire for adults (Cattell, 1972; Cattell, Coan, & Beloff, 1969; Coan & Cattell, 1972; Porter & Cattell, 1968).

Despite test limitations, standardized personality scales can aid in the understand-ing of adjustment variability in pediatric conditions. Objective scales allow for descriptions of client populations for comparative purposes, can function as pre-post measures of change and are useful in the exploration of personality trait-treatment interactions (Evans & Nelson, 1977).

Self-Concept Measures

Self-concept is an important aspect in the evaluation of handicapped and chronically ill children, especially as it is often difficult to predict the impact that a handicapping condition will have for any individual child. For example, research with arthritic children (McArney *et al.*, 1974) indicated that children with mildly handicapping conditions may have greater difficulty adjusting than those with moderate to severe handicaps.

Informal methods that have been used to assess children's perceptions about themselves include human figure drawings and negative self statements. Several formal self-concept scales, with more adequate reliability and validity, are currently available, for example, the Pies-Harris Self Concept Scale (1969), the Self-Esteem Inventory (Coopersmith, 1959), and the Tennessee Self-Concept Scale (Fitts, 1965). However, despite the necessity of adequately measuring self-perceptions, these scales are not typically used in assessment or treatment studies.

The abilty to describe self-concept is a function of age and therefore, few of the scales are designed for children below 8 to 10 year of age (Hess & Bradshaw, 1970). The Piers-Harris Self Concept Scale (Piers, 1969) and the Self-Esteem Inventory (Coopersmith, 1959) are the most widely used scales available for school-age children. The Tennessee Self-Concept Scale (Fitts, 1965) is designed for use with older adolescents and adults. All three instruments have been utilized in studies with chronically ill children and adolescents (Korsh, Negrette, Gardner, Weinstock, Mercer, Gruskin, & Fine, 1973; Pless, Cherry, Douglas, & Wadsworth, 1975); however, none is adequately developed to warrant use without other supporting measures. An interesting adaptation of direct assessment is the use of the Q-sort technique to assess the discrepancy between self-concept and ideal-self. This technique is used to measure the difference between a child's perception of "himself as he/she is" and ratings of "how he/she would like to be" (Cowen, Pederson, Babigian, Izzo, & Trost, 1973).

Behavior Rating Scales

Numerous behavior rating scales have been developed for use with children and adolescents. Information about behavior is usually derived from parents, teachers, or other caretakers who are familiar with a child's daily functioning. The scales discussed here have been standardized on children who are presumed to be at least within the average range cognitively, as compared wih the adaptive behavior scales designed primarily for mentally retarded and more significantly handicapped populations. In addition, most of the scales discussed here have also been applied to clinical populations. The primary purpose of behavior rating scales is the screening and identification of behavior disorders (Edelbrock, 1979), which, because of the scale format, involves little expenditure of professional time. Wright *et al.* (1979) and Creer and Christian (1976) recommend the use of behavior rating scales with chronically ill children in order to screen for possible behavioral difficulties, determine priorities for treatment, and monitor behavior change or follow-up. For a more comprehensive presentation of behavior checklists, refer to Walls, Werner, Bacon, and Zane's (1977) listing of both descriptive and prescriptive instruments.

For routine pediatric practice, parent ratings probably provide the most accessible broad-range assessment of children's behavior problems. There are several adequate scales derived for this purpose.

The Walker Problem Behavior Identification Checkist (Walker, 1970) is a 50-item parent report measure that has been standardized for elementary school childen and has been effectively utilized as part of a behavioral assessment package with asthmatic children (Creer & Christian, 1976).

Achenbach (1979) has developed the Child Behavior Checklist and Profile to assess patterns of both behavioral problems and competencies through parent report. It is standardized separately for boys and girls at three age ranges: 4 to 5 years, 6 to 11 years, and 12 to 16 years. Current research efforts are in progress to differentiate disturbed children according to profile patterns and determine differences in prognosis and treatment response.

Other behavior rating scales that utilize parent reports include The Behavior Problem Checklist (Quay, 1977), the Louisville Behavior Checklist (Miller, 1967), and the Connor's Parent Rating Scale (Connors, 1970).

The Connors Scale for Teachers ratings of child hyperactivity deserves special mention (Connors, 1969); Goyette, Connors, & Ulrich, 1978; Weery, Sprague, & Cohen, 1975). The teacher scale was developed for psychopharmacological studies of children and has extensive normative data for both normal and hyperactive populations. It is sensitive to changes in hyperactivity subsequent to medication and behavioral modification intervention (O'Leary & Pelhon, 1978; Sprague & Sleator, 1973).

Behavioral Assessment Questionnaires

A thorough discussion of applied behavioral analysis assessment and the role it plays in behavioral medicine will not be attempted here. The interested reader is referred to McNamara (1979), Russo, Bird, and Masek (1980), and Doyles, Meredith, and Ciminero (in press) as well as relevant journals such as the *Journal of Behavioral Medicine, Behavioral Medicine Abstracts,* and *Behavioral Assessment.*

Several formal and informal questionnaire techniques that can be used to evaluate components of handicapped and medically involved children and adolescents' behavior will be briefly mentioned. These scales have direct relevance to design of treatment programs. For example, reinforcement schedules have been devised for use with children that enable professionals to generate potentially rewarding items, activities, and events which can be utilized in intervention attempts (Cautela, 1977; Walker, 1979).

Fear surveys (Walker, 1979), anxiety scales (Bendig, 1956; Spielberger, Edwards, Lushener, Montuori, & Plazek, 1972; Spielberger, Gorusch, & Lushenie, 1970; Watson & Friend, 1969), and depression scales (Anton, 1971; Levitt & Lubin,1975; Nowlis, 1965; Zung, 1965), are especially useful in determining the impact that a handicapping or medical condition has had on specific aspects of a child's or adolescent's psychological functioning. Correspondingly, their use in research on psychosocial effects of pediatric conditions appears to be increasing (Kellerman, Zeltzer, Ellenberg, Dash, & Rigler, 1980; Koocher, O'Malley, Gogan, & Foster, in press).

Although behavioral questionnaires are convenient and efficient, caution is recommended in their selection since currently available scales vary widely in their empirical validity and utility. Wright (1978) and Haynes (1978) review many of the useful scales in this area.

Medically Oriented Scales

Several measures have been developed especially for the assessment of medically oriented issues and their impact on childrens' functioning. The Waechter Hospital Picture Test has been mentioned earlier in this chapter. The Magrab-Bronheim Hospital Sentence Completion Test (Magrab, 1975) is another technique that assesses overall concerns about disease, body image, family, and self. It has been used with normal, chronically ill, and acutely ill children, adolescents, and young adults, to differentiate levels of preoccupation with disease-related concerns and the general level of adaptive functioning.

Techniques that have also been developed to assess specific areas of functioning include the Wallston Health Locus of Control Scale (Wallston, Wallston, Kaplan, & Maides, 1976), which assesses the relationship between perception of control in the presence of disease and aspects of health behavior, and the Death Anxiety Questionnaire (Conte, Bakur-Weiner, Plutchnik, & Bennett, 1975), which has been utilized to assess the level of anxiety concerning death in healthy children (Koocher et al. 1976) and pediatric cancer survivors (Koocher et al., in press).

Interviews

Interviewing is an almost universal method for gathering information in clinical settings. In pediatric psychology practice, interviews may fulfill a variety of functions including establishing rapport, supplementing medical history, assessing the developmental status of a child, determining the behavioral aspects of a developmental or medical condition, and evaluating the coping strategies and adjustment of a child and the child's family.

The reliability of retrospective report data, especially from parents about their children's development and their own parenting, has been studied extensively (Chess, Thomas, & Burch, 1966; Yarrow, Campbell, & Burton, 1970). Interview data have been found to be distorted in the direction of age-expected behavior, stereotypic sex-appropriate behavior, and dominant cultural attitudes about childbearing. The unpleasantness of events as well as the level of associated emotion also affect reliability of recall (Evans & Nelson, 1977). However, information about current behavior correlates fairly well with independent assessment, especially if the information requested is relatively objective and quantifiable (Haggard et al., 1966; Lapouse & Monk, 1958; Yarrow et al., 1970). Not only adults but children also can be reliable sources about current behavior and possible symptoms (Herjanic, Herjanic, Brown, & Wheatt, 1975; Rutter & Graham, 1968).

Structured interviews have often been utilized in research on the social/emotional aspects of handicapping or medically related conditions (Money & Pollitt, 1966; Rutter, Graham, & Yule, 1970; Sterky, 1963; Swift, Seidman, & Stein, 1967). Purcell (1963) developed a structured interview that has proven helpful in differentiating rapidly remitting asthmatic patients from those who are steroid dependent. Other formats, such as the Sickness Impact Profile Questionnaire (Bergner, 1974) and the Illness Impact Questionnaire (Zeltzer, Kellerman, Ellenberg, Dash, & Rigler, 1980), have been developed to assess the behavior, feelings, and attitudes related to the experience of illness. Although interviews have the potential for yielding a great deal of information that is directly relevant to the understanding of pediatric conditions, the need for independent validation, especially through observation, as well as interpretive caution limits the exclusive use of interviews in information gathering.

Parent and Family Measures

Having a handicapped or chronically ill child places a great deal of stress not only on the sick child but also on the parents and siblings. In comparison with the large literature on handicapped and chronically ill children, comparatively little research has involved the impact that handicapping conditions can have on parent attitudes, parenting style, or parent and sibling coping abilities (Bogan, 1970; Dorner, 1973; Sourkes, 1980; Tew & Lawrence, 1973; Travis, 1976). For some chronic medical conditions, such as asthma and diabetes, parent and family functioning may be related to degree of disease control (Purcell, Brady, Chai, Muser, Molk, Gordon, & Means, 1969; Wright et al., 1978). Although this can be a complex area for assessment, especially due to the interactional nature of family data, several relatively time-efficient instruments are available, including measures of both parent and child perceptions of aspects of family functioning.

Parent attitude scales, such as the Parental Attitude Research Instrument (Schaefer & Bell, 1958), the Childrearing Attitude and Behavior Instrument (Wright, 1976), and the Maryland Parent Attitude Survey (Pumroy, 1962), assess parents' child rearing practices and attitudes toward their children. The scale can be used to compare parents' attitudes toward their handicapped and normal children, as well as to assess parenting skills in general.

The Family Relations Test (Bene & Anthony, 1957) is designed to assess relationships within the family. It can be individually administered to one, several, or all family members from three years of age through adult, with a profile compiled for each member's perception of family relationships. The Child Report of Parental Behavior Inventory (Margolies & Weintraub, 1977; Schaefer, 1965) is another scale that can be useful in assessing children's (both handicapped and normal) perceptions of parent-child relationsips. Both of these scales are at an experimental level but deserve further exploration.

Social-Emotional Functioning of Children with Chronic, Terminal, and/or Handicapping Conditons

There have been many observations and studies of the psychosocial impact of chronic illness on children and their families. Magrab (1978), Travis (1976), Wright et al., (1979) present comprehensive reviews of the current understanding and knowledge in this area, While it is reasonable to assume that chronic illness has an impact on the social and emotional development of children, the relationship between emotional precipitants of illness and emotional concomitants of illness are often difficult to differentiate. Earlier theories of psychosomatic conditions, particularly asthma, presumed an emotional precipitant to the disease in general, as well as for specific episodes of asthma attacks. Researchers have often assumed that children affected by a particular chronic illness would share similar, often pathological, personality patterns that could be distinguished both from patterns typical of other medical conditions and from the personality patterns of normal children (Knowles, 1971; Mattson, 1972). In the light of better controlled research, many of these assumptions have not been upheld. Rather, there appear to be no overall social-emotional characteristics for children with chronic illnesses, and the impact of emotional interaction in ''psychosomatic'' conditions is more complex than previously proposed. Instead, chronic illness appears to act primarily as a specific stress situation for both the child and his family (Pless & Pinkerton, 1975). Research on the psychosocial aspects of chronic illness has recently focused on distinguishing those children and families who cope well with chronic illness from those who have a variety of coping difficulties, and on differentiating those aspects of chronic illness that are especially stressful (Koocher, O'Mally, Gogan, & Foster, in press; Korsh et al., 1973; Morse, 1972; Sourkes, 1977; Sultz, 1972; Thomas, Millman, & Rodriguez-Torres, 1970; Zeltzer et al., 1980).

Although there is little research to support the hypothesis that chronic illness causes pathological personality development, the experience of chronic illness is often correlated with impaired psychological functioning. As Pless and Pinkerton (1975) state, ''No longer can there be any doubt that a a group, children with chronic disorders are more likely to experience psychosocial difficulties than their healthy peers. There is also no doubt that when such difficulties supervene, they frequently prove to be more disabling than the underlying physical disorder'' (p. 13). Wright et al. (1979) identify six concomitants of psychosocial difficulties that are important to assess in chronically ill children and adolescents:

1. Low self-esteem (and maladaptive compensation for it).
2. Discrepancy between child's self-concept and ideal self-image.
3. Discrepancy between child's functional capacities, and aspirations or perceptions of others' expectations.
4. Feminine identification in boys.
5. Depression.
6. Sexual concerns.

Difficulties in establishing positive self-concept and depression, at times involving suicidal attempts, are the areas that have been identified most frequently through informal observation and formal studies. Although chronic illness poses specific psychological adjustment challenges at every developmental level, adolescence is an especially crucial period. Chronically ill adolescents may risk medical complications and a greater degree of physical impairment in order not to be perceived as different from their peers (Jacobstein & Magrab, 1980; Kellerman & Katz, 1977; Kellerman *et al.,* 1980).

The overrepresentation of chronically ill children with behavioral or emotional diffiulties may be attributed to that portion of the population chosen for study. Children may have been identified because they were referred to mental health profesionals and thereby skew the impression of pathology as a function of chronic illness. One of the approaches for attaining a more balanced view of the psychosocial impact of chronic illness is to screen all affected children, not only those referred for evaluation. Wright *et al.* (1979) recommend a brief routine screening procedure that could be completed in the waiting room during outpatient clinic visits. Drawings, sentence completion forms, and behavior problem checklists can all be completed with a minimal investment of professional time. In this way, potential difficulties could be identified and treated before they become severe enough to interfere with development. Thorough evaluations, including self-concept, and projective techniques, are essential for those children experiencing psychosocial difficulties. Periodic evaluation, at 6- to 12-month intervals, are also recommended for those childen and adolescents who are experiencing severe or terminal medical conditions, such as leukemia and other cancers, or children experiencing chronic dialysis and renal transplant.

For the child with a significant sensory deficit multiple handicapping condition, or mental retardation, assessing social and emotional well-being is increasingly complicated. Determining what "healthy and normal" emotional and social behaviors are for these children is neither well documented in the literature nor fully understood. The standard projective techniques often yield spurious results. Play interviews and clinical observations are the best avenue to understanding the dynamics of the child, but these must be conducted with a full understanding of the condition and the normative behaviors and reactions developmentally appropriate for the particular child. Discerning emotional disturbances in these children should not be the sole goal of these procedures. Of equal importance is assessing the ways in which the handicapped child is coping with his or her condition and the special resources the child has or needs. Unfortunately, there are currently no well-constructed assessment tools to assist in this process.

FUTURE DIRECTIONS

The role of psychological assessment in pediatric care is continuously expanding. The application of existing techniques to define and to plan intervention in pediatric conditions has become, in many instances, routine. The more the relationship between health and mental status is understood, the need for psychological assessment will continue to expand. Yet, in some cases, existing tools are not, and will not be, sufficient to answer the questions being raised, either because the measures have an inappropriate philosophic bias, have inadequate standardization for pediatric populations, or have not yet been developed. For example, new techniques to assess behavioral management aspects of medical conditions such as dietary and medication compliance, pain relief, and aversive treatments are currently being developed. These may serve as major beakthroughs in the field of pediatric psychological assessment. The broader implications of repeated psychological assessments as a part of various intervention processes will also necessitate new measures and adaptation of traditional techniques for special uses.

In developing assessment strategies, pediatric psychologists must be creative in examining the various psychological processes that are related to specific medical conditions. There is an important need for research into the psychological components of pediatric conditions. Although in the last decade we have significantly expanded this understanding for diseases such as diabetes, pulmonary disorders, oncology, and renal conditions, there still is more that is unknown than is known. At times, new psychological assessment tools will be required for this research, and their development may necessitate substantial concomitant research. Research needs for assessment will not always be commensurate with clinical needs, and pediatric psychologists will have to devote their efforts to both arenas.

In managing children with pediatric conditions, health and health-related professionals are increasingly working together in a team approach to care. Psychological assessment usually represents one aspect of the comprehensive assessment process. As other professionals such as social workers, psychiatrists, occupational therapists, physical therapists, speech and language specialists, and special educators continue to define and expand their role in assessment as well as improve the tools available to them, pediatric psychologists will have to continuously reevaluate their role in the assessment process. To some extent, the pediatric psychologist is the generalist who cuts across all these areas and attempts to synthesize the various aspects of the assessment process. The major contribution the pediatric psychologist will always make to the health team is in developing an objective overview of the social, emotional, and intellectual aspects of the patient. For the future, the pediatric psychologist will have to look toward new strategies of continuing to make pediatric psychological assessment compatible with new advances in other professional areas.

The challenge ahead of us lies in continuing to develop psychological assessment approaches that will improve pediatric care. Research into psychological components of pediatric conditions, new assessment techniques and collaborative assessment approaches with other disciplines wil be needed. Pediatric psychological assessment is a young field that must respond to a growing need for documenting and further understanding the relationship of the mind and the body in health care.

REFERENCES

Achenbach, T. M. The Child Behavioral Profile: An empirically based system for assessing children's behavioral problems and competencies. *International Journal of Mental Health,* 1979, **7,** 24–42.

Ack, M., Miller, I., & Weil, W. B. Intelligence of children with diabetes mellitus. *Pediatrics,* 1961, **28,** 764–770.

Aleksandrowicz, M. K., & Aleksandrowicz, D. R. Obstetrical pain-relieving drugs as predictors of infant behavior variability. *Child Development*, 1974, **45**, 935–945.

Allain, J. P. A boarding school for hemophiliacs: A model for the comprehensive care of hemophiliac children. *Annals of the New York Academy of Sciences*, 1975, **240**, 226–237.

Allen, J. C The effects of cancer therapy on the nervous system. *Journal of Pediatrics*, 1978, **3**, 903–909.

Ambrus, C., Weintraub, D., Niswander, K., Fisher, L., Fleishman, J., Bross, I., & Ambrus, J. Evaluation of survivors of the respiratory distress syndrome. *Journal of Pediatrics*, 1970, **120**, 296–302.

Anton, R. D. An exploration into dimensions of depression in early adolescence. *Dissertation Abstracts International*, 1971, **32**(B), 1202.

Apgar, V. A proposal for a new method of evaluation of the newborn infant. *Current Researches in Anesthesia and Analgesia*, 1953, **32**, 260–267.

Bauman, M. K., & Kropf, C. A. Psychological tests used with blind and visually handicapped persons. *School Psychology Digest*, 1979, **8**, 257–270

Bayley, N. *Manual for the Bayley Scales of Infant Development*. Berkeley, CA: The Psychological Corporation, 1969.

Bellak, L. *The Thematic Apperception Test, The Children's Apperception Test, and the Senior Apperception Test in Clinical Use*, 3rd ed. New York: Grune & Stratton, 1975.

Bench, J., & Parker, A. On the reliability of the Graham/Rosenblith behavior test for neonates. *Journal of Child Psychology and Psychiatry*, 1970, **11**, 121–131.

Bendig, A. W. The development of a short form of the Manifest Anxiety Scale. *Journal of Consulting Psychology*, 156, **20**, 384–389.

Bene, E., & Anthony, J. A technque for the objective assessment of the child's family relationships. *Journal of Mental Sciences*, 1957, **103**, 541–555.

Bergner, M. Theoretical and conceptual issues in the development of a measure of health. In G. D. Grave & I. B. Pless (Eds.), *Chronic childhood illness: Assessment of outcome*. Bethesda, MD: Department of Health, Education and Welfare, 1974.

Berry, D. H. The child with acute leukemia. *American Family Physician*, 1974, **10**, 129–135.

Blok, J., Jennings, P. H., Harvey, E., & Simpson, E. Interaction between allergic potential and psychopthology in childhood asthma. *Psychosomatic Medicine*, 1964, **26**, 307–320.

Bogan, J. B. The child-rearing attitudes of parents of cerebral palsy children and their relationships to child adjustment factors in habilitative therapies. *Dissertation Abstracts International*, 1970, **31**(B), 2976–2977.

Boll, T. J. *The effect of age at onset of brain damage on adaptive abilities in children*. Paper presented at the American Psychological Association Convention, Montreal, August 1973.

Boll, T. J. Behavioral correlates of cerebral damage in children aged 9 through 14. In R. M. Reitan & L. A. Davison (Eds.), *Clinical neuropsychology: Current status and applications*. New York: Wiley, 1974.

Boll, T. J. Diagnosing brain impairment. In B. B. Wolman (Ed.), *Clinical diagnosis of mental disorders*. New York: Plenum, 1978.

Boll, T. J., & Berent, S. *Psychological aspects of coping with epilepsy*. Paper presented at the meeting of the American Psychological Association, San Francisco, August 1977.

Brazelton, T. B. Neonatal Behavioral Assessment Scale. *Monograph of the National Spastics Society*. Philadelphia: Lippincott, 1973.

Brazelton, T. B., Robey, J. S., & Collier, G. A. Infant development in the Zinacanteco Indians of southern Mexico. *Pediatrics*, 1969, **44**, 274−293.

Brazelton, T. B., & Tryphonopoulou, Y. A. *A comparative study of the Greek and U.S. neonates*. Unpublished manuscript, referred to in Brazelton, T. B. *Neonatal Behavioral Assessment Scale*. Philadelphia: Lippincott, 1973.

Brown, E., & Warner, R. Mental development of phenylketonuric children on or off diet after the age of six. *Psychological Medicine*, 1976, **6**, 287−296.

Brown, J. V., Bakeman, R., Snyder, P. A., Frederickson, W. T., Morgan, S. T., & Hepler, R. Interaction of black inner-city mothers with their newborn infants. *Child Development*, 1975, **46**, 677−686.

Burgemeister, B. B., Blum, L. H., & Lorge, I. *Columbia Mental Maturity Scale*, 3rd ed. New York: Harcourt Brace Jovanovich, 1972.

Buros, O. K. (Ed.) *Tests in print II*. Highland Park, NJ: Gryphon Press, 1974.

ain, L., Levine, S., & Elzey, F. *Cain-Levine Social Competency Scale*. Palo Alto, CA: Consulting Psychologists Press, 1963.

Cattell, P. *The measurement of intelligence of infants and young children*. New York: Psychological Corporation, 1940.

Cattell, R. *Sixteen P-F*. Champaign, IL: Institute for Personality and Ability Testing, 1972.

Cattell, R. B., Coan, R. W., & Beloff, H. *Junior-Senior High School Personality Questionnaire*. Champaign, IL: Institute for Personality and Ability Testing, 1969.

Cautela, J. R. *Behavior analysis forms for clinical intervention*. Champaign, IL: Research Press, 1977.

Cavanaugh, M. C., Cohen, I., Dunphy, D., Ringwall, E. A., & Goldberg, I. D. Prediction from the Cattell infant scale. *Journal of Consulting Psychology*, 1957, **21**, 33−37.

Chess, S., Thomas, A., & Birch, H. G. Distortions in developmental reporting made by parents of behaviorally disturbed children. *Journal of the American Academy of Child Psychiatry*, 1966, **5**, 226−231.

Chisholm, J. J. Management of increased lead absorption and lead poisoning in children. *New England Journal of Medicine*, 1973, **289**, 1016−1018.

Chodorkoff, J., & Whitten, C. F. Intellectual status of children with sickle cell anemia. *Journal of Pediatrics*, 1963, **63**, 29−35.

Ciminero, A. R., Calhoun, K. S., & Adams, H. E. (Eds.) *Handbook of behavioral assessment*. New York: Wiley, 1977.

Clements, P. R., Bates, M. U., & Hafer, M. Variability within Down Syndrome (Trisomy-21): Empirically observed sex differences in IQs. *Mental Retardation*, 1976, **14**, 30−32.

Cleveland, S. E., Reitman, E. E., & Brewer, E. J., Jr. Psychological factors in juvenile rheumatoid arthritis. *Arthritis and Rheumatism*, 1965, , 1152−1158.

Coan, R., & Cattell, R. *Early school personality questionnaire*. Champaign, IL: Institute for Personality and Ability Testing, 1972.

Cone, J. D., & Hawkins, R. P. (Eds.) *Behavioral assessment: New directions in clinical psychology*. New York: Brunner/Mazel, 1977.

Connors, C. K. Symptoms patterns in hyperkinetic, neurotic and normal children. *Child Development*, 1970, **41**, 667−682.

Connors, C. K. A teacher rating scale for use in drug studies with children. *American Journal of Psychiatry,* 1969, **126,** 884–888.

Conte, H. R., Bakur-Weiner, M., Plutchnik, R., & Bennett, R. Development and evaluation of a death anxiety questionnaire. *Proceedings of the 83rd Annual Meeting of the American Psychological Association,* 1975.

Coopersmith, S. A method of determining types of self esteem. *Journal of Abnormal and Social Psychology,* 1959, **59,** 87–94.

Corman, H. H., & Escalona, S. K. Stages of sensorimotor development: A replication study. *Merrill-Palmer Quarterly,* 1969, **15,** 351–361.

Coulter, W. A., & Morrow, T. (Eds.) *Adaptive behavior: Concepts and measurement.* New York: Grune & Stratton, 1978.

Cowen, E. L., Pederson, A., Babigian, H., Izzo, L. D., & Trost, M. A. Long term follow-up of early detected vulnerable children. *Journal of Consulting and Clinical Psychology,* 1973, **41,** 438–444.

Creer, T. L., & Christian, W. P. *Chronically ill and handicapped children: Their management and rehabilitation.* Champaign, IL: Research Press Co., 1976.

Criticos, A. K. Psychological assessment of multihandicapped children. In P. Ziring (Ed.), *Diagnosis and management of the multihandicapped child.* New York: Dekker, in press.

Davison, L. A. Current status of clinical neuropsychology. In R. M. Reitan & L. A. Davison (Eds.), *Clinical neuropsychology: Current status and applications.* New York: Wiley, 1974.

Dicks-Mireaux, M. Mental development of infants with Down's syndrome. *American Journal of Mental Deficiency,* 1972, **77,** 26–30.

Dikman, S., Matthews, C. G., & Harley, J. P. The effects of early versus late onset of major motor epilepsy upon cognitive-intellectual performance. *Epilepsia,* 1975, **16,** 73–81.

DiVitto, B., & Goldberg, S. The effects of newborn medical status of early parent-infant interaction. In T. M. Field, A. M. Sostek, S. Goldberg, & H. H. Shuman (Eds.), *Infants born at risk.* New York: Spectrum, 1979.

Dodrill, C. Diphenylhydantoin serum levels, toxicity, and neuropsychological performance in patients with epilepsy. *Epilepsia,* 1975, **16,** 593–600.

Doll, E. A. *Vineland Scale of Social Maturity.* Minneapolis: American Guidance Service, 1965.

Dorner, S. Psychological and social problems of families of adolescent spina bifida patients: A preliminary report. *Developmental Medicine and Child Neurology,* 1973, Supplement **29,** 24–26.

Dorner, S. & Elton, A. Short, taught and vulnerable. *Special Education,* 1973, **62,** 12.

Doyles, D. M., Meredith, R. S., & Ciminero, A. R. (Eds.) *Behavioral psychology in medicine: Assessment and treatment strategies.* New York: Plenum, in press.

Dubowitz, L. M. S., Dubowitz, V., & Goldberg, C. Clinical assessment of gestational age in the newborn infant. *Journal of Pediatrics,* 1970, **77,** 1.

Edelbrock, C. Empirical classification of children's behavior disorders: Programs based on parent and teacher ratings. *School Psychology Digest,* 1979, **8,** 355–369.

Eiser, C. *Effects of chronic illness on intellectual development: A comparison of normal children with those treated for childhood leukemia and solid tumors.* Unpublished paper, 1979, Hospital for Sick Children, London, England.

Eiser, C. Intellectual abilities among survivors of leukemia as a function of CNS irradiation. *Archives of Disease in Childhood,* 1978, **53,** 391–395.

Ellis, D. Methods of assessment for use with the visually and mentally handicapped: A selective review. *Child Care Health Development,* 1978, **12,** 397–411.

Escalona, S. K., & Moriarty, A. Prediction of school age intelligence from infant tests. *Child Development,* 1961, **32,** 597–605.

Evans, I. M., & Nelson, R. O. Assessment of child behavior problems. In A. R. Ciminero, K. S. Calhoun, & H. E. Adams (Eds.), *Handbook of behavioral assessment.* New York: Wiley, 1977.

Exner, J. E., Jr. *The Rorschach: A comprehensive system,* Vols. 1 and 2. New York: Wiley, 1974, 1978.

Feldt, R. H., Ervert, J. C., Stickler, G. B., & Weidman, W. H. Children with congenital heart disease. *American Journal of Diseases of Childhood,* 1969, **117,** 281–287.

Field, T., Hallock, N., Ting, G., Dempsey, J., Dabiri, C., & Shuman, H. A first year follow-up of high risk infants: Formulating a cumulative risk index. *Child Development,* 1978, **49,** 119–131.

Finley, K. H., Fitzgerald, L. H., Pichter, R. W., Riggs, N., & Shelton, J. T. Western encephalitis and cerebral ontogenesis. *Archives of Neurology,* 1967, **16,** 140–164.

Fisch, R., Bilek, M., Miller, L., & Engel, R. Physical and mental status at four years of age of survivors of the respiratory distress syndrome. *Journal of Pediatrics,* 1975, **86,** 497–503.

Fish, B., Shapiro, T., Halpern, F., & Wile, R. The prediction of schizophrenia in infancy: Ten year follow-up report of neurological and psychological development. *American Journal of Psychiatry,* 1965, **121,** 768–775.

Fishler, K., & Fogel, B. *Psychological correlates in children with ulcerative colitis.* Paper presented at the American Psychological Association Convention, Montreal, 1973.

Fishman, M. A., & Palkes, H. S. The validity of psychometric testing in children with congenital malformations of the central nervous system. *Developmental Medicine and Child Neurology,* 1974, **16,** 180–N185.

Fitts, W. H. *Tennessee Self-Concept Scale.* Nashville: Counselor Recordings and Tests, 1965.

Fitzelle, G. T. Personality factors and certain attitudes towards childrearing among parents of asthmatic children. *Psychosomatic Medicine,* 1959, **21,** 208–217.

Flick, G. L., & Duncan, C. Perceptual-motor dysfunction in children with sickle cell trait. *Perceptual and Motor Skills,* 1973, **36,** 234.

Ford, F. R. *Diseases of the nervous system.* Springfield, IL: Charles C. Thomas, 1944.

Fox, C., Davidson, K., Lighthall, F., Waite, R., & Sarason, S. B. Human figure drawings of high and low anxious children. *Child Development,* 1958, **29,** 297–303.

Francis-Williams, J., & Davies, P. A. Very low birth weight and later intelligence. *Developmental Medicine and Child Neurology,* 1974, **16,** 709–728.

Franz, W. K., Self, P. A., & Franz, G. N. *Individual differences and auditory conditioning in neonates.* Paper presented at the Southeastern Conference on Human Development, Nashville, 1976.

Frazer, F. C., & Sadovick, A. D. Correlation of IQ in subjects with Down syndrome and their parents and siblings. *Journal of Mental Deficiency Research,* 1976, **20,** 79–82.

Freedman, D. G., & Freedman, N. Behavioral differences beween Chinese-American and European-American newborns. *Nature,* 1969, **24,** 1227.

Friedman, H., & Orgel, S. A Rorschach developmental scores and intelligence level. *Journal of Projective Techniques and Personality Assessment,* 1964, **28,** 425−428.

Gallagher, J. Clinical judgement and the Cattell intelligence scale. *Journal of Consulting Psychology,* 1953, **17,** 303−305.

Garner, A. M., & Thompson, C. W. Facts in management of juvenile diabetes. *Pediatric Psychology,* 1974, **2,** 6−7.

Gayton, W. F., & Friedman, S. Psychosocial aspects of cystic fibrosis. *American Journal of Diseases of Children,* 1973, **126,** 856.

Gellert, E. Children's conceptions of the content and function of the human body. *Genetic Psychology Monographs,* 1962, **65,** 293−405.

Gerken, K. C., Hancock, K. A., & Wade, T. H. Comparison of the Stanford-Binet Intelligence Scale and the McCarthy Scales of Children's Abilities with preschool children. *Psychology in the Schools,* 1978, **15,** 468−472.

Goggin, E. L., Lansky, S. B., & Hassanein, K. Psychological reactions of children with malignancies. *Journal of the American Academy of Child Psychiatry,* 1976, **14,** 314−325.

Golden, C.J. *Diagnosis and rehabilitation in clinical neuropsychology.* Springfield, IL: Charles C. Thomas, 1978.

Goldfried, M. R., Strickler, G., & Weiner, I. *Rorschach handbook of clinical and research applications.* Englewood Cliffs, NJ: Prentice-Hall, 1971.

Goldstein, G., & Shelly, C. H. Neuropsychological diagnosis of multiple sclerosis in a neuropsychiatric setting. *Journal of Nervous and Mental Disease,* 1974, **158,** 280−290.

Gottfried, A. W., & Brody, D. Interrelationships between and correlates of psychometric and Piagetian scales of sensorimotor intelligence. *Developmental Psychology,* 1975, **11,** 379−387.

Goyette, C. H., Connors, C. K., & Ulrich, R. F. Normative data on revised Connors Parent and Teacher Rating Scales. *Journal of Abnormal Child Psychology,* 1978, **6,** 221−236.

Graham, F., & Berman, P. Current status of ehavior tests for brain damage in infants and preschool children. *American Journal of Orthopsychiaty,* 1961, **4,** 713−N727.

Green, J. B., & Hartlage, L. C. Comparative performances of epileptic and non-epileptic children and adolescents. *Diseases of the Nervous System,* 1971, **32,** 418.

Griffiths, R. *The abilities of babies.* New York: McGraw-Hill, 1954.

Grossman, H. J. *Manual on terminology and classification in mental retardation.* Washington, DC: American Association of Mental Deficiency, 1973.

Guthrie, G. M., Masangkay, Z., & Guthrie, H. A. Behavior, malnutrition and mental development. *Journal of Cross-Cultural Psycholog,* 1976, **7,** 169−180.

Haggard, E. A., Breksted, A., & Skard, A. G. On the reliability of the anamnestic interview. *Journal of Abnormal and Social Psychology,* 1966, **61,** 311−313.

Harris, D. B. *Goodenough-Harris Drawing Test and Manual.* New York: Harcourt, Brace & Co., 1965.

Harrod, J. R., L'Heureaux, P., Wagensteen, D. O., & Hunt, C. D. Long-term follow-up of severe respiratory distress syndrome treated with IPPV. *Journal of Pediatrics,* 1974, **84** 277.

Haskin, R., Ramey, C., Stedman, D., Blacher-Dixon, J. & Pierce, J. Effects of repeated assessment on standardized test performance by infants. *American Journal of Mental Deficiency,* 1978, **83,** 233−239.

Hathaway, S., & McKinley, J. *Minnesota Multiphasic Personality Inventory: Manual for administration and scoring.* New York: Psychological Corporation, 1967.

Haynes, S. N. *Principles of behavioral assessment.* New York: Gardner Press, 1978.

Hayes, S. *Interim Hayes-Binet Intelligence Tests for the Blind.* Watertown, MA: Perkins School for the Blind, 1949.

Herbert, M. The concept and testing of basic damage in children: A review. *Journal of Child Psychology and Psychiatry,* 1964, **5,** 197−216.

Herjanic, B., Herjanic, M., Brown, F., & Wheatt, T. Are children reliable reporters? *Journal of Abnormal Child Psychology,* 1975, **3,** 41−48.

Hess, A. L., & Bradshaw, H. L. Positiveness of self-concept and ideal-self as a function of age. *Journal of Genetic Psychology,* 1970, **117,** 57−61.

Hindly, C. B. The Griffiths Scale of Infant Development: Scores and predictions from 3 to 18 months. *Journal of Child Psychology and Psychiatry,* 1960, **1,** 99−112.

Hiskey, M. S. *Hiskey-Nebraska Test of Learning Aptitude.* Lincoln. NE: Union College Press, 1966.

Horowitz, F. D., & Brazelton, T. B. Research with the Brazelton Neonatal Scale. In T. B. Brazelton (Ed.), Neonatal Behavioral Assessment Scale. *Monograph of the National Spastics Society,* 1973.

Hughes, H. E. Norms developed at the University of Chicago for the neuropsychological evaluation of children. *Journal of Pediatric Psychology,* 1976, **1,** 11.

Hunt, J. V., & Rhodes, L. Mental development of preterm infants during the first year. *Child Development,* 1977, **48,** 204−210.

Ireton, H., Thwing, E., & Grave, H. Infant mental development and neurological status, family socioeconomic status, and intelligence at age four. *Child Development,* 1970, **41,** 937−945.

Jacobstein, D., & Magrab, P. The adolescent coping with cancer. In P. Ahmed (Ed.), *Coping with cancer.* New York: Elsevier North-Holland, in press.

Johnson, K., & Kopp, C. *An analysis of tests for infants.* Unpublished manuscript, 1980.

Johnson, J. D., Malachowski, N. C., Grobstein, R., Dailey, W. J. R., & Sunshine, P. Prognosis of children surviving with the aid of mechanical ventillation in the newborn period. *Journal of Pediatrics,* 1974, **84,** 272−276.

Katz, A. H. *Hemophilia—A study in hope and reality.* Springfield, IL: Charles C. Thomas, 1970.

Kaufman, A. S. WISC-R research: Implications for interpretation. *School Psychology Digest,* 1979, **8,** 5−27. (a)

Kaufman, A. S. *Intelligence testing with the WISC-R.* New York: Wiley, 1979. (b)

Kaufman, A. S., & Kaufman, N. L. *Clinical evaluation of young children with the McCarthy Scales.* New York: Grune & Stratton, 1977.

Kellerman, J., & Katz, E. The adolescent with cancer: Theoretical, clinical, and research issues. *Journal of Pediatric Psychology,* 1977, **2,** 127−131.

Kellerman, J., Zeltzer, L., Ellenberg, L., Dash, J., & Rigler, D. Psychological effects of illness in adolescents I. Anxiety, self-esteem, and perception of control. *Journal of Pediatrics,* 1980, **97,** 126−131.

Kennell, J H., Soroker, E., Thomas, P., & Wasman, M. What parents of rheumatic fever patients don't understand about the disease and its prophlactic management *Pediatrics,* 1969, **43,** 160−167.

Khan, A. V., Herndon, C. H., & Ahmadian, S. Y. Social and emotional adaptations of children with transplanted kidneys and chronic hemodialysis. *American Journal of Psychiatry,* 1971, **127,** 1194–1198.

King, W. L., & Seegmiller, B. Performance of 14 to 22 month old black, firstborn male infants on two tests of cognitive development: The Bayley Scales and the Infant Psychological Development Scale. *Developmental Psychology,* 1973, **8,** 317–326.

Klein, R. E., Freeman, H. E., & Yarbough, C. Effects of protein-caloric malnutrition on mental development. *Advances in Pediatrics,* 1971, **18,** 75–91.

Klonoff J., & Low, M. Disordered brain function in young children and early adolescents: Neuropsychological and electroencephalographic correlates. In R. M. Reitan, & L. A. Davison (Eds.), *Clinical neuropsychology: Current status and applications.* New York: Wiley, 1974.

Klonoff, H., & Paris, R. Immediate, short-term and residual effects of acute head injuries in children: Neuropsychological and neurological correlates. In R. M. Retan & L. A. Davison (Eds.), *Clinical neuropsychology: Current status and applications.* New York: Wiley, 1974.

Klopfer, W. G., & Taulbee, E. S. Projective tests. In *Annual Review of Psychology.* Palo Alto, CA: Annual Reviews, 1976.

Knoblock, H., & Pasamanick, B. *Gesell and Amatruda's Developmental Diagnosis,* 3rd ed. New York: Harper & Row, 1974.

Knowles, H. C. Diabetes mellitus in childhood and adolescence. *Medical Clinics of North America,* 1971, **55,** 1007–1012.

Koff, E., Kammerer, B., Boyle, P., & Pueschel, S. M. Intelligence and phenylketonuria: Effects of diet termination. *Journal of Pediatrics,* 1979, **94,** 534–537.

Koocher, G. P., O'Malley, J. E., Gogan, J. L., & Foster, D. J. Psychological adjustment among pediatric cancer survivors. *Journal of Child Psychology and Psychiatry,* in press.

Koocher, G. P., O'Malley, J. E., Foster, D. I., & Gogan, J. L. Death anxiety in normal children and adolescents. *Psychiatric Clinics,* 1976, **9,** 220–229.

Kopp, C. Measurement issues: The mild to moderately handicapped child. In T. Black (Ed.), *Perspectives of measurement.* Chapel Hill, NC: Frank Porter Graham Child Development Center, 1979.

Koppitz, E. *Psychological evaluaton of children's human figure drawing.* New York: Grune & Stratton, 1968.

Korsh, B., Cobb, K., & Ashe, B. Pediatricians appraisals of patient's intelligence. *Pediatrics,* 1961, **27,** 990–1003.

Korsh, B. M., Negrette, V. F., Gardner, J. E., Weinstock, C. L., Mercer, A. S., Gruskin, C. M., & Fine, R. M. Kidney transplanation in children: Psychosocial follow-up on child and family. *Journal of Pediatrics,* 1973, **89,** 399–407.

Kron, R. E., Finnegan, L. P., Kaplan, S. L., Litt, M., & Phoenix, M. D. The assessment of behavioral change in infants undergoing narcotic addiction withdrawal: Comparative data from clinical and objective methods. *Addictive Diseases,* 1975, **2,** 257–275.

Kucera, J. Leukemia and twinning tendency in families of children with Down's syndrome. *Journal of Mental Deficiency Research,* 1971, **15,** 77–80.

Landtman, B., Valanne, E., Pentti, & Aukee, M. Psychosomatic behavior of children with congenital heart disease: Pre- and post-operative studies of eighty-four cases. *Annales Paediatrical Fennial,* 1960, **6,** 1–78.

Lapouse, R., & Monk, M. A. An epidemiologic study of behavior characteristics in children. *American Journal of Public Health,* 1958, **48,** 1134–1144.

Lawler, R. H., Nakielny, W., & Wright, N. Y. Psychological implications of cystic fibrosis. *Canadial Medical Association Journal,* 1966, **94,** 1043–1046.

Lawson, D., Metcalfe, M., & Pampiglione, G. Meningitis in childhood. *British Medical Journal,* 1965, **1,** 557–562.

Lee Painter, S., Lewis, M. *Mother-infant interaction and cognitive development.* Paper presented at Eastern Psychological Association Meeting, 1974.

Leiter, R. *Leiter International Performance Scale.* Chicago: C. H. Stoelting., 1966.

Levin, H. S., & Eisenberg, H. M. Neuropsychological outcome of closed head injury in children and adolescents. *Child's Brain,* 1979, **5,** 281–292.

Levitt, E. E., & Lubin, B. *Depression: Concepts, controversies, and some new facts.* New York: Springer, 1975.

Levitt, E. E. & Truumaa, A. *The Rorschach techniques with children and adolescents: Applications and norms.* New York: Grune & Stratton, 1972.

Levitt, J. & Taran, L. M. Some of the problems in education of rheumatic children. *Journal of Pediatrics,* 1963, **32,** 553–557.

Lewis, M. & McGurk, H. Evaluations of infant intelligence. *Science,* 1972, **178,** 1174–1177.

Lezak, M. D. *Neuropsychological assessment.* New York: Oxford University Press, 1976.

Linde, L. M., Rasof, B. & Dunn, O. J. Mental development in congenital heart disease. *Journal of Pediatrics,* 1967, **71,** 198–203.

Linde, L. M., Rasof, B., Dunn, O. J. & Rabb, E. Attitudinal factors in congenital heart disease. *Pediatrics,* 1966, **38,** 92–101.

Livingstone, J. *An evaluation of a photographically enlarged form of the revised Stanford-Binet Intelligence Scale for use with the partially seeing child.* Doctoral dissertation, New York University, 1957, University Microfilm No. 21–712.

Lubchenco, L. O., H., Goldman, A. L., Coyer, W. E., McIntyre, C. & Smith, D. M. Newborn intensive care and long-term prognosis. *Developmental Medicine and Child Neurology,* 1974, **16,** 421–431.

Magrab, P. R. Psychological management and renal dialysis. *Journal of Clinical Psychology,* 1975, **4,** 38–41.

Magrab, P. R. (Ed.) *Psychological management of pediatric problems,* Vol. 1. *Early life conditions and chronic disease.* Baltimore: University Park Press, 1978.

Magrab, P. R., & Papadopoulou, Z. L. Renal disease. In P. R. Magrab (Ed.), *Psychological management of pediatric problems,* Vol. 1. *Early life conditions and chronic disease.* Baltimore: University Park Press, 1978.

Margolies, P. J., & Weintraub, S. The revised 56-item CRPBI as a research instrument: Reliability and factor structure. *Journal of Clinical Psychology,* 1977, **33,** 472–476.

Mash, E. J., & Terdal, L. G. (Eds.) *Behavior therapy assessment: Diagnosis, design and evaluation.* New York: Springer. 1976.

Massry, S. G., & Sellers, A. L. *Clinical aspects of uraemia and dialysis.* Springfield, IL: Charles C. Thomas, 1976.

Matheny, A. P. Twins concordant for Piagetian equivalent items derived from the Bayley Mental Tests. *Developmental Psychology,* 1975, **11,** 224–227.

Mattson, A. Long-term physical illness in childhood: A challenge to psychosocial adaptation. *Pediatrics,* 1972, **50**, 801–811.

Maxfield, K., & Buchholz, S. *A social maturity scale for blind children.* New York: American Foundation for the Blind, 1961.

McArney, E. R., Pless, I. B., Satterwhite, B., & Friedman, S. B. Psychological problems of children with chronic juvenile arthritis. *Pediatrics,* 1974, **53**, 523–528.

McCarthy, D. *The McCarthy Scales of Children's Abilities.* New York: Psychological Corporation, 1972.

McCluskey, K. A., & Horowitz, F. D. A. *A comparison of neonatal assessment scores with laboratory performance in auditory and visual discrimination tasks between the ages of one and four months.* Paper presented a the biennial meeting of the Society for Reserch in Child Development, 1975.

McFie, J. *Assessment of organic intellectual impairment.* London: Academic Press, 1975.

McNamara, J. R. (Ed.) *Behavioral approaches to medicine Application and analysis.* New York: Plenum Press, 1979.

Meadows, P. T., & Evans, A. E. Effects of chemotherapy on the central nervous system: A study of pariental methotrexate in long-term survivors of leukemia and lymphoma in childhood. *Cancer,* 1976, **1**, 1079–1085.

Merkel, F. K., Ing, T. S., Ahmadian, Y., Lewy, P., Ambruster, K., Oyama, J., Sulieman, J. S., Belman, A. B., & King, L. R. Transplantation in and of the young. *Journal of Urology,* 1974, **111**, 679–686.

Miller, L. C. Louisville Behavior Checklist formales 6 to 12 years of Age. 4Psychological Reports, 1967, **21**, 85–896.

Money, J., & Pollitt, E. Studies in the psychology of dwarfism II. Personality maturation and response to growth hormone treatment in hypopituitary dwarfs. *Journal of Pediatrics,* 1966, **68**, 381–390.

Morse, J. Aspiration and achievement— study of one hundred patients with juvenile rheumatoid arthritis. *Rehabilitation Literature,* 1972, **33**, 290–295.

Murawski, B. J., Chazan, B. I., Balodimos, M. C., & Ryan, J. R. Personality patterns in patients with diabetes mellitus of long duration. *Diabetes,* 1970, **19**, 259–263.

Nagle, R. J. The McCarthy Scales of Children's Abilities: Research implications for the assessment of young children. *School Psychology Digest,* 1979, **8**, 319–326.

Nelson, K. B., & Ellenberg, J. Predictors of epilepsy in children who have experienced febrile seizures. *New England Journal of Medicine,* 1976, **295**, 1029–1033.

Neman, R. S., Neiman, J. F., & Sells, S. B. *Language and adjustment scales for the Thematic Apperception Test for Children 6 to 11 years.* Washington, DC: U.S. Government Printing Office, Vital and Health Statistics. Series 2-No. 58, DHEW Pub. No. (HRA) 74–1332, 1973.

Newland, T. E. *The Blind Learning Aptitude Test.* Urbana: University of Illinois Press, 1969.

Nichols, P. L. & Broman, S. H. Famipial resemblance in infant mental development. *Developmental Psychology,* 1974, **10**, 442–446.

Nihira, K., Foster, R., Shellhaas, M., & Leland, H. *AAMD Adaptive Behavior Scale, 1970.* Washington, DC: American Association of Mental Deficiency,1974.

Nowlis, V. Research with the mood adjective checklist. In S. Tomkins & C. E. Izard (Eds.), *Affect, cognition and personality.* New York: Springer, 1965.

Oakland, T. *Psychological and educational assessment of minority children.* New York: Brunner/Mazel, 1977.

Olch, D. Effects of hemophilia upon intellectual growth and academic achievement. *Journal of Genetic Psychology,* 1971, **119,** 63−74. (a)

Olch. D. Personality characteristics of hemophiliacs. *Journal of Personality Assessment,* 1971, **35,** 72−79. (b)

O'Leary, S. G., & Pelham, W. E. Behavior therapy and withdrawal of stimulant medication with hyperactive children. *Pediatrics,* 1978, **61,** 211−217.

Oski, F. A., & Honig, A. S. The effects of therapy in the developmental scores of iron-deficient infants. *Journal of Pediatrics,* 1978, **92,** 21−25.

Parmelee, A., Kopp, C., & Sigman, M. Selection of developmental assessment techniques for infants at risk. *Merrill-Palmer Quarterly,* 1976, **22,** 177−197.

Petrovich, D. V. The Pain Apperception Test: Psychological correlates of pain perception. *Journal of Clinical Psychology,* 1958, **14,** 367−374.

Petrovich, D. V. The Pain Apperception Test: A preliminary report. *Journal of Psychology,* 1957, **44,** 339−346.

Peylan-Ramu, N., Poplack, D. G., Pizzo, P. A., Adornato, B. T., & DiChiro, G. Abnormal CT scans of the brain in asympomatic children with acute lymphocytic leukemia after prophylactic treatment of the central nervous system with radiation and intrathecal chemotherapy. *New England Journal of Medicine,* 1978, **298,** 815.

Phatak, P., & Phatak, A. T. Application of the Bayley Scales of Infant Development (BSID) to neurological cases. *Indian Pediatrics,* 1973, **10,** 147−154.

Phillips, B. L., Pasewark, R. A., & Tindall, R. C. Relationship among McCarthy Scales of Children's Abilities, WPPSI and Columbia Mental Maturity Scales. *Psychology in the Schools,* 1978, **15,** 352−356.

Piers, E. V. *Manual for the Piers-Harris Children's Self ConceptScale (The way I feel about myself).* Nashville Counselor Recordings and Tests, 1969.

Pless, I. B., Cherry N. M., Douglas, J. W. B., & Wadsworth, M. E. J. *Psychological and social aspects of long-term illness in childhood: Results from a longitudinal national survey.* Unpublied manuscript, 1975.

Pless, I. B., Pinkerton, P. *Chronic childhood disorder: Promoting patterns of adjustment.* Chicago: Year Book Medical Publishers, 1975.

Porter, R., & Cattell, R. *Children's Personality Questionnaire.* Champaign, IL: Institute for Personality and Ability Testing, 1968.

Posey, R. A. Creative nursing care of babies with heart disease. *Nursing,* 1974, **4,** 40−45.

Prechtl, H. F. R., & Beintema, D. The neurological examination of the fullterm newborn infant. *Little Club Clinics in Development Medicine,* No. 12, London: Spastics Society, 1964.

Pueschel, S. M., Kopito, L., & Schwachman, H. Children with increased lead burden: A screening and follow-up study. *JAMA,* 1972, **222,** 462−466.

Pumroy, D. *Maryland Parent Attitude Survey.* College Park: University of Maryland, 1962.

Purcell, K. Distinctions between subgroups of asthmatic children: Children's perceptions of events associated with asthma. *Pediatrics,* 1963, **31,** 486−494.

Purcell, K., Brady, L., Chai, H., Muser, J., Molk, L., Gordon, N., & Means, J. The effect of asthma in children of experimental separation from the family. *Psychosomatic Medicine,* 1969, **31,** 144−164.

Purcell, K., Weiss, J., & Hahn, W. Certain psychosomatic disorders. In B. Wolman (Ed.), *Manual of child psychopathology*. New York: McGraw-Hill, 1972.

Quay, H. C. Measuring dimensions of deviant behavior: The Behavior Problem Checklist. *Journal of Abnormal Child Psychology*, 1977, **5**, 277–289.

Ramey, C. T., Campbell, F. A., & Nicholson, J. E. The predictive power of the Bayley scales of infant development and the Stanford-Binet intelligence scale in a relatively constant environment. *Child Development*, 1973. 790–795.

Ramey, C., & Smith, B. Assessing the intellectual consequences of early intervention with high risk infants. *American Journal of Mental Deficiency*, 1976, **81**, 318–324.

Ratcliffe, K. J., & Ratcliffe, M. W. The Leiter Scales: A review of validity findings. *American Annals of the Deaf*, 1979, **124**, 38–45.

Reitan, R. M. Psychological effects of cerebral lesions in children of early school age. In R. M. Reitan & L. A. Davison (Eds.), *Clinical neuropsychology: current status and applications*. New York: Wiley, 1974.

Reitan, R. M. *Manual for administration of neuropsychological test batteries for adults and children*. Indianapolis: Privately published by author, 1969.

Reitan, R. M., & Boll, T. J. Neuropsychological correlates of minimal brain dysfunction. *Annals of the New York Academy of Sciences*, 1973, **205**, 65–88.

Reitan, R. M., & Davison, L. A. *Clinical neuropsychology: Current status and applications*. New York: Wiley, 1974.

Reite, M., Davis, K., Solomons, C., & Ott, J. Osteogenesis imperfecta: Psychological function. *American Journal of Psychiatry*, 1972, **128**, 90–98.

Reynolds, W. M., & Sundberg, N. D. Recent research trends in testing. *Journal of Personality Assessment*, 1976, **40**, 228–233.

Rie, H. E., Hilty, M. D., & Cranblitt, H. G. Intelligence and coordination following California encephalitis. *American Journal of the Disabled Child*, 1973, **125**, 824–827.

Robach, H. B. Human figure drawings: Their utility in the clinical psychologist's armamentation for personality assessment. *Psychological Bulletin*, 1968. **70**, 1–6.

Rorschach, H. *Psychodiagnostics*. Bern: Bircher, 1921.

Roberts, J. A. F., & Sedgley, G. Intelligence testing of full term and premature children by repeated assessments. In C. Banks & P. L. Broadhurst (Eds.), *Studies in psychology*. London: University of London Press, 1965.

Rosenblith, J. F. Prognostic value of neonatal behavioral tests. In B. Z. Freidlander, G. M. Sterritt, & G. E. Kirk (Eds.), *Exceptional infant*, Vol. 3. *Assessment and intervention*. New York: Brunner/Mazel, 1975.

Rosenblith, J. F. Relations between neonatal behaviors and those at eight months. *Developmental Psychology*, 1974, **10**, 779–792. (a)

Rosenblith, J. F. *Relations between newborn and four year behaviors*. Paper presented at the meeting of the Eastern Psychological Association, 1974. (b)

Rosenblith, J. F. The modified Graham behavior test for neonates: Test-retest reliability, normative data and hypotheses for future work. *Biologia Neonatorium*, 1961, **3**, 174–192.

Russo, D. C., Bird, B. L., & Masek, B. S. Assessment issues in behavioral medicine. *Behavioral Assessment*, 1980, **2**, 1–18.

Rutter, M., & Graham, P. The reliability and validity of the psychiatric assessment of the child. I, Interview with the child. *British Journal of Psychiatry*, 1968, **114**, 563–579.

Rutter, M., Graham, P. J., & Yule, W. *A neuropsychiatric study in childhood*. Clinics in Developmental Medicine, No. 35/36. London: Spastics International Medical Publications in association with Heineman Medical Books, 1970.

Rutter, M., Tizard, J., & Whitmore, K. *Education, health and behavior*. London: Longmans Green, 1970.

Salvia, J., & Ysseldyke, J. E. *Assessment in special and remedial education*. Boston: Houghton Mifflin, 1978.

Salvia, J., Ysseldyke, J., & Lee, M. 1972 revision of the Stanford-Binet: A farewell to the mental age. *Psychology in the Schools*, 1975, **12**, 421—422.

Sattler, J. *Assessment of children's intelligence*. Philadelphia: Saunders, 1974.

Scarr-Salapatek, S., & Williams, M. L. The effects of early stimulation on low birth-weight babies. *Child Development*, 1973, **44**, 94—101.

Schaefer, E. S. Children's reports of parent behavior. *Child Development*, 1965, **36**, 413—424.

Schaefer, E. S., & Bell, R. Q. Development of a parental attitude research instrument. *Child Development*, 1958, **29**, 339—361.

Schoenfeld, W. A. Body image disturbances in adolescents with inappropriate sexual development. *American Journal of Orthopsychiatry*, 1964, **34**, 493—498.

Seidenfeld, M. A. The psychological sequelae of poliomyelitis in children. *Nervous Child*, 1948, **7**, 14—21.

Sigman, M., & Parmalee, A. H. Longitudinal evaluation of the preterm infant. In T. Field, A. M. Sostek, S. Goldberg, & H. H. Shuman (Eds.), *Infants born at risk*. New York: Spectrum, 1979.

Smith, I., Lobascher, M. E., Stevenson, J. E., Wolff, O. H., Schmidt, H., Grubel-Kaiser, S., & Bickel. Effect of stopping low-phenylalanine diet on intellectual progress of children with phenylketonuria. *British Medical Journal*, 1978, **2**, 723—726.

Smith, R. E. A Minnesota Multiphasic Personality Inventory profile of allergy. *Psychosomatic Medicine*, 1962, **29**, 203—209.

Sostek, A. M., Quinn, P.O., & Davitt, M. K. Behavior, development, and neurologic status of premature and full term infants with varying medical complications. In T. Field, A. M., Sostek, S. Goldberg, & H. H. Shuman (Eds.), *Infants born at risk*. New York: Spectrum, 1979.

Soule, A. B., III, Standley, K., Copans, S. A., & Davis, M. Clinical uses of Brazelton Neonatal Scale. *Pediatrics*, 1974, **54**, 583—586.

Sourkes, B. Siblings of the pediatric cancer patient. In J. Kellerman (Ed.), *Psychological aspects of childhood cancer*. Springfield, I: Charles C. Thomas, 1980.

Sourkes, B. Facilitating family coping with childhood cancer. *Journal of Pediatric Psychology*, 1977, **2**, 65—67.

Sprague, R. L., & Sleator, E. E. Effects of psychopharmacological agents on learning disabilities. *Pediatric Clinics of North America*, 1973, **20**, 719—735.

Spielberger, C. D., Edwards, C. S., Lushene, R., Montuori, J., & Plazek, D. *Manual for the State-Trait Anxiety Inventory children (How I feel questionnaire)*. Palo Alto, CA: Consulting Psychologists Press, 1972.

Spielberge, C. D., Gorusch, R. L., & Lushenie, R. E. *State-trait anxiety inventory manual*. Palo Alto, CA: Consulting Psychologists Press, 1970.

Spreen, O., & Gaddes, W. H. Developmental norms for 15 neurological tests ages 6 to 15. *Cortex,* 1969, **5,** 170.

Spungin, S., & Swallow, R. Psychoeducational assessment: Role of the psychologist to teacher of the visually handicapped. *Education of the Visually Handicapped,* 1975, **7,** 67–75.

Standley, K., Soule, A. B., Copans, S. A., & Duchowny, M. S. Local-regional anesthesia during childbirth: Effects on newborn behaviors. *Science,* 1974, **186,** 634–635.

Sterky, G. Family background and state of mental health in a group of diabetic school children. *Acta Paediatrica,* 1963, **52,** 377–381.

Stevenson, J. G., Stone, E. F., Dillard, D. H., & Morgan, B. C. Intellectual development of children subjected to prolonged circulatory arrest during hypothermic open heart surgery in infancy. *Circulation,* 1974, **50,** 54–59.

Stillman, R. D. *Assessment of deaf-blind children: The Callier-Azusa Scale.* Dallas: Collier Hearing and Speech Center, 1975.

Stores, G. Behavioral effects of anti-epileptic drugs. *Developmental Medicine and Child Neurology,* 1975, **17,** 647–658.

Strauss, M. E., Lessen-Firestone, J. K., Starr, R. H., & Ostrea, E. M. Behavior of narcotic addict newborns. *Child Development,* 1975, **46,** 887–893.

Stutsman, R. *The Merrill-Palmer Scale of Mental Tests.* New York: Harcourt, Brace, & World, 1948.

Sullivan, P. M., & Vernon, M. Psychological assessment of hearing impaired children. *School Psychology Digest,* 1979, **8,** 271–290.

Sultz, H., Schlesinger, E. R., Mosher, W. E., & Feldman, J. G. *Long-term childhood illness.* Pittsburgh: University of Pittsburgh Press, 1972.

Swallow, R. Assessment for visually handicapped children and youth. *American Foundation for the Blind Practice Report,* 1977.

Swenson, C. H. Empirical evaluations of human figure drawings. *Psychological Bulletin,* 1968, **70,** 20–44.

Swift, C. R., Seidman, F., & Stein, H. Adjustment problems in juvenile diabetes. *Psychosomatic Medicine,* 1967, **29,** 555–571.

Tarter, R. E. Intellectual and adaptive functioning in epilepsy. *Diseases of the Nervous System,* 1972, **33,** 763–770.

Terman, L. M., & Merrill, M. A. *Stanford-Binet Intelligence scale, Form L-M, Third Revision.* Boston: Houghton Mifflin, 1973.

Tew, B. J., & Lawrence, K. M. Mothers, brothers and sisters of patients with spina bifida. *Developmental Medicine and Child Neurology,* 1973, Supplement 29, 69–76.

Thatcher, L. G. Treatment of acute leukemia in children. *Wisconsin Medical Journal,* 1968, **67,** 530–533.

Thomas, L. A., Milman, D. H., & Rodriques-Torres, R. Anxiety in children with rheumatic fever. Relation to route of prophylaxis. *Journal of the American Medical Association,* 1970, **212,** 2080–2085.

Travis, G. *Chronic illness in children: Its impact on child and family.* Stanford CA: Stanford University Press, 1976.

Uzgiris, I. C. Organization of sensorimotor intelligence. In M. Lewis (Ed.). *Orgins of Intelligence.* New York: Plenum Press, 1976.

Uzgiris, I. C., & Hunt, J. *Toward Ordinal Scales of Psychological Development in Infancy.* Champaign: University of Illinois Press, 1975.

Vernon, M. Psychologic evaluation of hearing impaired chidren. In L. Llyod (Ed.), *Communication assessment and intervention strategies.* Baltimore: University Park Press, 1976.

Vernon, M. Meningitis and deafness: The problem, its physical, audiological, psychological, and educational manifestations in deaf children. *Laryngoscope,* 1967, **77,** 1856−1974.

Vernon, M., Bair, R., & Lotz, S. Psychological evaluation and testing of children who are deaf-blind. *School Psycology Digest,* 1979, **8,** 291−295.

Vietze, P. M., & St. Clair, K. *Infant tests: Measures of cognitive development in the study of high risk infants.* Paper presented at the Georgia Warm Springs Conference. Princeton, NJ, 1976.

Wachs. T. D. Relation of infants' performance on Piaget scales between twelve and twenty-four months and their Stanford-Binet performance at thirty-one months. *Child Development,* 1975, **46,** 929−935.

Waechter, E. H. Childrens awareness of fatal illness. *American Journal of Nursing,* 1971, **7,** 1168−1172.

Walker, C. E. Behavioral intervention in a pediatric setting. In J. R. McNamara (Ed.), *Behavioral approaches to medicine: Application and analysis.* New York: Plenum Press, 1979.

Walker, H. M. *Walker Problem Behavior Identification Checklist.* Los Angeles: Western Psychological Services, 1970.

Walls, R. T., Werner, T. J., Bacon, A., & Zane, T. Behavior checklists. In J. O. Cone & R. P. Hawkins (Eds.), *Behavioral assessment: New directions in clinical psychology.* NEW York: Brunner/Mazel, 1977.

Wallston, B. S., Wallston, K. A., Kaplan, G. D., & Maides, S. A. Development and validation of the health and locus of control scale. *Journal of Consulting and Clinical Psychology,* 1976, **44,** 580.

Watson, D. L., & Friend, R. Measurement of social-evaluative anxiety. *Journal of Consulting and Clinical Psychology,* 1969, **33,** 448−457.

Wechsler, D. *Manual for the Wechsler Adult Intelligence Scale.* New York: Psychological Corporation, 1955.

Wechsler, D. *Manual for the Wechsler preschool and primary scale of intelligence.* New York: Psychological Corporation, 1967.

Wechsler, D. *Manual for the Wechsler Intelligence Scale for Children—Revised.* New York: Psychological Corporation, 1974.

Weiss, J. R., Quinlan, D. M., O'Neill, P., & O'Neill, P. C. The Rorschach and structured tests of perception as indices of intellectual development in mentally retarded and non-retarded children. *Journal of Experimental Child Psychology,* 1978, **25,** 326−336.

Weery, J. S., Sprague, R. L., & Cohen, M. N. Connors Teacher Rating Scale for use in drug studies with children: An empirical study. *Journal of Abnormal Child Psychology,* 1975, **3,** 217−229.

Whitehouse, D. Psychological and neurological correlates of seizure disorders. *Johns Hopkins Medical Journal,* 1971, **129,** 36−42.

Whitman, V., Drotar, D., Lamberti, S., VanHeecheren, D. W., Borkat, G., Ankeney, J., & Liebman, J. Effects of cardiac surgery with extracorporal circulation in intellectual functioning in children. *Circulation,* 1973, **48,** 160−163.

Willerman, L., Broman, S. H., & Fiedler, M. Infant development, preschool IQ, and social class. *Child Development,* 1970, **41,** 69−77.

Williams, H., & McNichol, K. N. Prevalence, natural history and relationship of wheezy bronchitis and asthma in children. An epidemiological study. *British Medical Journal,* 1969, **4,** 321−325.

Wilson, R. S. Twins: Mental development in the preschool years. *Developmental Psychology,* 1974, **10,** 580−588.

Wright, L. Assessing the psychosomatic status of children. *Journal of Clinical Child Psychiatry,* 1978, **7,** 94−112.

Wright, L. Indirect treatment of children through principles-oriented parent consultation. *Journal of Consulting and Clinical Psychology,* 1976, **44,** 148.

Wright, L. Intellectual sequelae of Rocky Mountain spotted fever. *Journal of Abnormal Psychology,* 1972, **80,** 315−316.

Wright, L., & Fulwiler, T. L. Sequelae of lead poisoning in children. *Oklahoma State Medical Association Journal,* 1972, **65,** 372−375.

Wright, L., & Jimmerson, S. Intellectual sequelae of hemophilus influenzal meningitis. *Journal of Abnormal Psychology,* 1971, **77,** 181−183.

Wright, L., Schaefer, A. B., & Solomons, G. *Encyclopedia of Pediatric Psychology.* Baltimore: University Park Press, 1979.

Wysocki, B. A., & Whitney, E. Body image of crippled as seen in Draw-a-Person test behavior. *Perceptual and Motor Skills,* 1965, 499−504.

Yarrow, M. R., Campbell, J. D., & Burton, R. V. Recollections of childhood: A study of the retrospective method. *Monographs of the Society for Research in Child Development,* 1970, **35,** (Serial No. 138).

Zeltzer, L., Kellerman, J., Ellenberg, L., Dash, J., & Rigler, D. Psychological effects of illness in adolescence. II, Impact of illness in adolescents—Crucial issues and coping styles. *Journal of Pediatrics,* 1980, **97,** 132−138.

Zubin, J., Eron, L., & Schumer, F. *An experimental approach to projective techniques.* New York: Wiley, 1965.

Zung, W. W. K. A self-rating depression scale. *Archives of General Psychiatry,* 1965, **12,** 63−70.

CHAPTER 4

Intervention Techniques in Pediatric Psychology

Gary B. Mesibov
Melissa R. Johnson

The diverse backgrounds of pediatric psychologists (Routh, 1977) and the clinical problems they confront have stimulated the development of many different intervention strategies. These strategies have been adapted to meet the needs of children from birth through adolescence, with many different problems, and in a variety of settings. The purpose of this chapter is to review the intervention techniques that have evolved from the practice of pediatric psychology and to illustrate their uses. The intervention techniques that have been most widely applied by pediatric psychologists can be classified under the broad headings of prevention, consultation, psychotherapy, and behavioral therapy.

PREVENTION

Preventive efforts of pediatric psychologist have been directed at three major targets. The first is parent education. If one assumes that parents are the most important influences on their developing children, then the more they know and understand about child development, the better they will be able to avoid potential difficulties. The second major thrust of prevention efforts has been in the areas of early assessment and intervention for behavioral and developmental problems. This work has been aimed primarily at high-risk populations, including children with developmental problems, and those from families of lower socioeconomic backgrounds. The third area of intervention has been the development of social competence in children, which, as Kent and Rolf (1979) have noted, encompasses much of the prevention research. Because the social competence approach has, in fact, been one of the major interventions with high-risk populations, there is considerable overlap between these last two categories.

Parent Education

Parent education has been the most frequently used of the preventive approaches. Salk (1975) has strongly advocated parent training, arguing that parents are the most neglected population in America in terms of the support and assistance they receive. Moreover, Salk argues that parenthood is one of the most important roles any human can assume in life and that pediatric psychologists must assume the major responsibility for training in this area.

Other experts have supported the need for parent training (Murphy & Frank, 1979; Zigler & Hunsinger, 1978). Zigler and Hunsinger claim that the tendency to have fewer children provides less opportunities for older children to observe younger ones and help care for them, thus increasing their need for training in parenting when they become parents themselves. Others have argued the need for parent training based on the growing isolation of the nuclear family and the lack of adequate support and information in local communities (Mesibov, Schroeder, & Wesson, 1977; Woodward & Malamud, 1975).

Pediatric psychologists have met the need for preventive parent education primarily in two ways. The first has been through the popular literature, as exemplified by the work of Salk (1973). The second approach has involved parent education groups, conducted in private psychological practices, pediatric offices, universities, and other settings.

Parent Education Books

Written guides for parents represent the most common source of parenting information and have recently become important commercially. Clarke-Stewart's (1978) study has revealed some characteristics of this literature and its consumers. Overall, most parents read at least one childrearing book and a substantial proportion read more than five. Those who read such books are relatively young, caring for their first child, and isolated from ongoing family support.

The books can be divided into several major types. First are books on behavioral principles and their application to childrearing issues. Prominent among these are *Living with Children* (Patterson & Gullion, 1968), *Parent Power* (Wright, 1979b), *Parents Are Teachers* (Becker, 1971), and a more detailed summary of behavioral principles entitled *Changing Children's Behavior* (Krumboltz & Krumboltz, 1972). Although other theoretical approaches are sometimes advanced in childrearing books such as Dreikurs's popularization of Adlerian childrearing principles (Dreikurs & Grey, 1970), behaviorism is the orientation most commonly espoused.

A second kind of childrearing book involves discussions of normal developmental issues and strategies for dealing with problems. Spock (1946) and Salk (1973) are the two most prominent examples of this approach. Others include Brazelton (1969, 1974) and White (1975) on infants, and Gesell (Gesell & Ilg, 1945) on older children. Wright has also made significant contributions to this literature (1979b).

The third kind of book focuses primarily on communication between parent and child. Gordon's *Parent Effectiveness Training* (1970), Dodson's *How to Parent* (1970) and Ginott's *Between Parent and Child* (1965) and *Between Parent and Teenager* (1971) are the best examples of these approaches.

In addition, several books on specific topics have appeared and gained wide acceptance. Azrin and Foxx's *Toilet Training in Less Than a Day* (1974) and Beck's *How to Raise a Brighter Child* (1967) are two popular examples.

In general, the evidence suggests that these books have had an important influence on parents of young children and that this influence is increasing as our society becomes more mobile (Clarke-Stewart, 1978). The contributions of pediatric psychologists in these efforts have been significant and should increase in the coming years.

Parent Groups

Preventive parent education is also provided through parent groups. Arnold (1978) describes guidance for parents as a continuum from simple information-giving or education to psychotherapeutic tactics. The preventive education groups discussed here will fall along the information-giving end of the continuum.

One model for providing parent training has been described by Schroeder (1979). These groups focus on the normal developmental issues that occur during specific age groups. The role of the group leader is to provide information and support. These groups are reinforced by a call-in/come-in service where parents may receive assistance for more individual problems (Mesibov, 1977; Mesibov et al., 1977). Another such program has been described by Jackson and Terdal (1978), which also tries to give parents a clear understanding and appropriate expectations of their children. The Jackson and Terdal model, however, provides more direct experience and also uses videotapes and films where appropriate.

Several parent training programs focus exclusively on teaching behavior management skills. Lindsley (1978) presents one such program, which includes teaching parents to count, chart, and ultimately change behaviors in their children. Forgatch and Toobert (1979) find that parents who received training in behavior modification techniques are more effective in altering whining and noncompliant behaviors in their children than those in an untreated control group.

Parent groups show considerable promise as an important preventive technique. They combine the advantages of parent education books (information dissemination) with a more personalized, individualized, and supportive approach. Future efforts should explore more creative formats for conducting these groups as well as a greater variety of theoretical approaches (Ellis, 1978; McGuiness & Glasser, 1978).

Early Assessment and Intervention

A second way in which pediatric psychologists have furthered preventive efforts is through intensive work with high-risk children and their families. A child is considered high-risk when some aspect of the child or his/her environment suggests the likelihood of social, behavioral, or intellectual difficulties. High-risk populations include children whose parents are mentally retarded, economically disadvantaged, divorced, and/or potentially abusive, in addition to children who are premature and/or developmentally delayed.

Children of Economically Disadvantaged and Mentally Retarded Parents

Rolf and Hasazi (1977) initiated one of the most elaborate early intervention programs for high-risk children. The risk factors they studied included mental disability, developmental lags, social problems, family problems, and problems with the physical environment. Their intervention, consisting of an intensive day-care program, resulted in many fewer problems for the children compared with a group of untreated controls.

The effectiveness of an intensive day-care program for high-risk children has also been demonstrated by Heber (1978) in the well-known Milwaukee project. This program, starting at birth, focused on high-risk children of mothers with IQs of 75 or less. The children spent their first five years in a day-care center receiving intensive instruction. This was supplemented by a home teacher who taught mothers how to care for their children as well as other everyday skills. By age 7, the high-risk children in the experimental group had a mean IQ of 121 compared with a mean of 87 for the control group.

Johnson (1976) used a similar model in a Houston program for bilingual Mexican-American families with extremely low incomes, little schooling, and children under age 5. As with the Heber studies, the intervention consisted of an intensive day-care program and home training for the mothers. Local people, trained as paraprofessionals to teach the mothers and to work with the children, were able to produce long-term changes at relatively low cost.

The classroom intervention model for high-risk children has also been used effectively without the home training component (Ramey, Holmberg, Sparling, & Collier, 1977). As with the Heber program, this intervention focused on single mothers whose social, economic, and intellectual backgrounds made their children at risk for mental retardation. The intervention consisted of an intensive day-care program but did not have the additional home training component described by Heber. Nonetheless, the children in this study showed normal intellectual performance at age 5 as compared to the borderline performance of the control children.

Other early intervention programs have focused solely on parent training without a day-care or school component. Maisto and German (1979) showed substantial gains on both cognitive and language development for 32 high-risk infants after a 1-year intervention program. Their degree of success related to how early the child was identified and treated and to the initial severity of the problem. Heifeitz (1977) initiated a behavioral training program for parents of retarded children, using self-contained instructional materials plus direct professional intervention.

Children of Divorce

Wallerstein and Kelly (1977) have recently outlined the needs of children of divorce for preventive intervention. After following large numbers of families over 10 years, they concluded that divorce can have negative effects on children for at least 5 years. They advocate preventive counseling for these children and have demonstrated its effectiveness as an intervention tool. With the recent increase of divorce in our society, and its recognition as a significant social problem, the quantity and quality of intervention approaches with these children is certain to increase dramatically.

Premature Infants

There is considerable evidence that children born prematurely have a higher incidence of numerous physical, behavioral, and intellectual handicaps during their lives (Schafer & Maersh, 1977; Tjossem, 1976). Moreover, these children are also more likely to be battered and abused.

Intervention efforts with these children have been directed at increasing general stimulation, parent-child contact, and parental participation in the caretaking role, all of which are related to improved child outcomes (Field, 1977). For example, Scarr-Salapatek and Williams (1973) combined added visual, tactile, and kinesthetic stimulation with weekly home visits for 1 year to produce IQ increases in a group of premature infants as compared with a control group. Other investigators have found similarly positive results with these same general intervention strategies (Brown & Hepler, 1976; Powell, 1974). Current work with premature infants is attempting to implement these effective techniques by changing restrictive hospital policies (Klaus & Kennell, 1976) and identifying ways of working with different socioeconomic groups (Elmer & Gregg, 1967).

Abused Children

Another high-risk population that has received considerable attention has been children of abusing parents. With this group, the general strategy has been to get assistance to potentially abusing parents as quickly as possible. Willis (1976) advocates four ways in which hospitals should provide this early assistance. These include, first, working with high-risk mothers in the obstetrician's office. Such a program requires obstetricians to refer mothers who appear to lack mothering skills for further training and intervention. Second, premature babies who are known to be at risk for abuse should be followed very carefully from birth. Third, a parent assistance center should be set up within the hospital to help abusive and potentially abusive parents. Finally, each hospital should have a policy abuse team to coordinate plans, treatment efforts, and training of hospital staff.

Several volunteer prevention programs have also been developed for potential child abusers (Johnstone, 1973; Pike, 1973). These programs include volunteer staffs who are available by telephone on a 24-hour-a-day basis. Parents unable to endure the stresses of daily childrearing are able to call these volunteers for support and specific assistance. Most of the programs work closely with community agencies and are able to help coordinate the delivery of assistance for those who are eligible. Volunteer programs of this kind have been extremely effective in communities willing to commit the time and resources for ther development.

Finally, there are a number of people who feel the problem of child abuse is a broad societal one and that prevention efforts must be undertaken on a broader basis than some of the programs already described. Gil (1976) and Zigler and Hunsinger (1978) have most recently advanced this position. They argue that child abuse is an outgrowth of our society's attitudes concerning children's rights. Any society that allows corporal punishment of children and that prevents them from exercising most human and legal rights should expect to have a group who become devalued. Once this occurs, child abuse is a consequence that should be expected.

According to Zigler, the role of the pediatric psychologist, along with all child advocates, in preventing child abuse needs to include advocacy on the local, state, and national levels. Policies allowing children to be devalued through corporal punishment and other forms of social and political inequity must be changed. In addition, policies advancing child rights and allowing for equal opportunities must be promoted. Only after our society recognizes the needs and rights of children can we expect that they will be treated in a more dignified way.

In summary, early intervention strategies have been developed by pediatric psychologists to serve a wide range of needs. Overall, these strategies are designed to provide additional stimulation, instruction, and support to children and families who by history or life situation are likely to encounter difficulties in the future. Many believe this to be the best use of professional time and energy because of accumulating evidence that preventive efforts are much more effective than are remedial strategies that are applied after a problem has already developed (Albee & Joffee, 1977).

Development of Social Competence

Training children in social competence is another important preventive technique. Advocates of this training assume it will make children more successful, and therefore less likely to be disruptive and to develop significant problems. Social competence interventions have focused on problem-solving strategies, understanding others' perspectives, and social skills training.

The most widely used preventive training program for social competence was developed by Spivack and Shure (1974). This program is designed to teach problem-solving skills to preschool and school-aged children. The program emphasizes developing alternative solutions to specific social problems and also evaluating the consequences of each potential solution. For example, a child might be confronted with a situation in which another child hits him/her. The child is then asked to generate possible responses such as hitting back, walking away, or getting the teacher. The consequences of each response are then evaluated such as getting into a fight for hitting back, being called a sissy for walking away, or solving the problem by getting the teacher. Children are then asked to select the best course of action based on this analysis. The goal of the Spivack and Shure program is to have children apply these problem-solving skills in their everyday interaction.

The Spivack and Shure program for preschool and early school-aged children takes about three months of daily 20-minute sessions to complete. One advantage is that an entire classroom can participate together. The program is one of the most effective available for teaching social skills to a large group of children. It has been used effectively with problem children as well.

Another potentially useful approach to teaching social competence is by sensitizing children about how their behaviors affect others. Unfortunately, this approach has not been widely implemented, although one study (Ross & Ross, 1976) did explore this idea with an active sixth grader. The child and his class were shown a series of three skits illustrating the adverse effect that a very active child can have on a classroom, a small group game, and a birthday party. These skits were then discussed with the very active child, followed by the child's rehearsing more appropriate behaviors with adults, and then role-playing with peers. During this process, much discussion was encouraged. The goal of the procedure was to have the active child learn to evaluate his own as well as other people's behavior, and to increase his skill in observational learning. As a result of this procedure, the boy was reportedly much improved.

Another approach to social competence training has been direct teaching of specific social skills. LaGreca and Santogrossi (1980) have demonstrated one application of this relatively new and potentially useful technique. Using socially shy first and second graders, they developed a social skills program to teach basic interpersonal and communication skills. Their procedure was very effective in developing these skills in the children. Because social skills training has been more frequently utilized as a therapeutic intervention rather than a preventive technique, it will be described in more detail in a later section.

Summary

Considering that a new trend in the delivery of mental health services has been an emphasis on prevention (Albee & Joffe, 1977), it is encouraging that pediatric psychologists are already strongly committed to this endeavor. Preventive efforts show great potential for reaching more people in a cost-effective way. To date, most of the pediatric psychology preventive efforts have emphasized parent education and high-risk children. Future efforts should be directed at more children, themselves, so that pediatric psychologists can play a direct role in improving the life situations and growth potential of large groups of children.

CONSULTATION

Because pediatric psychologists frequently work in multidisciplinary and group care settings, they often function by teaching or directing others who deliver services, or by interacting with a system for the indirect benefit of the child. Therefore, consultation is another important intervention technique. The literature offers several models of consultation, some of which are specific to particular settings and some of which are more general. This section will review consultative intervention techniques in three types of settings: medical settings, school settings, and residential institutions.

Medical Consultation

As the role of the pediatric psychologist in medical settings has expanded in recent years, so has the literature on many aspects of this role. Three issues are of primary concern to those writing on this topic. The first is how pediatric psychologists function professionally in medical settings and how these functions differ from traditional roles. The second is the relationship between pediatric psychologists and the health care team. The other issue involves the specific intervention techniques that are most effectively used by pediatric psychologists consulting in medical settings.

Several writers have described the development and history of psychological involvement in medical settings (Drotar, 1976; Routh, 1975; Wright, 1976, 1979a; Schowalter, 1979). Because this involvement is relatively new, there are no clear role definitions as yet. However, the most useful generalization is that pediatric psychologists participate in most of the traditional consultative activities, but also go far beyond them in many new and different ways.

For example, Koocher and Sallan (1978), in describing the role of the pediatric psychologist on a pediatric oncology team, note that the frequency and intensity of intervention are likely to vary from hours of intensive therapeutic and supportive contact to weeks or months with only occasional consultations. They emphasize that in addition to possessing crisis intervention and more traditional therapeutic skills, these consultants must be "team players," who are able to facilitate communication among a large number of professionals as well as between the child and family.

Several authors have helped to clarify the various consultative roles in pediatric settings through classification schemes describing different levels of consultation. Schowalter (1979), though writing from the perspective of a psychiatrist, offers a distinction between "indirect" and "direct" consultation. In the role of indirect consultant, the psychiatrist or psychologist seeks to "improve the emotional climate for patients in the hospital" by functioning as a "resource person for issues of child development, group dynamics, crisis intervention, and policy formation" (p. 37). Direct consultation refers to the more traditional role of consultation around an individual case in response to a request from the primary physician. Schowalter sees direct consultation as the traditional function of the child psychiatrist, with the complications being limited time and space as well as limited comprehension on the part of most families concerning the consultant's role. Most pediatric psychologists try to provide both direct and indirect consultation.

Stabler (1979) has emphasized the teaching role of the psychological consultant. He has identified three models by which liaison with pediatricians in both inpatient and outpatient settings may occur. His resource model corresponds closely with Schowalter's direct consultation, relying on the transmission of a limited set of data through formal channels around a particular case. Stabler's second model, process consultation, increases the involvement for psychologists by a "collaborative liaison in which patient care and treatment responsibilities are shared" (p. 310) over time. Stabler identifies the most sophisticated model as the process-educative approach, which casts the psychologist in the role of "supportive source of information and technical skill" (p. 311) for the physician.

Other aspects of the pediatric psychologist's role are described by workers in a variety of specialized settings. Pediatric oncology appears to provide especially valuable opportunities for consultative interventions as demonstrated by the work of Koocher and Sallan (1978), O'Malley and Koocher (1977), Lewis (1978), Lansky (1974), and Humphrey and Vore (1974). These authors describe a number of roles for pediatric psychologists in oncology settings. One involves limiting the stress, to the extent possible, that children in these settings must endure. Humphrey and Vore

(1974) advocate delaying procedures if adequate therapeutic preparation has not occurred. The pediatric psychologist is also viewed as a source of information about the psychology of chronically ill and dying children. Lewis (1978) suggests developing a curriculum based on empirical psychological knowledge in this area for medical care givers. A third role described in this literature is as a resource for the staff to help them cope with the stress of working with fatally ill children and managing the maladaptive responses that this stress may produce.

Similar roles are outlined by workers on pediatric burn units and surgical wards. Bernstein, Sanger, and Fras (1969) emphasized the role of the mental health practitioner as a facilitator of communication between staff and families. In order to successfully fill this role, pediatric psychologists have to be especially skillful in handling the negative feelings of the staff and families in these stressful circumstances. The educative function is also described. Bernstein et al. (1969) discussed the tendency of medical staff to emphasize medical concerns without similar involvement or understanding of important psychological issues. As an example, they write that "epithelialization of a skin graft or dehydration are debated, rather than the problems of depression and separation which produced refusal to eat and drink, thus causing dehydration and failure of grafts" (p. 633). Geist (1977) suggests that the emotional well-being of both patients and staff is an appropriate responsibility for pediatric psychologists to assume.

The dual role of the pediatric psychology consultant as both a provider of direct services to children and a catalytic educational and supportive figure within the ward or clinic has been emphasized in all of the literature summarized above. In order to fulfill this dual role, relationships with staff are obviously important, yet quite complex, and the literature on consultation in medical settings gives these relationships considerable attention. The most thorough discussion focuses on the nursing and psychiatric relationships rather than the psychological mental health consultant (Petrillo & Sanger, 1980); however, the principles are applicable to pediatric psychologists as well. Changes from crisis-oriented, case-centered interventions by the consultants to a more environmental approach have been marked by considerable resistance from many sources. Physicians tend to be biologically oriented and lack motivation to develop behavioral, diagnostic, and therapeutic skills. Nurses want relief from the aggravation caused by difficult problems rather than to be potential behavior managers. Related personnel such as recreation therapists, educators, and other staff have been unaccustomed to contributing their valuable observations and innovations to the professionals with more influence. Finally, territorial conflicts have been encountered among staff with overlapping roles, such as social workers, psychiatrists, and psychologists.

Although assuming a more comprehensive and effective role can cause some conflicts among staff involved, the problems are not insurmountable. However, more than simple consultative services are required if these expanded roles are to evolve. Petrillo and Sanger (1980) describe the successful process: "The most effective mental health personnel participated directly in the clinical management of psychological crises, serving as role models and demonstrating that their work promoted staff development and efficient operation of the department; they demonstrated that their presence or absence made a difference" (p. 30).

Others have also written of the necessity of being "more than a consultant", by being a dependable part of the milieu and effecting change at the systems level as well. Geist (1977) uses the term "sculpting of a milieu" (p. 433) to describe the consultants' relationships. He maintains that the consultant must have an element of being a "good mother" who is available, provides empathetic verbal and nonverbal support to the staff, is capable of tolerating anger and complaints, and has the confidence to give the staff "permission to be helpless." Similar arguments are advanced by Patenaude, Szymanski, and Rappaport (1979), who feel that the consultant must "provide a context for emotional consideration" and be a "lightning rod of sorts" (p. 400) for the staff's intense but sometimes unrecognized emotions. They note that in order to be accepted by a pediatric bone-marrow transplant team, the mental health workers have to prove themselves "tough enough" to tolerate anger and to display the depths of commitment to the patients that the team feels is appropriate.

This enlarged role of helping, creating an environment in which improved handling of emotional issues allows for more effective coping by the staff as well as the patient, has been widely recognized (Drotar, 1975, 1977, 1978; Magrab & Papadopoulou, 1978; Vore & Wright, 1974). Schneider (1978) has emphasized the delicacy of such relationships. He cautions that psychologists in medical settings must "tread with a very gentle interpretive step" (p. 7), as they interact with the group of professionals in which "we are least likely to have our expertise taken for granted" (p. 6). Yet in many settings it is imperative for the psychologist to be incorporated into the team as a functional equal (Brewer, 1978) to be effective in working with families and physicians as an integral part of the service delivery team. While there are no simple formulas for achieving a position in which one can be effective, it seems clear that two initial elements are demonstrating one's practical usefulness and showing flexibility in accommodating to medical norms on such basic issues as writing concise notes and operating within tight time constraints (Poznanski, 1979).

Finally, a third important area for consultations in medical settings has involved the selection of intervention techniques. A sampling of problems in need of intervention is provided by Bolian (1971), who found that 32% of referrals were for psychological reactions to physical disorders, 20% were for psychological reactions with associated changes in bodily functions, 14% were for psychophysiological disorders, 19% resulted from self-inflicted injury, suicide attempts, or drug abuse, 6% were for mixed conversion and psychophysiological reactions, and only 9% were considered to be purely psychological reactions. While more recent information from a number of centers would be helpful, these data emphasize the differences between consultative interventions in pediatric settings and other forms of clinical activities with children.

Many different intervention techniques have been recommended in this unique situation. Not surprisingly, most authors emphasize communication with children, though often with special caution. For example, Bernstein et al. (1969) suggest that while children's feelings of hopelessness, anxiety, and despair must be discussed, they must also be helped to express these in a controlled and modulated form so as not to be overwhelmed.

Petrillo and Sanger (1980) stress the need to call upon a variety of interventions with the child and family. Their clinical vignettes illustrate how behavioral techniques, short- and long-term contacts with the child and family members, and play techniques must be combined in order to meet the complex needs of children in medical settings. O'Malley and Koocher (1977) point out that the consultant must often go beyond the expectations of the consultees, who may have psychotherapy on their minds when in fact environmental manipulations may be a more appropriate and effective form of therapy. Geist (1979) suggests various necessary environmental conditions which the consultant may be able to facilitate, including continuity of care in the hospital and the home, a chance for the patient to feel valued, useful, and accepted on the ward, and the honest presentation of permanent losses, so that mourning can begin.

In summary, the pediatric psychologist who consults in a medical setting has the opportunity to combine interdisciplinary teaching and intervention with a wide variety of services to children and their families in what is a demanding but potentially satisfying role.

School Consultation

Another common area of consultation for pediatric psychologists has been with the public schools. Although psychologists have assumed a variety of roles in the public schools for several decades (Blanco, 1972), the role of the pediatric psychologist has differed somewhat from the traditional school psychologist's role. This section will focus on the unique contributions of pediatric psychologists consulting public schools and provide an overview of the relevant literature.

The most important distinction between the roles of school and pediatric psychologists involves their functions in the school and surrounding community. School psychologists function primarily within the school system as an integral part of that milieu. They are generally funded by their school systems and have the primary responsibility of meeting their schools' needs for assessment, placement, and management of children within the system. On the other hand, pediatric psychologists more frequently relate to schools as external agents, visiting them from their more permanent settings in clinics, hospitals, community mental health centers, developmental evaluation centers, or private practices. Although both groups of psychologists consult with school staff, the relationship of a pediatric psychologist to the school personnel is more consistent with the traditional consultative role (Berkowitz, 1975) in that the consultant is an outsider who must gain entry into the school system and must be especially sensitive to issues of communication, hierarchy, ownership of the problem, and professional role, in order to be effective.

For the pediatric psychologist in a school system, the consultation may be one of two types: it may involve an individual child, or it may involve more general questions such as how the school can meet the needs of a group of children or improve the general organization of a classroom environment. After examining these two roles, this section will then explore how they have changed with the enactment of PL 94-142, which has made the public schools more accessible to pediatric psychologists as well as to a number of other professionals.

Recent workers have developed approaches to school consultation, which are especially relevant for pediatric psychologists consulting about individual children. These approaches follow a behavioral framework similar to the one used for many short-term therapeutic interventions. This approach is outlined by Schroeder and Schroeder (1979), who define it as "a problem-solving approach that systematically looks at how behavior relates to its environment and through the use of learning principles brings about change in the behavior and/or the environment" (p. 1). This behavioral approach to consultation involves four steps: defining the desirable and undesirable behaviors, gathering baseline data, planning an intervention program, and continuing to evaluate the effectiveness of the intervention program. The effectiveness of this approach is in the systematic way that the consultant assesses need, designs interventions, and measures results. In this behavioral approach to consultation, the intervention may or may not be behavioral; however, the process by which the consultant approaches the problem certainly is.

A similar general approach is outlined in detail by Bergan (1977). The Bergan approach systematically outlines problem identification, analysis, solution, and evaluation as the necessary components of a successful consultation experience. Specific case examples, including discussions of developmental and speech problems, emphasize the applicability of this approach to pediatric psychology.

Although the behavioral approach to consultation is widely used, there are several potential problems of concern to pediatric psychologists. Kauffman and Vincente (1972) have outlined these, emphasizing the importance of communication, sensitivity to both spoken and unspoken issues, and adequate follow-up. The behavioral approach neither precludes nor guarantees attention to these important issues. Another concern is that short-term changes will not persist in the long -run. O'Leary (1977) offers several suggestions for enhancing the long-term effects of classroom intervention. He suggests the gradual withdrawal of any reinforcement procedures, systematic programming of generalization, and understanding and utilizing the entire chain of authority in the school system as necessary to produce long-term changes.

Although the literature on school consultation by pediatric psychologists to help groups of children is not large, there are some examples of consultations for children with developmental delays, learning disabilities, hyperactivity, medical illness, and physical handicaps. This literature tends to highlight both the multiple services needed by these children and the important role of the psychological consultant in educating the school personnel about these needs.

Schroeder (1978) provides an example of how her behavioral approach to consultation was used in the case of a moderately retarded 13-year-old child who had returned to a regular seventh-grade classroom after a long-term placement in a residential setting. The consultants used a variety of strategies to build both socially appropriate behaviors in the child and acceptance of the child by his peer group. After using peer support groups, film presentations, and classroom discussions, the consultant found that several of their interventions led to more positive attitudes toward handicapped individuals in girls but more negative attitudes in boys.

Schroeder suggests that these findings highlight the critical importance of systematic and continuous follow-up of interventions in this relatively new and uncharted area.

A consultation program with learning-disabled children is reported by Pihl, Parkes, and Stevens (1980), who defined a professional role of "modulator." The modulator was defined as a combination of child advocate and consulting therapist, whose task it was to coordinate, stimulate, and work in the community on behalf of learning-disabled children. Like Schroeder, the authors report mixed results with improvement in some areas (social acceptance) and actual decrements in others (teacher ratings). The authors point out that no matter how face valid a program may seem, it should not be accepted as effective without systematic evaluation.

Although the literature on hyperactivity contains proportionately few studies on consultation, the standard works (Ross & Ross, 1976; Safer & Allen, 1976) do describe the need for combining educational programs with other interventions. Safer and Allen suggest that various models for coordination of management are possible, which vary as to the distribution and location of responsibility. The consultant managing the hyperactive child in the school needs to not only be familiar with the literature on various intervention approaches, but also with how these approaches can be integrated into the school setting. Models for this activity are still emerging and further exploration and research are needed.

The challenge of integrating seriously medically ill and physically handicapped children into school settings presents a different set of consultation problems. These have recently been explored by those responsible for integrating these populations into public school programs under the mandate of PL 94-142. For example, Cyphert (1973) suggests organizing information according to a matrix considering the needs and contributions of the child, medical personnel, the teacher and other school personnel, the family, and the child's peers. According to Cyphert, each of these groups has certain knowledge, skills, and attitudes that can facilitate or impede the child's integration into the school setting. Katz, Kellerman, Rigler, Williams, and Siegel (1977) describe the process of consulting around pediatric cancer patients. They have outlined four major categories of referral for school consultation: requests to assist in evaluation and arrangement of school placement, preventive intervention for newly diagnosed patients, assistance in school reintegration after a prolonged absence, and counseling for anxiety related to secondary effects of cancer treatment such as hair loss. The role of the pediatric psychologist in coordinating these programs and providing direct intervention is a large one, yet few techniques for implementing these four functions are suggested.

One of the most serious problems that can arise when consulting around seriously ill children is discussed by Kaplan, Smith, and Grobstein (1974). They point out that seriously ill children create anxieties in the healthy majority by reminding them of their own vulnerability. Thus adults, such as school personnel, may protect themselves by isolating or rejecting these sick children in the name of protecting either the children or their classmates. They suggest that teachers should allow open discussions of these situations so that classmates can cope in ways that will be helpful to both themselves and the seriously ill children. They maintain that the other children in the class are not hurt by their exposure to the reality of illness in their peers. Further research confirming this idea would be a valuable adjunct to the integration of seriously ill children into classroom programs.

Finally, Lansky, Lowman, Vats, and Gyulay (1975) note a relatively high rate of school phobias in their pediatric cancer population. They find similar dynamics to those noted in school phobia in healthy children, with separation anxiety in both mother and child playing a major role, and the illness as a crisis that precipitates the school avoidance. They note the problem is difficult to treat once established, but are encouraged by preventive approaches utilizing school visits by psychologists and parent-child groups.

Although the literature on consultation in the public school setting is somewhat limited, this whole area has grown significantly with the passage of PL 94-142, which requires public schools to educate all children, regardless of handicap. Now that the schools have the legal mandate to serve all children, the pediatric psychologist's role should change significantly from advocate to consultant in helping the school to effectively meet this mandate. Schroeder (1978) outlines these changes and points to the need to understand the provisions of the law and to respond to its requirements. She describes three levels of consultation: information or task-oriented consultations, training consultations, and ongoing collaborative consultations. She suggests that the last model is the one required to meet the needs of the handicapped child and the school system.

The importance of this task and the extent that remains to be done is emphasized by Brick and Scheiner (1978), who have found significant shortcomings in programs for handicapped children in the school districts they have investigated. They raise many important issues such as the extent of the school system's responsibility, cost, and the need for knowledge about the effectiveness of various intervention approaches and services. While pediatric psychologists cannot be expected to answer all of these questions alone, their input should be considerable and their involvement with these questions is inevitable. As Zigler and Muenchow (1979) point out, "It takes more than legislation to create a social revolution in the school" (p. 93). The pediatric psychologist functioning as a school consultant may be in a crucial role to help create this revolution.

In summary, there is an important role for the pediatric psychologist in the public school system, and this role has recently expanded with the exactment of PL 94-142. Unfortunately, there is little research available to direct this most important role.

Consultation to Residential Settings

In addition to medical and educational settings, pediatric psychologists also commonly consult to residential facilities. Institutions for the mentally retarded are the most common settings of this kind, although other possibilities include residential institutions for chronically ill and handicapped children (Creer & Christian, 1976) and, increasingly, small group homes in the community (Schinke

& Wong, 1977). Consulting for residential settings shares many common characteristics with the already described medical and educational consultation. Pediatric
psychologists who consult must enter and learn a new system, decide how to best
meet the needs of the clients, and work through the staff within the existing
program. However, there are also several unique aspects of consultation to
residential settings. They tend to include more severely handicapped clients, more
limited resources, and more clients totally dependent on staff. In addition, there is
an opportunity to bring about more enduring changes because of the potential for
creating a total therapeutic milieu.

Considering the unique aspects of consulting for residential settings, and the great
potential for development within these programs, there is surprisingly little material
in the pediatric psychology literature about this kind of consultation. However,
some trends and guidelines do emerge based on the literature on interventions with
mentally retarded persons. This literature suggests that the role of the consulting
pediatric psychologist is to participate in the development of long-term treatment
plans, assist in staff development, facilitate staff communication, and disseminate
new information as it becomes available.

Helping to develop short- and long-term goals for clients, along with specific
techniques for implementing these goals, is a major function of a pediatric
psychologist consulting to a residential setting. This role is particularly important
because the direct care staff in these programs are generally less adequately trained
and prepared than those working in medical or educational settings. Pediatric
psychologists assist in the establishment and maintenance of behavior programs to
teach residents new skills and reduce problem behaviors. For example, comprehensive instructional booklets on teaching a variety of skills to institutional populations
have been developed (Baroff, 1974). Another example of consultation to develop
new skills is the establishment of a sheltered workshop within an institution, to train
institutional residents in work skills that might be appropriate for later community
living (Tate & Baroff, 1966).

The second role of pediatric psychologists in these settings is the training,
development, and motivation of existing staff. The importance of adequate planning
for staff training is especially important in residential institutions, given the
three-shifts-daily structure of these programs. McInnis (1976) emphasizes the
importance of specifying programs and goals precisely to both maximize the staff's
chances for success and to allow for adequate evaluation. In consulting with a
residential staff, the role of the pediatric psychologist is both to design appropriate
programs and to train staff on appropriate procedures while implementing these
programs.

Kazdin (1973) feels that motivating a staff is an important part of the consultation
process. He argues that the principles of behavior change, especially positive
reinforcement for correct performances, must be applied to staff as well as clients.
For example, a staff member who successfully carries out a client's program should
receive a special privilege such as extra time off or some other meaningful
recognition. Kazdin cites evidence that the success of the behavioral program alone
is often not enough to maintain staff behavior, but that rewards for staff members
are often necessary as well.

Nay (1978) highlights the facilitation of staff communication as an additional role for the pediatric psychologist in a residential setting. Communication blocks within various programs and between levels of administration are among the obstacles that consultants must be able to confront. A consultant in these settings must be able to analyze the amount of flexibility evidenced by employees in different positions and the existing avenues for communication. In some settings, according to Nay, a consultant may need to change institutional structures before being able to implement programs. Nay also discusses sources of resistance that must be understood and avoided if possible. These include such factors as individual resistance to change, investment in customary patterns of behavior, and emotional responses to various situations in the institution. As in most other settings, Nay advocates the gradual introduction of change so that it can comfortably fit within the existing setting and communication structure.

A final role of the residential consultant is to disseminate new information as it becomes available. This was an important role a decade ago when behavior modification principles were being discovered and had to be integrated into existing residential programs. Although dramatic new techniques are not as common today, there are still many new ideas that can benefit residential programs.

One example of a new approach has been recent work applying ecobehavioral analysis to residential institutions as well as other treatment settings. This approach addresses "the importance of specific environments in which selective behaviors are performed, the completeness of behavioral description required to understand antecedent conditions, and an impact statement which takes into account long- and short-range therapeutic objectives" (Schroeder, Rojahn, & Mulick, 1978, p. 81). In short, these authors argue for an understanding of the interactions between behaviors and the individual's environment. The role of a consultant may be to help residential settings to understand the implications of this emphasis and to alter their environments in beneficial ways that will improve the behavior of the residents. Schroeder *et al.* (1978) have shown how this approach led to a combination of self-protective devices and medication to reduce the incidence of self-injurious behaviors in institutionalized clients.

In summary, consultation to residential institutions allows for a wide range of intervention techniques. Pediatric psychologists in these programs participate in the development of individualized objectives, behavior management plans, innovative programs, and training opportunities. Residential settings provide intensive intervention opportunities with severely handicapped clients.

Summary

Because pediatric psychologists work in a variety of settings, consultation has become a major intervention technique. Consultative interventions have to be adjusted to meet the needs of individual clients in such settings. To be successful in this role, pediatric psychologists must learn to delicately balance the needs of their clients with the demands and procedures of the settings in which they are functioning.

PSYCHOTHERAPY

Despite the emergence of many new techniques in recent years, the individual verbal therapy session, more or less modified by the limitations of the situation, still plays a very important role in the activity of the pediatric psychologist. In fact, when medically ill children alone are considered, there is more literature describing this intervention than any other (Johnson, 1979). Also relevant to the pediatric psychologist is the use of this modality with children who have developmental delays, brain damage, or sensory handicaps, as well as children with psychosomatic disorders and abused children. This section will review the literature on therapy with each of these populations.

Individual Verbal Therapies

Children with a variety of conditions including malignancies, burns, mutilating accidents, surgical procedures, and others are discussed in the literature on verbal therapy with medically ill children. While many of those who have worked in this area are pediatric psychologists, important contributions from the fields of psychiatry, social work, child care, and nursing also exist. The paucity of controlled research is especially striking because the clinical literature is extensive; testable hypotheses are, however, abundant, and it is to be hoped that new contributions will take the form of experimental tests of the many techniques available.

Individual Verbal Therapies for Medically Ill Children

One area that has received considerable attention in the recent literature is intervention with the child who has a malignancy or other terminal illness. Individual verbal techniques are the most frequently used with this population, and authors generally emphasize the importance of communication, especially indirect communications (Howarth, 1974; Kellerman, Rigler, Siegel, & Katz, 1977; Koocher, 1974; Kubler-Ross, 1974). Kubler-Ross, a pioneer in this area, discusses the importance of understanding the "languages of dying," which include symbolic nonverbal, symbolic verbal, and direct English communication. She advocates clinicians seek the true meaning of the symbolic messages and offer, but not force, the opportunity to continue to explore the issue (Kubler-Ross, 1974). Vernick (1973) similarly emphasizes open communication, using the "life-space interview" technique to offer therapeutic assistance when and where it is needed in the child's daily life in the hospital. He also points out that discomfort felt by professionals about discussing such painful topics as dying may be projected onto children, with the professional rationalizing to himself that it is the child who is uncomfortable with the discussion.

Useful data relevant to this issue are provided by Kellerman *et al.* (1977), who found a tendency for children who spoke openly about their cancer to be less depressed; Koocher (1974) who found that normal children were quite comfortable in discussing death with a researcher; and Spinetta (1974, 1977), who found that children as young as 6 were aware that they were dying, and could express this awareness directly. Bluebond-Langer (1974), using anthropological techniques, found that children not given the opportunity for direct discussion communicated their knowledge and concerns through behavior, play, and other metaphoric means.

Despite this information, there still exists disagreement on how much frankness is advisable and how much children should be encouraged in denial. Some therapists advocate supporting denial to varying extents (Howarth, 1974) while others move relatively aggressively to thwart denial, even deliberately creating "therapeutic anxiety" to facilitate this (Kagen, 1976).

Case histories can be cited supporting many sides of this question. For example, Binger (1973) writes of a boy who, before he died of leukemia at the age of 12, admitted that he had secretly known about his disease for several years, unable to discuss his knowledge with anyone. Although no simple answer can be expected to the question of how best to deal therapeutically with the emotional needs of dying children, empirical research is obviously needed.

Different issues are raised in working with children having difficulty confronting or recovering from surgery. Problems of confusion and misinterpretation of reality arc often mentioned. In these instances, a major activity of the therapist is to clarify the situation to the child in a manner that can be accepted without excessive anxiety, often by eliciting fantasies from the child about what is wrong and what will be done, and correcting the frequent notion that the child or significant other is at fault (Ack, 1976).

The correction of misconceptions is mentioned in other contexts, and may be very important to the child's psychological recovery. An example of this is a case in which part of the psychologist's intervention involved reassuring a terrified child that his abdominal incision, closed with new "tape" stitches, was not really closed with Scotch tape that would pop open at any moment (Oremland & Oremland, 1973).

Other interventions with child surgery patients have been more lengthy and complex. Drotar (1975b) describes a case in which psychiatric hospitalization and lengthy psychotherapy were needed to help an adolescent renal transplant patient work through his fear of sexual inadequacy, guilt, body image problems, and longing for continued dependency. Several cases requiring psychotherapy for cardiac surgery patients have also been described (Cline & Rothenburg, 1974; Toker, 1971). This therapy often involves the working through of anxiety which can be intense enough to cause loss of contact with reality (Danilowicz & Gabriel, 1971) but which can often be dealt with successfully in short-term work.

Another medical problem in which individual verbal therapy has an important role is the burned child. Much of the writing in this area is by Seligman (1974, 1976), who writes from a psychiatric and strictly clinical perspective but who presents interesting case histories and theoretical support for her position that emotional needs require as much attention as physical needs for these children. For example, she notes an excellent outcome in a case where ego-building, relationship-oriented psychotherapy was seen as lifesaving in a child who cngaged in self-mutilative behavior and was originally given a very poor prognosis.

Bernstein (1976) and Woods (1975) make similar points, also emphasizing the importance of therapy in rehabilitation for individuals with lifelong and often obvious disfigurement.

Special Individual Therapeutic Techniques

The authors discussed so far have placed more emphasis on the particular medical problem affecting their therapy clients than on the processes and techniques they employed, limiting the degree to which their ideas can be applied in different settings. However, several authors have described the application of a specific technique to medically ill children in general.

For example, Gardner (1971) has written about the use of his well-known Mutual Storytelling Technique with a child suffering a traumatic reaction to seven operations before the age of 5. The technique consists of a game in which the child tells a fantasy story for a "television progam" which the therapist then uses as the basis for his own story. This story is designed to introduce new ways of thinking about the problems presented in the child's story, including alternative solutions, and different interpretations of the reasons for others' behavior. In the case presented, the main focus of the storytelling was the child's anger against doctors and his father, and his self-loathing for having such feelings. However, the technique would be readily adaptable to other problems, since the child's own story provides the thematic material.

A technique called "story-making" (Robertson & Barford, 1970) has some similarities, although this method employs stories written by the psychologist and read to the child. The authors of this technique discuss a child who has spent a year on a respirator. In this case it was a challenge to provide avenues for socialization, expansion of the child's contact with the world of reality, and opportunities to express feelings through fantasy. This technique would seem to have special usefulness for children whose use of speech is curtailed in some way.

Johnson, Martin, Whitt, and Weisz (1980) have provided experimental evidence suppoting the effectiveness of such techniques. They found that a two-week exposure to verbal imagination games played with the mother resulted in measurable reductions in anxiety in chronically ill children, compared to a control group of children who played skill games. All of the children in the experimental group received the same set of games, with no attempt to individualize the content. One would expect that individualized games and stories would be even more effective.

Another verbal technique, also specifically designed for sick children, has been labeled the "three-step process" (Rothenberg, 1974). The therapist asks the child to relate his ideas and feelings about six crucial questions: What do I have? How did I get it? Why did I get it? When will I get well? Why did my parents leave me in he hospital? What do my parents think about what has happened? Next, the "third-person" technique is used, which explores the child's feelings through questions phrased, "Lots of times kids feel. . . ." The child is allowed to accept, reject, or ignore interpretations through what the authors call the "option play" approach. Finally, factual information and reassurance is provided to correct misconceptions. Case presentations illustrate how the processes may need to be repeated over time, especially in the presence of the "FAGS syndrome"—fear, anger, guilt, and sadness (Kohlberg & Rothenberg, 1970).

Individual Verbal Therapies for Developmentally Disabled and Brain Damaged Children

Another situation in which pediatric psychologists employ individual verbal therapy techniques is with the mentally retarded and brain-damaged children. Despite the heavy emphasis on the application of behavioral interventions with these groups, there is a long, if not large, tradition of verbal therapy (Stacey & DeMartino, 1957). Three recent articles review the use of verbal psychotherapy with mentally retarded children, each emphasizing the potential place of this intervention technique within a total treatment plan, and each clearly stating that mental retardation does not rule out the use of "talk therapy." Lott (1970) reviews the early literature extensively, arguing that even though Carl Rogers claimed that psychotherapy was not relevant for mentally retarded people, Sternlicht (1965) offerred an extensive bibliography of successful examples of such therapy. Lott states that although mentally retarded individuals have fewer intellectual resources, they have the same "varied emotional quirks, inhibitions, frustrations, guilt feelings, conflicts, and erroneous self-concepts" as do others (Lott, 1970, p. 246) and need successful defense mechanisms more, not less, than do normal individuals. Lott suggests looking at the mentally retarded individual in terms of level of personality maturity, using such frameworks as Anna Freud's or Erik Erickson's, and being especially conscious of the difficulties these children and adolescents have with issues of emancipation and dependency.

LaVietes (1978) places special emphasis on integrating psychotherapy into a total treatment program and offers a number of concrete suggestions for accomplishing this. She advocates taking an active role in defining the limits, structure, and goals of treatment. She emphasizes the potential usefulness of therapy in improving self-acceptance by providing a relationship that counteracts the mentally retarded person's usual experience of having little attention paid to his or her individuality or dignity. Another major aspect of therapy, strengthening ego functions, is seen as developing as the therapist helps the child to clarify and label feeling states, thus gaining some control over emotions. Postponement of gratification, ways of coping with frustration, and taking responsibility for one's behavior are also important themes.

Bernstein (1979) discusses the potential role of therapy in helping the mentally retarded child to operate at a higher level of social functioning in order to counter the argument that therapy with mentally retarded people is a poor use of valuable therapist time. He argues that verbal psychotherapy is appropriate with mentally retarded persons who show psychiatric symptoms based on conflicts comparable to those of persons with normal intelligence. In keeping with this argument, he advocates the extensive use of verbal communication, with the therapist giving the retarded child maximum opportunity to verbalize fantasies. This may be especially difficult, Bernstein suggests, because families of mentally retarded children often discourage the verbalization of negative emotions. Thus the child may need slow, patient, and repeated reassurance that such feelings are acceptable.

Many similar points are made by those few authors who have written specifically on the use of verbal intervention with the brain-damaged child. Christ (1978) and Gardner (1979) suggest the use of considerable structure with this group. Christ suggest that these children's defense mechanisms are fragile, and that they need much help in building such defenses as rationalization and intellectualization to add to such primitive defenses as denial and projection. Both authors advocate straightforward, instructive, verbal interventions that clarify the environment and teach the child alternative behaviors. For example, Gardner may help a child deal with impulsive, angry outbursts by warning the child before he makes a challenging move in a checkers game and suggesting ways that the child will be able to control his feelings about it. In addition to impulsivity, he notes that major issues in therapy with brain-damaged children include denial, distortion, and ignorance of unpleasant realities about limitations, problems in social perception, immaturity, perseveration, low self-esteem, fear of and withdrawal from others, and chronic feelings of anger and resentment.

Individual Verbal Therapies for Psychophysiological Disorders

The last major group with whom individual verbal therapy is used includes children with a variety of psychophysiological disorders. While the major contribution of pediatric psychology to the treatment of these disorders has come in the behavioral realm, individual verbal therapy, extensively used in these disorders (Prugh & Eckhardt, 1979), should be mentioned.

While the individual psychotherapeutic approach to these disorders sees them as stemming from neurotic conflicts, communication among members of the treatment team, and coordination of care are frequently emphasized (Prugh & Eckhardt, 1979). The range of diseases for which individual therapy has been applied is wide (Wright, Schaeffer, & Solomons, 1979) and includes such diverse conditions as bronchial asthma (Bentley & Wilmerding, 1977), ulcerative colitis, various dermatological disorders, and rheumatoid arthritis. Typical of the approach taken in these conditions is that outlined by Bruch (1977) in her treatment of anorexia nervosa. She works with her patients in individual therapy over a period lasting several years, in addition to working with the family on communication issues. She maintains that behavioral programs, while helpful in inducing weight gain, are dangerous because they do not affect the underlying personality dynamics and often rob the patients of control, already a major issue in the disorder. She attempts to focus on her patients' distorted self-concepts and difficulties with achieving independent identities; and finds profound underlying feelings of emptiness and despair which, in some of her patients, must be dealt with in a long-term therapeutic relationship.

In summary, the traditional verbal therapies have been used with most of the children pediatric psychologists see. Although intelligent and verbal children are often more responsive to these techniques, all children have a need to understand

and express their concerns on a level that is meaningful to them. The many innovations in the traditional verbal therapies cited here have made these techniques useful to an increasing group of children in a wide variety of settings.

PLAY THERAPY

Judging from the literature, pediatric psychologists are most likely to use play therapy with medically ill children, especially in hospital settings, although there are a few articles on the use of play therapy with abused and developmentally handicapped children. Definitional problems arise in discussing this topic, because while the use of play in medical settings with the goal of better emotional health is increasing (Oremland & Oremland, 1973; Petrillo & Sanger, 1980), play activities vary along a continuum from traditional play therapy models to straightforward recreation. This section will focus on individual and group play activities that possess the following characteristic of therapy: the participation of a mental health professional, the use of play to express fears or conflicts or to master anxiety, and the use of identifiable therapeutic goals. It is hoped that this selection will provide a useful sampling of techniques and applications.

Petrillo and Sanger (1980), who have made such important contributions in humanizing pediatrics wards, discuss the use of play for a wide variety of purposes, applying the basic principles of good play therapy flexibly and creatively in the hospital environment. They suggest that play is especially useful in the preparation of children for medical procedures, and in facilitating their integration of these traumas afterward. This is because play permits the miniaturization of these experiences and, by allowing the child to experiment with perceived dangers, strengthens the ego to cope with these stresses. In addition, it might be suggested that such play reduces anxiety by allowing a process similar to systematic desensitization to occur, as the child is exposed to feared situations while feeling relaxed and supported. Regardless of one's interpretation, Petrillo and Sanger's use of small models of treatment rooms and of real medical equipment for teaching individuals and groups should provide numerous ideas for the pediatric psychologist.

Other authors have described the use of play therapy to help children who have had special difficulties coping with unusually traumatic medical histories. Oremland and Oremland (1973) cite a case of a 5-year-old, who after four operations for hypospadias, was seen for symptoms of severe hyperactivity and aggression. His therapist helped him to play out his fears of being destroyed and his difficulty in deciding whether he, himself, was a good guy or a bad guy.

In a different kind of situation, Oremland and Oremland (1973) describe another 5-year-old facing medical therapy and several surgical procedures for a malignancy. Tinker toys and stuffed animals were used to represent the large and terrifying cobalt machine, with the animals expressing the child's terror for him. The therapist described the importance of helping the child to structure the play, and of explaining and interpreting medical procedures and the behavior of doctors and parents.

An example of the use of unique materials is offered by Plank and Horwood (1977), who helped a 4-year-old girl cope successfully with a leg amputation through the use of a "prosthesis doll" prepared with the same degree of leg loss that the child would suffer.

The case of a 6-year-old renal transplant patient is an example of how postoperative play therapy allowed for an understanding of difficult family dynamics (Bernstein, 1971). The child was able to communicate in play her awareness of her father's ambivalence toward the donation of his kidney, as well as playing out aggression that she had totally repressed while hospitalized.

Cline and Rothenberg's (1974) report of play therapy with a 7-year-old facing open heart surgery is notable for a useful description of a possible therapeutic error. In this case, therapist responded with reassurance to the child's worry about a doll patient's dying; in retrospect, he felt that his own discomfort caused him to gloss over the child's concern about this issue.

The question of how much to pursue points raised by the child in play therapy is never an easy one, but perhaps is even more important when issues such as death and mutilation are real and salient. Lewis (1978) has addressed this question, advocating the usual kind of expressive play therapy for the seriously ill child, but asserting that any expression of concern about pain, loneliness, fear, and related issues should be silently noted. They suggest that reassurance should then be offered at another time, without reference to the play session, to avoid causing the child to feel tricked and exposed, and thus inhibiting future play. They also advocate allowing a significant amount of denial but controlling regression.

Several authors have presented ingenious specialized play techniques. Linn (1977) and Cassell and Paul (1967) have both used puppetry for hospitalized children. Cassell and Paul used puppets specifically with children who faced cardiac catheterization, while Linn proposes their use for leading to open-ended conversations with children about a variety of feelings and situations. While she permits the child to control the theme and outcome of the play, she interjects new ideas into the scenarios when they seem therapeutically important. Linn has observed that when using puppets in follow-up to preoperative teaching carried out by nurses, many fears and confused feelings are often revealed, even after doll play with the nurse.

Rae and Stieber (1976) see plants as having special usefulness as therapy materials with hospitalized children. They note that the plants allow reverse dependency to be played out, as the plant is dependent on the child. In caring for the plant, the child is able to deal with the constant requirement of receiving care. Terrariums are used as analogues of oxygen tents, grafting and rooting is related to the healing of broken bones, and the infusion of fertilizing "medicine" into the soil with syringes helps children understand the function of injections. Another nontraditional approach, called "paraverbal therapy," is described by McDonnell (1979), who uses music and art media to engage children who have difficulty with verbalization in expressive therapy. She has found that children will sometimes sing about feelings or traumas that they will not discuss in spoken words, and that the use of a variety of materials permits many children to discharge painful affect and communicate feelings and fantasies that would otherwise remain inhibited.

The literature on the use of individual play therapy with developmentally handicapped children is very limited, although Cowen (1955) described its use over 25 years ago. Moustakas (1959) describes his work with such children in deeply humanistic terms, although the lack of clear goals makes it understandable why a larger literature on this application of play therapy has not developed. Nevertheless, Moustakas's report of improvements in communication and trust using the most nondirective form of play therapy suggests that perhaps further exploration of this approach, modified by our current understanding of social learning, is warranted.

Interestingly, Guerney (1979) has recently reported on experiments with filial therapy, in which parents are taught nondirective play therapy techniques to use with their learning-disabled children, as well as children with other handicaps. Guerney reports marked improvement, especially in the children's sense of control over themselves and their actions.

Abused children are yet another group that has recently begun to receive systematic therapeutic attention from pediatric psychologists. Individual play therapy for these children is only a small part of the total management program necessary (Williams, 1978). However, our awareness of and sensitivity to this problem are increasing steadily (Kempe & Kempe, 1978), and it is to be hoped that a wide variety of resources wil be made available to child victims, including individual therapy when indicated. Beezley, Martin, and Alexander (1976) have reported on children's responses to play therapy and found it to be helpful in an initial study of approximately 25 children. They reported that the establishment of trust was, not surprisingly, a major issue with these children, and that younger children were able to develop a therapeutic alliance more quickly. The children also demanded enormous amounts of nurturance and demonstrated immature relationships. They tended to regress noticeably in play, especially in situations such as water play, and needed much help in coming to a point where they could relax and have fun. As Beezley, Martin, and Kempe (1976) poignantly describe, "They seemed surprised that the therapist demonstrated pleasure and enjoyment from games and play" (1976, p. 207). The therapists also found that children acted out their own injuries with surprising accuracy in their play.

While group play activity is becoming commonplace on modern pediatrics wards, literature on specifically psychotherapeutic play by pediatric psychologists is limited. The work of pioneers in the fields of child life, recreation therapy, and nursing has, however, described a number of programs in which group play is used as preparation for procedures for coping with stressful long-term hospitalization, for expressing hostility appropriately, for forming supportive relationships with staff and other children, and for mastering developmental tasks that otherwise might be missed because of hospitalization (Azarnoff & Flegal, 1975; Oremland & Oremland, 1973). Many of the activities and functions of individual play methods are similar to the approaches taken in these groups, the main difference being the support and socialization value of peer interaction and the greater freedom of expression that may be achieved by a group of children playing together.

The application of group play techniques to problems faced by specific medical conditions has been carried out in several very different settings. Hoffman and Futterman (1971) have developed a program in the waiting room of a pediatric oncology clinic that makes creative use of otherwise wasted and stressful time, when separation and mutilation anxiety are especially intense. A number of activities were instituted involving the entire family, including play sessions for the children that were designed to support the child's self-image and sense of trust. The program was judged to be successful in improving the atmosphere of the clinic as well as the adjustment of the children and families.

Two group psychotherapeutic play programs whose major emphasis was on speech development have been found effective with cleft palate children and in children with multiple physical handicaps. Irwin and McWilliams (1974) involved cleft palate preschoolers in a year-long program of creative dramatics, which they felt led to significant improvements in speech and overall behavior. They attributed improvement in part to a reduction of fears and inhibitions brought about by the group play experiences, as well as to the more direct focus on speech and communication as a source of pleasure and enjoyment. Colman, Dougher, and Tanner's (1976) project involved young, multiply handicapped preschoolers in group play activities, emphasizing awareness and response to sounds and speech. These authors, too, felt that the emotional freedom brought about by group play was an important part of the treatment.

In summary, the literature on play therapy, though not containing many experimentally controlled studies, offers some creative and innovative techniques for pediatric psychologists to consider. Although these techniques have primarily been utilized with medically ill children, there are indications that they could be extended to developmentally disabled children as well. Future work in this area should include controlled outcome studies as well as the extension of these techniques to other populations of children.

VERBAL GROUP THERAPY FOR CHILDREN

While the use of traditional therapy groups has been reported with children having psychosomatic illnesses for several decades (Groen & Pelser, 1960), the increasing use of group therapy with a wide range of chronically and acutely ill children is of special interest to pediatric psychologists. Reports can be found on the use of this intervention in inpatient and outpatient hospital settings (Gratzick, 1973; Heffron, 1975), in schools or rehabilitation settings (Bayrakal, 1975), in a renal dialysis program (Magrab, 1975), and in therapeutic camping (Adler, 1973). There are also reports—unfortunately, very few in number—on the use of group therapy with mentally retarded children.

Daily meetings with all pediatric patients aged 5 and over were begun in one setting as a means of improving self-esteem in hospitalized children (Sheridan, 1975) but evolved to encompass broader goals. The authors noted that peer support and influence, modeling by confident children, and mutual helping relationships among the children helped them work through such issues as separation and loss, physical self-image problems and discomfort, and troubling fantasies. Sheridan notes that the group leader needs to be aware of the presence of ambivalent and displaced hostile feelings in the group, and also suggests directness about the issue of death.

In contrast, Schowalter (1971) has described a weekly group for adolescents, in which the topic of death was generally taboo. Frightening details of surgery tended to be discussed at length, although the adolescents seemed to derive some reassurance from such discussions. The leaders of the group noted the importance of following up individually with youngsters who had particular fears, especially on the issue of death. They also discuss, as an outgrowth of this experience, the useful technique of having children describe their fears and expectations about upcoming surgery on tape, and then describe what actually transpired after the procedure. This was found to be beneficial for the child who made the tape as well as for other children who could then listen to the recording.

Groups of children with similar disease processes have recently been found useful by several authors. Thomas (1980) contacted eight major pediatric cancer centers, and found that six ran play groups, one for pediatric cancer specifically, and seven offered adolescent discussion groups. The issues of whether to mix diagnoses, whether to include medical staff, and which ages to include were all of concern to these centers, as was the question of how children would be affected by deaths within the groups and whether those deaths might be anxiety provoking, More research is obviously needed on all of these questions as the clinical use of these groups expands.

Heffron (1975) has tried several group approaches with oncology patients, ranging from general discussion groups, through personal growth groups, to "minimarathons." The discussion groups, it was found, engendered close supportive relationships among the children. The growth groups emphasized emotional reactions, using encounter techniques, and were felt to be of benefit in helping the children deal with such issues as loneliness and meaning in their lives.

Gardner (1977) has advocated a number of uses for a group approach with adolescent oncology patients, including a focus on skill training and problem solving around such issues as dealing with one's family and peers, accepting limitations, and the use of relaxation, hypnosis, and imagery.

Another disease for which groups have been found helpful is cystic fibrosis. Gratzick (1973) has reported on this approach for various age groups, noting interesting age-related differences. Winder and Medalie (1973) worked with a time-limited adolescent group with goals of helping the children cope with the tasks of adolescence, and helping their parents allow growth in the children. They found that their first goal was met with considerably more success than the second, and that a longer series of sessions with a heavier emphasis on parental contact would have been helpful.

Group therapy with chronically ill or physically handicapped adolescents in school and rehabilitation settings involves a different set of problems and goals. Bayrakal (1975) reported on a group experience with adolescent muscular dystrophy patients, which was seen as resulting in significantly improved attitudes and functioning in severely handicapped children who faced progressive deterioration. She took an analytic approach with a relatively inactive leader and intensive discussions over the course of a year, and noted that the group passed through a series of stages including struggles with dependence and independence, open recognition of anxiety and despair, and finally a phase of greater maturity characterized by intimacy and the sharing of appropriate affect.

Group therapy can also be used to meet more concrete, short-term needs in the rehabilitation of disabled adolescents, as illustrated by the work of Salhoot (1974). She points out the advantages of a group approach for such a population, including the opportunity to give rather than accept help, the development of relationships in socially isolated youngsters, the opportunity to learn from the self-expression of others in the group, the sharing of solutions to common reality problems, and the development of communication skills.

Magrab's (1975) use of weekly meetings for patients in a pediatric renal dialysis program exemplifies a similar focus but with a different population. These children, who faced an ongoing medical stress, used the groups for discussions of feelings, peer relationship building, and the development of an improved sense of normalcy. Such groups were also seen as necessary by Korsch, Fine, Grushkin, and Negrete (1971) in another renal disease program, where such interactions were noted to be taking place informally and spontaneously among the patients and families.

A short-term but intensive group experience was studied under relatively controlled conditions by Adler (1973), who worked with child muscular dystrophy patients in a camp setting. She interacted with an experimental group of children in ways designed to improve social interactions and acknowledge and encourage talents and abilities. Multiple assessment methods indicated that the experimental children made more gains in emotional state and interpersonal behavior than did a control group.

Finally, the use of traditional group psychotherapy techniques was reported with retarded adolescents (Slivkin & Bernstein, 1970). Short-term, structured groups were conducted using similar approaches to those employed with schizophrenic patients, including activity, the reinforcing of reality, clear limit-setting, and active teaching. The groups were seen as especially useful in diminishing hyperactivity in response to emotional stress, and many detailed suggestions for their operation are offered.

Because pediatric psychologists often deal with rare and serious diseases, group therapy has been an important intervention technique. Only through talking with others experiencing similar difficulties can afflicted children fully define their feelings and begin to deal with them.

FAMILY THERAPY

Family therapy, one of the newer interventions to come into general use, has been applied to a number of problems with which pediatric psychologists are concerned, including children with psychophysiological disorders, chronically ill and dying children, abused or neglected children, and children with developmental handicaps. However, formal family therapy does not seem to be one of the modalities more extensively used by the pediatric psychologist.

Some of the pioneers in family therapy have focused on psychophysiological diseases in children, viewing these disorders as being, in part, expressions of the family structure, with the ill child serving an important function in the operation of the family system (Minuchin, 1974; Minuchin, Rosman, & Baker, 1978). These authors have worked extensively with children having anorexia nervosa, juvenile onset diabetes, chronic asthma, and other conditions. While a review of their well-known and pioneering work is beyond the scope of this chapter, their extensive writings should serve as a resource for pediatric psychologists who are being called upon with increasing frequency to participate in the management of such conditions.

The pediatric psychologists who have used family therapy with these children (Lask & Kirk, 1979; Bauer, Harper, & Kenny, 1974) have found them to be most helpful. Lask and Kirk have focused on the operation of a circular interaction pattern in the families of chronic asthmatics that leads to progressively poorer medical and psychosocial functioning unless interrupted by therapy, and Bauer *et al.* have emphasized working with two-person communication patterns to facilitate conflict resolution.

An application of therapeutic efforts to strengthen family systems, which may or may not involve structured, regular family therapy sessions, has been found helpful by several workers involved with chronically ill and dying children. Sourkes (1977) has found that the role of "family facilitator" for the pediatric psychologist can be especially helpful in pediatric oncology settings. Through ongoing and often informal availability, the therapist works to facilitate communication in the family and models skills for the parents to use in interacting with their children. She points out that it is easy to develop an involvement with a dying child that supplants the parents, which may be highly dysfunctional for child, parents, and therapist alike. Drotar (1977) echoes this concern and also suggests that, with adolescent patients especially, the therapist may help the family by negotiating the intensity of the parent's involvement from his or her role as a supportive individual available to the entire family.

Gogan, O'Malley, and Foster (1977) suggest further study of interventions targeted at the entire family, which would be responsive to families from the point of diagnosis onward through the entire course of the disease. Munson (1978) has found that careful analysis of the family structure of new cancer patients, using the systems theories of Minuchin and others, can be most helpful to the staff in deciding on appropriate interventions. At times, it is noted, the family may have been chronically dysfunctional even before diagnosis, while in other cases the family system is responding to stress in identifiable ways that may be more easily remediated through the selection of specific interventions, such as clarification with each spouse of their perceptions of the situation.

The area of child abuse and neglect has been the target of increasing attention in recent years, first from pediatricians and later from other disciplines including psychology, social work, and psychiatry (Kempe & Kempe, 1978; Williams, 1978). While reviews such as those of Williams have pointed out the many obstacles to the use of family therapy with abusing families, including the danger of exposing the child to reactivated rage in the parent, innovative family-oriented approaches continue to be tried. Beezley *et al.* (1976) describe a combination of approaches with abusing families, placing a high premium on flexibility and availability. These approaches include not only casework, individual, and group treatment efforts, but also marital therapy and lay therapist family intervention. Alexander, McQuiston, and Rodenheffer (1976) have made substantial use of family techniques in their intensive residential approach to child abuse at the National Child Abuse Center. The treatment focuses on the parent-child relationship, beginning by intensive efforts to meet the needs of the parents and child separately, and gradually bringing the parents and child back together with support, supervision, and direct teaching.

Finally, family therapy has been used with developmentally handicapped children, although, as we have found in considering the other nonbehavioral intervention modalities, this literature is very small.

Howell (1973) has advocated the use of family therapy with mentally retarded children when the child is capable enough to engage in some abstract conceptualization, and when family relationships are a major problem, especially when the parents have a difficult time determining what their child cannot do as opposed to what he will not do.

Kaslow and Cooper (1978) and Kaslow and Abrams (1979) have described their work using family therapy with families of learning-disabled children, relating the child's educational difficulties to his related problems with ego-functioning, in the context of the family and their reactions to the handicap.

In summary, family therapy techniques seem to hold promise for the growing field of pediatric psychology. As with the other therapeutic approaches described in this section, family therapy can be most useful for pediatric psychologists if utilized along with some of the preventive, consultative, and behavioral interventions described in other sections of this chapter.

BEHAVIOR THERAPY

The intervention technique most commonly used by pediatric psychologists has been behavior therapy. This is because the settings in which they work generally require efficient, short-term interventions rather than long-term treatments (Routh, 1977). In addition, behavior therapy approaches are more effective with the less verbal populations (such as handicapped and younger children) frequently served by pediatric psychologists. In defining behavior therapy techniques for the purpose of this section, the broad definition of Craighead, Kazdin, and Mahoney (1976) will be used. They define behavior therapy as a broad set of clinical procedures whose description and rationale often rely on experimental findings of psychological research. Moreover, these procedures result from an analytic approach to clinical data and rely on objective and measurable outcomes. Under this section, the following areas will be discussed: behavioral programs emphasizing contingent reward and/or punishment, overcorrection, self-control, biofeedback and relaxation training, modeling, and social skills training.

Behavioral Programs Emphasizing Contingent Reward and/or Punishment

The systematic manipulation of consequences for specific appropriate and inappropriate behaviors has been the most widely used of the behavior therapy techniques by pediatric psychologists as well as other mental health professionals. These techniques have been used to manage a wide range of behaviors from toileting to seizures, and with a wide variety of children including those with severe behavior disorders and mental retardation. Pediatric psychologists have applied these techniques directly to the children having difficulties, as well as through consultation with parents, teachers, and others caring for the children.

The earliest use of behavior therapy techniques was for the treatment of enuresis. The original technique (Mowrer & Mowrer, 1938) involved a mechanical device which gave a signal strong enough to wake the child whenever the bed was wet. The goal was to teach the child to wake up before urinating.

Although the Mowrer and Mowrer apparatus was somewhat primitive, the basic technique is still in use and accepted by most as the most effective treatment for nighttime enuresis (Walker, 1978). The major differences in modern treatment approaches are the more sophisticated ways of evaluating their effectiveness and more sophisticated techniques for analyzing the component behaviors responsible for producing the desired results.

Doleys and Ciminero (1976) effectively summarize the current research in behavioral treatments of enuresis, identifying the following techniques as proven helpful in improving enuretic behavior: dietary restrictions, baseline recording, advice and encouragement, positive reinforcement, staggered awakening, and retention control training. In their review, they cite studies demonstrating the effectiveness of each of these techniques.

To summarize briefly, the Doleys and Ciminero review shows how each of the five intervention techniques has brought about positive behavioral changes in the treatment of enuresis. Dietary restrictions, eliminating milk and dairy products, citrus fruit, tomato products, chocolate, and coloring agents, were found successful in a study by Esperanca and Gerrard (1969). Baseline recording has been shown to be an effective strategy for a wide variety of behavior problems (Maletzky, 1974). Simply recording the incidence of a behavior seems to provide important feedback which is helpful in reducing the behavior's occurrence. Collins (1973) found this to be an effective treatment for enuresis without any other intervention, as did Doleys and Ciminero (1976). Advice and encouragement for both children and their families have also produced positive results (Kimmel & Kimmel, 1970; Mesibov, 1977). Systematic delivery of more tangible positive reinforcements has also decreased the frequency of nighttime wetting (Doleys & Ciminero, 1976).

The other two techniques that have been effective with enuresis have been staggered awakening and retention control training. Awakening a child at variable intervals throughout the night has been associated with a decrease in bed wetting (Creer & Davis, 1975). The retention control technique was devised by Kimmel and Kimmel (1970). During this procedure the parents chart the child's daytime toileting behavior and have the child retain urine for successively longer periods of time in an attempt to increase bladder capacity. Starfield (1967) has used this technique effectively in the training of enuretic children.

In addition to working with the problem of enuresis, pediatric psychologists have assisted parents with the toilet training of their normally developing children, which recent studies suggest is one of the most common of normal childrearing problems (Mesibov et al., 1977). In this effort, most of the general behavior principles are usually applied including baseline recording, advice and encouragement, and systematic administration of tangible reinforcers. Azrin and Foxx's (1974) technique, discussed later, has been an especially popular toilet training program.

Treatments for encopresis have been similar to those for enuresis. The major difference has been that the treatment programs for encopresis have emphasized medical factors to a greater extent, because encopresis has frequently been found to have more physical sequelae than enuresis. This has necessitated the use of somewhat different treatment techniques as well as closer collaboration with pediatricians.

The most widely used treatment program for encopresis was developed by Wright and Walker (1976). Their program consists of the following sequence:

1. A physician performs a careful physical examination to rule out organic etiology.
2. The psychologist interviews the parents and child to rule out serious emotional disturbance.
3. Instruction is given to the parents in the program who then explain the procedures to the child.
4. The child's colon is thoroughly evacuated.
5. The child is sent to the bathroom at a specific time each day.

If the child produces any feces at this point, he or she is praised and given a small reward. If the child does not produce any feces, the parents insert a suppository and the child is taken back to the bathroom. If the child is successful after the suppository, a reward is received, though not as large as if the child had evacuated on her or his own.

The above program is supplemented by periodic checks of the child's clothing for soiling throughout the day. Use of rewards and punishments are also recommended during these checks. This regimen is continued on a daily basis. Weekly telephone contact is made by the professional who is monitoring the program. After two weeks in which no soiling has occurred, a phase-out procedure is initiated. The authors report close to 100% effectiveness when this program is carefully implemented.

The Wright and Walker procedure was replicated by Christophersen and Rainey (1976) through a pediatric outpatient clinic. They found equally successful results with a minimum of staff time, leading them to the conclusion that the technique is practical for implementation in any pediatric setting.

Contingent reward and punishment programs have also been used by pediatric psychologists for a wide variety of feeding problems. Brown (1975) reports on a feeding clinic in a University Affiliated Program, where infants are rewarded for appropriate feeding behaviors with small bits of flavored food, fluids, or social reinforcers. Social reinforcement is highlighted in this program though the withdrawal of attention for inappropriate behaviors is also emphasized.

Contingent rewards and punishment have also been used with failure-to-thrive infants in a case described by Linscheid (1978). After a two-week hospitalization, the investigators noted several subtle problems which were interfering with the mother-child interactions. Interventions focused on reinforcing the mother's positive interactions with her child through positive comments until these interactions became longer and more pleasurable. In addition to their behavior modification approach, information was given to the mother concerning the child's needs and appropriate ways of meeting them. Behavioral techniques were also supplemented by information in the treatment of a failure-to-thrive infant by Roberts and Horner (1979).

Linscheid, Oliver, Blyler, and Palmer (1978) used contingent rewards and punishments for the feeding problems of developmentally disabled preschoolers. In a case of a 4-year, 7-month-old female with spina bifida, preferred food such as peanut butter and chocolate milk were given contingent upon eating nonpreferred foods. For another multihandicapped 2-year-old-child, a bottle plus verbal praise for appropriate behaviors, combined with time-out and withdrawal of the bottle following undesired behaviors, produced increases in consumption of desired foods and decreases in noncompliant behaviors.

Epstein, Wing, Steranchak, Dickson, and Michelson (1980) used contingency contracting, self-monitoring, social reinforcement, and therapist contact in the treatment of overweight adolescents. The contingency contracting consisted of a $65.00 family deposit which was to be returned during the treatment and follow-up sessions if the clients carried out their programs. Self-monitoring involved self-observation and recording of caloric intake. The social reinforcement consisted of praise from other family members when the adolescent successfully made changes in eating and exercise behaviors. The rewarded behaviors included removal of environmental stimuli that promoted eating and the slowing down of the eating rate. Therapist contact consisted of phone calls during treatment and follow-up. Parents were an integral part of this treatment program and were used as models for other family members. The difference between this and most other behavior modification techniques (Kingsley & Shapiro, 1977; Wheeler & Hess, 1976) is the greater family involvement. The Epstein et al. procedure was very effective in treating adolescent obesity.

Contingent reward and punishment techniques have also been utilized by pediatric psychologists for another adolescent eating problem, anorexia nervosa (Garfinkel, Garner, & Moldofsky, 1977). Studies from the Philadelphia Clinic (Barcai, 1971) suggest that operant techniques combined with family therapy can have a positive outcome with this disorder. Although operant behavior modification techniques are very effective with this condition, Garfinkel et al. (1977) cautioned that these techniques can be used only as a part of the total management program, and concomitant psychotherapy is also necessary.

Contingent reward and punishment programs have also been used by pediatric psychologists with specific populations of handicapped children. These techniques have most commonly been applied to those with developmental disabilities because of the nature of these disorders. Developmentally disabled children typically have less language and ability to abstract than other groups of children and the more verbal, traditional forms of therapy are less effective for them. In general, these techniques involving the application of contingencies have been more commonly used with children who are more severely and profoundly handicapped, both for severe behavior problems and for developing educational skills.

An early and classic example of the use of contingent rewards and punishments with a severely mentally retarded child was reported by Wolf, Risley, and Mees (1964). The child, a 3½-year-old boy, presented a number of behavior problems including severe tantrums. One of the major difficulties addressed by the investigators was this child's refusal to wear his glasses, even though he was nearly blind without them.

At first, the child was reinforced for playing with or touching the frames. Later on, he was reinforced for bringing them closer to his eyes. By using food as a reinforcer and this shaping technique, the authors were eventually able to have the child keep his glasses on for most of the day.

Repp and Dietz (1976) reduced the frequency of severe aggression and disruptive behaviors in several mentally retarded children. Their procedure involved reinforcements for units of time during which no aggressive behavior occurred. Initially the time interval was very short, only about 5 seconds, but it was gradually increased to over 15 minutes. During the course of training, aggressive behaviors decreased dramatically. Other investigators have reported the use of operant techniques for reducing severe self-injurious behaviors (Schroeder, Mulick, & Schroeder, 1980; Tate & Baroff, 1966).

In addition to decreasing inappropriate behaviors, these techniques have also been utilized to increase the incidence of appropriate behaviors. Neisworth and Smith (1974) taught a severely retarded woman to pay attention in a classroom setting. She was given praise and attention for sitting with her head up and paying attention, and was sent to a time-out room for having her head down and not paying attention. After 19 days of treatment, the amount of attention she paid in a classroom was dramatically increased. Neisworth and Smith (1974) improved the cafeteria behavior of retarded children with similar techniques. They identified three target behaviors: using quiet, conversational voices when talking, staying seated until excused, and lining up quietly and waiting for the teacher after completing their meal. These goals were accomplished by giving each child three tokens before going to the cafeteria. Every time a child violated one of the three rules, a token was taken away. Those children who retained tokens were able to play on monkey bars or with various toys after lunch was completed.

Contingent reward and punishment techniques have also been widely used with autistic children. Ferster (1961) first used these techniques to broaden the response repertoires of severely autistic children. Lovaas and Koegel (1973) have used various forms of negative reinforcement to decrease self-destructive behaviors in autistic children. Lovaas (1966) has also used reward techniques to develop rudimentary language and attention skills in these children. Dodge and Harris (1969) have increased appropriate social skills and verbalization of two autistic children through contingent reward and punishment tehniques. In addition to the programms already described, these techniques have been used to teach self-help skills (Marshall, 1966) and speech (Lovaas, 1966), and have been used for the establishment of classrooms (Rincover & Koegel, 1977) and for parent training (Schreibman & Koegel, 1975).

Contingent reward and punishment procedures have also been used for children with seizure disorders. Several successful instances of seizure control being achieved through these techniques have been reported. Gardner (1967) treated a 10-year-old female by instructing her parents to reward appropriate behaviors and ignore seizures or other inappropriate behaviors. Seizures were eliminated within two weeks following the use of this technique. Similar techniques, carried out in a classroom, were also found to be effective by Balaschak (1976). Other successful treatments have been reported for a 17-year-old retarded female (Zlutnick, Mayville, & Moffat, 1975) and a 15-year-old with severe family turmoil (Dollinger, 1980). In most of these cases, contingent reward and punishment techniques are most effective if the seizures have a strong psychological component; however, many argue that they can also be effective if organic etiology is involved.

A final use of contingent reward and punishment procedures has involved token economies, which allow children to earn tokens for appropriate behaviors. The earned tokens are then exchanged for back-up reinforcers.

Token economies have most typically been used with moderately retarded children in classrooms and residential institutions (Baroff, 1974; Robinson & Robinson, 1976). In addition to developing academic and self-help skills, token programs have been used to improve eating behaviors (Brown, 1975), increase compliance behaviors (Magrab, 1975), and teach interpersonal skills (Mesibov & Fontaine, 1975). Token programs have been effective because they are clear, concrete, and highly reinforcing.

In summary, contingent reward and punishment techniques have been effective in a wide variety of situations. These techniques are the most popular of the intervention strategies uses by pediatric psychologists and are generally quite effective. They can be used by themselves or in conjunction with other treatment techniques.

Overcorrection

Overcorrection is a recently developed punishment procedure described by Foxx and Azrin (Foxx, 1978; Foxx & Azrin, 1972). It was developed as an alternative to physical punishment, and designed to be somewhat less aversive but equally effective as existing techniques. Like other forms of punishment, overcorrection is designed to follow an inappropriate behavior and to assure that the behavior will be less likely to occur in future situations.

Foxx and Azrin have described two types of overcorrection: restitution and positive practice. Restitution requires the individual to correct the consequences of an inappropriate behavior by making the disturbed situation significantly improved over that which existed prior to the inappropriate behavior. For example, restitution for a child who scribbles on a wall with chalk might involve thoroughly cleaning all of the walls in the room, not only correcting the problem caused by the child's scribbling on one wall, but also bringing the room to a status vastly improved over what existed prior to the disruption.

The other type of overcorrection, positive practice, consists of repeated direct or appropriate behaviors following an error. For example, a child who inappropriately interacts with a peer by hitting him is required to say something nice and appropriate to everyone in the room. The child thus repeatedly practices the appropriate response and is, therefore, more likely to perform that behavior in a similar future situation.

The two types of overcorrection, restitution and positive practice, have several common characteristics. First, they insure that the consequences are directly relevant to the misbehaviors. Second, the procedures require that children experience some of the effects of their misbehaviors, correcting the situation on their own rather than having another person correct a situation the child has created. Third, the punishment immediately follows the behavior, which is thought to be desirable with any behavioral therapy technique. Finally, the duration of the overcorrection procedure is generally lengthy, making it a somewhat aversive procedure.

Overcorrection has primarily been used by pediatric psychologists working with developmentally disabled individuals, especially those with mental retardation and/or autism. It has been popular with these populations because it does not emphasize verbal techniques and because it is thought to be a positive alternative to the more restrictive and aversive forms of punishment that these clients often require. It has been most commonly used for self-injurious behaviors (Bernard, Christopherson, & Wolf, 1977), property destruction (Foxx & Azrin, 1972), school problems (Foxx, 1978), noncompliance (Foxx, 1977), and toileting problems (Azrin & Foxx, 1974).

Foxx and Martin (1975) used overcorrection in the treatment of one type of self-injurious behavior, pica. Pica involves the ingestion of nonfood substances, such as trash, nails, or cigarette butts. Positive practice required the clients to throw away trash or empty and clean ashtrays, depending upon which had been ingested. The restitutional overcorrection procedure consisted of thoroughly cleaning the mouth and hands after the ingestion of an inappropriate item.

Another example of overcorrection is the Azrin and Foxx (1974) toilet training program that has been applied to both handicapped and nonhandicapped children. The positive practice procedure requires a child to walk repeatedly to the toilet and engage in the usual toileting procedures such as removing their clothes and sitting on the toilet. The restitutional overcorrection procedure involves mopping the floor where the accident occurred, washing the soiled clothing, and dressing oneself in clean clothing. This technique has been extremely effective in toilet training a wide variety of handicapped and nonhandicapped children.

Although relatively new, overcorrection has been used effectively as a punishment procedure. It has the advantages of being minimally aversive and intrusive. A major difficulty is the amount of one-to-one time needed for implementation. More research is needed on potential applications of this technique and their effectiveness.

Self-Control

Self-control techniques have recently been used by behavioral therapists (Mahoney & Thoreson, 1974) to help bring about and maintain behavior change. The techniques attempt to replace external means of controlling behavior (reinforcements or punishments) by internal processes. The goal of self-control programs is to bring the reinforcement contingencies under the control of the individual so that the behavior can be self-controlled as well.

Traditionally, the self-control techniques have been classified into four types (Glynn, Thomas, & Shee, 1973): (1) self-assessment, which involves observing one's own behavior, (2) self-monitoring, which involves collecting data on the frequency of one's own behavior, (3) self-determination of reinforcement, and (4) self-administration of reinforcement.

Although the traditionally described self-control procedures have been utilized in several laboratory investigations, evidence on their effectiveness in changing children's behaviors in interdisciplinary settings has been minimal. The few studies that have been done have focused on self-monitoring to reduce whining behavior (Kunzelman, 1970) and increase class participation (Gottman & McFall, 1972). The limited use of these techniques has been attributed to the limited cognitive ability of children to set standards, objectively observe their own behaviors, and strictly adhere to self-imposed reinforcement contingencies. However, a more recent self-control procedure involving self-verbalization has been effectively applied to several types of childhood difficulties.

The self-verbalization technique was first developed by Meichenbaum and Goodman (1971). They taught impulsive second-grade children to self-verbalize the phrase "slow down" as they were working on a task requiring reflective thinking. The children receiving this training made fewer mistakes on a task of cognitive impulsivity. Camp (1977) and Schneider and Robin (1975) have applied these self-verbalization strategies to clinical and educational settings.

The Schneider and Robin "turtle technique" involved a classroom application of the self-verbalization strategy. The technique is named for the analogy to a turtle, which withdraws when threatened, in the same way a child is taught to withdraw into himself when the child feels threatened by uncontrollable emotions or external events. In practice, the key word "turtle" is taught to the child, who then responds by pulling his or her arms and head in close to the body and closing her or his eyes. The child is taught relaxation procedures to use at these times. Finally, problem-solving strategies similar to the Spivack and Shure (1974) techniques are taught to help solve the problem that the child finds threatening. The combination of withdrawing, relaxing, and developing appropriate problem-solving strategies is advanced as an appropriate alternative to the more aggressive behaviors that children might practice at these times.

Friedman (1980) has used a similar self-control technique to modify the obscene vocalizations and verbal tics of an 11-year-old girl with Gilles de la Tourette syndrome, a childhood disorder consisting of vocal and bodily tics. This program involves close collaboration between the child, her parents, and the therapist. The child was encouraged to use the word "fun" whenever she felt the need to shout something out loud. The mother was also encouraged to substitute this word and to gently remind the daughter about using it whenever the daughter shouted obscenities. As a result of the program, the child's use of obscenities decreased dramatically within several weeks.

Although the literature on self-control techniques with children is limited, their potential utility seems great. Self-control techniques represent the goals most espouse for their children: the ability to monitor and control one's own behavior. Pediatric psychologists should explore potential applications of self-control techniques more thoroughly.

Biofeedback and Relaxation Training

Biofeedback and relaxation training procedures have recently been developed for treatment of various psychological problems, especially those with an organic component such as pain. Because many psychological and physical conditions are thought to result from extreme tension or the inability to relax, these techniques have been developed to facilitate the relaxation process. Although their use has been documented most carefully with adult patients, investigators have recently begun to examine their effectiveness with several childhood disorders, especially those that are thought to have an organic basis such as hyperactivity, learning disabilities, and seizure disorders.

Biofeedback is defined as a technique for acquiring control over internal processes: "Essentially, biofeedback is operant conditioning of autonomic, electrophysiological, and neuromuscular responses . . . this process may take place with or without awareness on the part of the organism as to exactly what manipulations must be performed to bring about such control" (Luber & Shouse, 1977, p. 204).

In one of the first controlled studies using biofeedback with children, Hunter, Russell, Russell, & Zimmerman (1976) demonstrated that learning-disabled children could learn biofeedback techniques as easily as their normal controls. In fact, the learning-disabled sample in this study even performed slightly better than the nonhandicapped controls. Russell and Carter (1978) reported academic gains and improved self-control, impulsivity, and distractibility in a group of learning-disabled children after 10 weeks of biofeedback training. Braud (1974) reports decreased out-of-seat behavior, emotionality, and aggressiveness in hyperactive children after biofeedback training.

In a more detailed study of the use of biofeedback with children, Russell and Carter (1978) gave a group of learning-disabled children three biofeedback training sessions a week for a total of four weeks. In addition, the children were asked to practice relaxation exercises at home using a prerecorded cassette tape containing muscle relaxation exercises. The children showed significant gains on a variety of academic and muscle coordination tasks. The authors identified the key aspects of biofeedback as facilitating the relaxation process. Their argument is that muscular tension prohibits learning-disabled children from learning more effectively and executing necessary motor and perceptual-motor functions.

Although the literature on biofeedback training is very new, there is evidence that this technique holds promise for a wide range of children. The need to relax is important for most children exhibiting problems, whether they are emotional or neurological. An additional benefit of this approach is its applicability to populations of children with communication problems, especially those with severe language disorders, autism, and severe mental retardation. Certainly more work should be done exploring this technique with these populations. The use of biofeedback by Schroeder et al. (1980) with a severely retarded, autistic, adolescent suggests that this technique can be effectively used with this population.

Specific relaxation training has also been an effective intervention technique, though it too has not been widely applied. Shaw and Walker (1979) used relaxation to treat an 8-year-old moderately retarded child with PKU for inappropriate and excessive sexual responses in the presence of barefooted women. The process began by teaching the child some basic relaxation techniques. The therapist modeled the relaxation exercises and then rewarded the child's sucessful replication of these with candy and praise. During the training the child was given considerable verbal encouragement and was urged to use this technique whenever he saw a woman's feet.

The technique was learned after approximately three days of intensive training. At this time, a female assistant entered the room barefooted and instructed the child to practice his relaxation exercises. Two daily sessions were held with rewards of candy and praise freely administered. The female assistant interacted positively with the client by playing games and puzzles. Engaging activities were initially used to help distract the client, but as the sessions progressed, less engaging games were used to put greater pressure on the child to practice the relaxation exercises. The results indicated that the technique was very effective and 6-, 12-, and 18-month follow-ups suggested no recurrence of the fetishistic behavior.

LaGreca and Ottinger (1979) also used a relaxation procedure effectively. Their client was a 12-year-old girl with cerebral palsy who had to complete a set of painful exercises to stretch her hip muscles. The relaxation combined with a self-monitoring procedure resulted in a significant increase in her exercising which was maintained at 3- and 6-month follow-ups. Relaxation techniques have also been used in treating psychosomatic disorders (Bauer, 1975) and supplemented the biofeedback training program described above (Russell & Carter, 1978).

In summary, there is increasing evidence that biofeedback and relaxation can be used for a variety of childhood difficulties. These techniques should be of particular interest to pediatric psychologists who serve many nonverbal clients who could be responsive to these approaches.

Modeling

As Bandura (1969) wrote, "One of the fundamental means by which new modes of behavior are acquired and existing patterns are modfied entails modeling and vicarious processes"(p. 118). He further stated that "virtually all learning phenomena resulting from direct experiences can occur on a vicarious basis through observation of other persons' behavior and its consequences for them." Because modeling is essentially an observational procedure and does not require much language ability, it has been an especially popular intervention technique with children. Modeling has been used to improve the social adjustment of children, modify fears, improve attention in distractable children, and develop skills in developmentally handicapped children.

Much of the earlier work using modeling with children focused on their social behavior. Several investigators have tried to reduce social withdrawal through modeling techniques. O'Connor (1969) showed a group of social isolates several scenes of a child initially observing interactions, and then joining in with the activities and experiencing positive consequences. As a result of this procedure, social withdrawal was sharply reduced in comparison to a control group of children. Other studies comparing modeling techniques with control groups have found similarly encouraging results (Evers & Schwarz, 1973; Keller & Carlson, 1974). In the Evers and Schwarz study, modeling was found to be effective by itself, and no additional improvement was found in children who were rewarded for performing the desired behavior. Ross, Ross, and Evans (1971) report another successful case study of the effective use of modeling with a severely withdrawn 6-year-old boy.

In addition to modifying social withdrawal, modeling has been used to modify social aggression. Although positive short-term effects of modeling have been noted with social aggression, these have not been as pronounced or long-term as the effects on social withdrawal. Chittenden (1942) did the original study in this area, attempting to teach children nonaggressive reactions to frustrations. After children observed aggressive and cooperative solutions to problems, a discussion followed pointing out the advantages of cooperation. Children observing the modeling scenes showed a decrease in aggressive behaviors in this nursery school setting.

Sarason and Ganzer (1973) used modeling with male juvenile delinquents. This group observed models applying for jobs, resisting peer pressure, and delaying gratification. In addition, they received feedback on their performance after observing the models. The results indicated improved behavior as a result of this procedure. Equally effective results with juvenile delinquents in group home settings have been reported by Thelen, Fry, Dollinger, and Paul (1976).

Modeling has also been used to reduce fears in children. Several studies have demonstrated the positive effect of a fearless model combined with some guidance on interacting with the feared object. Bandura, Grusec, and Menlove (1967) significantly increased the ability of dog-phobic preschool children to approach two dogs. This effect of modeling was replicated with dogs (Bandura & Menlove, 1968) and snakes (Ritter, 1968). Lewis (1974) has used modeling plus guidance to reduce children's fear of swimming.

Modeling techniques have also been used to reduce fears in dental and medical settings. Melamed, Weinstein, Hawes, and Katin Borland (1975) successfully reduced disruptive dental behavior by using a film depicting a 4-year-old child successfully coping with dental treatment. Melamed and Siegel (1975) have also used filmed modeling effectively in preparing young children for surgery. The film depicted certain common fears and ways in which children can successfully cope with them. The anxiety levels of the children who viewed the film were significantly reduced compared with those viewing a control film. Vernon (1973) demonstrated similar results using film models for children who were to receive dental anesthesia.

Modeling has also been used to teach a wide range of skills to developmentally disabled children. Lovaas's group has used modeling to improve behavior (Lovaas & Koegel, 1973) and language skills (Lovaas, 1966) in severely retarded, autistic children. Other investigators have also emphasized modeling techniques in teaching language skills to autistic children (Rincover & Koegel, 1977). Modeling has been widely used to teach self-help skills to mentally retarded children. A wide range of important skills have been taught through this technique, including eating behaviors (Butterfield & Parson, 1973), tooth brushing (Horner & Keilitz, 1975), and appropriate community behavior such as answering the telephone (Stephan, Stephano, & Talkington, 1973).

In summary, modeling is an easily used and very effective training technique in teaching a wide variety of behaviors to a wide variety of children. Its emphasis on observation as opposed to language makes it applicable to very low functioning and also very young children.

Social Skills Training

Social skills training is a more recently developed intervention technique that is becoming increasingly popular among pediatric psychologists and other service providers (Combs & Slaby, 1977). This behavioral intervention emphasizes teaching specific social and interpersonal skills to children whose main difficulty is in this area. Its use as a preventive technique (Spivack & Shure, 1974) has already been described. Its use as an intervention technique for children with difficulties will be described in this section.

Two of the most common social skills intervention training techniques have already been described: (1) contingent rewards and punishment and (2) modeling. Other techniques more specifically identified with social skills training have been coaching, behavior rehearsal, role-playing, and perspective-taking.

Oden and Asher (1977) were the first to describe coaching as a social skills training technique. They coached socially isolated third- and fourth-grade children on how to play with others and followed this with an opportunity to practice and obtain feedback on their play behavior. The six-session coaching program emphasized participating in play activities, cooperating with peers, communicating with peers, and giving peers attention and support. Children participating in the coaching procedure showed significant increases in their sociometric standings among their classmates. These results were maintained in a 1-year follow-up.

Behavior rehearsal was first successfully used by Bornstein, Bellack, and Hersen (1977), in teaching assertiveness to children. The authors stressed *in vivo* practice as a major component of their training program. Teachers rewarded appropriate cooperation or appropriate assertiveness in saying no to an unreasonable request. LaGreca and Santogrossi (1980) emphasized behavioral rehearsal, although modeling and coaching were also used in their treatment of 30 third- through fifth-grade children with low peer-acceptance ratings. The procedure involved rehearsal of specific interpersonal skills with videotaped feedback. Children participating in this program demonstrated increased skill in role-playing situations, a greater verbal knowledge of how to interact with peers, and more appreciation of peer interactions in school. LaGreca and Mesibov (1979) used the same technique in improving interpersonal skills in a group of learning-disabled children with severe peer problems.

Staub (1971) has used role-playing to improve children's social skills. In his study, pairs of children role-played situations in which one person needed help and another provided the help, and they subsequently exchanged roles. Children participating in his role-playing condition showed significantly more helping and sharing both immediately after treatment and one week later. Rathjen, Hiniker, and Rathjen (1976) also used role-playing to teach verbal skills such as expressing opinions, feelings, and feelings with criticism. Ross *et al*. (1971) used role-playing plus modeling to treat the extreme avoidance behaviors of a 6-year-old boy.

Although learning to take the perspective of another is thought to be an important social skill, most studies in this area have dealt with perceptual role-taking rather than role-taking in social situations. One exception is the study by Chandler (1973) of a group of 45 chronically delinquent boys. Chandler's role-taking procedure involved allowing the boys to make videofilms of themselves and others. The expectation was that making the films would require them to take the perspectives of other people. The results suggested that those in the perspective-taking condition improved significantly in their role-taking ability over those in control conditions. These changes were associated with a reduction in the number of criminal offenses committed during the next 18 months.

Although social skills training programs are relatively new, the success of those studies conducted to date suggest this is a potentially important and useful intervention technique for pediatric psychologists. Much more research is needed concerning the aspects of these techniques which are most effective and the types of populations that will be most likely to benefit from these techniques. In addition, as with most areas of therapy, more attention needs to be addressed to the generalization problem to be sure that improvements in the laboratory are translated to the everyday settings in which these children participate.

Behavior Therapy Summary

In addition to being the most frequently used intervention technique in pediatric psychology, behavior therapy approaches also seem to hold the most promise for future efforts. Their short-term emphasis and compatibility with the consultation process make them well-suited to the needs of pediatric psychologists and the settings in which they work. Although much recent research has been done on behavioral interventions in interdisciplinary settings, much more needs to be done.

SUMMARY

Despite its brief history, pediatric psychology has had a major impact on the field of intervention techniques with children. This has been accomplished by combining the more traditional one-to-one psychotherapeutic interventions with newer consultative, preventive, and behavioral techniques. If pediatric psychology continues the growth described in this chapter, the result will be more improved, refined, and sophisticated intervention techniques which will be well-suited to the multiple needs of the children they serve.

REFERENCES

Ack, M. New perspectives in comprehensive health care for children. *Journal of Pediatric Psychology*, 1976, **1**, 9–11.

Adler, S. N. M. The stigma of handicap and its unlearning: A social perspective on children with muscle disease and their families. *Dissertation Abstracts International*, 1973, **34**, 1266B–1267B.

Albee, G. W., & Joffe, J. M. (Eds.) *Primary prevention of psychopathology*, Vol. 1. Hanover, NH: University Press of New England, 1977.

Alexander, H., McQuiston, M., & Rodenheffer, M. Residential family therapy. In H. P. Martin (Ed.), *The abused child: A multidisciplinary approach to developmental issues and treatment*. Cambridge, MA: Ballinger, 1976.

Arnold, L. E. Strategies and tactics of parent guidance. In L. E. Arnold (Ed.), *Helping parents help their children*. New York: Brunner/Mazel, 1978.

Azarnoff, P., & Flegal, S. *A pediatric play program*. Springfield, IL: Charles C. Thomas, 1975.

Azrin, N. H., & Foxx, R. M. *Toilet training in less than a day*. New York: Simon & Schuster, 1974.

Balaschak, B. A. Teacher-implemented behavior modification in a case of organically based epilepsy. *Journal of Consulting and Clinical Psychology*, 1976, **44**, 218–223.

Bandura, A. *Principles of behavior modification*. New York: Holt, Rinehart & Winston, 1969.

Bandura, A., Grusec, J. E., & Menlove, F. L. Vicarious extinction of avoidance behavior. *Journal of Personality and Social Psychology*, 1967, **5**, 16–23.

Bandura, A., & Menlove, F. L. Factors determining vicarious extinction of avoidance behavior through symbolic modeling. *Journal of Personality and Social Psychology*, 1968, **82**, 99–108.

Barcai, A. Family therapy in the treatment of anorexia nervosa. *American Journal of Psychiatry*, 1971, **128**, 286–290.

Baroff, G. S. *Mental retardation: Nature, cause, and management*. New York: Halsted, 1974.

Bauer, R. Treatment strategies in psychosomatic disorders. *Pediatric Psychology*, 1975, **3**, 4–5.

Bauer, R., Harper, R., & Kenny, T. Treatment for uncontrolled juvenile diabetes. *Pediatric Psychology*, 1974, **2**, 2–3.

Bayrakal, S. A group experience with chronically disabled adolescents. *American Journal of Psychiatry*, 1975, **132**, 1291–1294.

Beck, J. *How to raise a brighter child*. New York: Simon & Schuster, 1967.

Becker, W. C. *Parents are teachers*. Champaign, IL: Research Press, 1971.

Beezley, P., Martin, H., & Alexander, H. Comprehensive family oriented therapy. In R. E. Helfer & C. H. Kempe (Eds.), *Child abuse and neglect: The family and the community*. Cambridge, MA: Ballinger, 1976.

Beezley, P., Martin, H. P., & Kempe, R. Psychotherapy. In H. P. Martin (Ed.), *The abused child: A multidisciplinary approach to developmental issues and treatment*. Cambridge, MA: Ballinger, 1976.

Bentley, J., & Wilmerding, J. W. Individual psychotherapy with asthmatic children as an adjunct to milieu therapy: Two case studies. *Journal of Asthma Research*, 1977, **15**, 163–170.

Bergan, J. R. *Behavioral consultation*. Columbus, OH: Charles C. Merrill, 1977.

Berkowitz, M. I. *A primer on school mental health consultation*. Springfield, IL: Charles C. Thomas, 1975.

Bernard, J. D., Christopherson, E. R., & Wolf, M. M. Parent-mediated treatment of children's self-injurious behavior using overcorrection. *Journal of Pediatric Psychology*, 1977, **2**, 56–61.

Bernstein, D. M. After transplantation—The child's emotional reactions. *American Journal of Psychiatry*, 1971, **127**, 1189–1193.

Bernstein, N. R. *Emotional care of the facially burned and disfigured*. Boston: Little, Brown, 1976.

Bernstein, N. R. Mental retardation. In J. D. Noslpitz (Ed.), *Basic handbook of child psychiatry*, Vol. 3. New York: Basic Books, 1979.

Bernstein, N. R., Sanger, S., & Fras, J. The functions of the child psychiatrist in the management of severely burned children. *Journal of the American Academy of Child Psychiatry*, 1969, **8**, 620–636.

Binger, C. M. Jimmy—A clinical case presentation of a child with a fatal illness. In E. J. Anthony & C. Koupernik (Eds.), *The child in his family*. Vol. 3, *The impact of disease and death*. New York: Wiley, 1973.

Blanco, R. F. *Prescriptions for children with learning and adjustment problems*. Springfield, IL: Charles C. Thomas, 1972.

Bluebond-Langer, M. I know, do you? A study of awareness, communication & coping in terminally ill children. In B. Schoenberg, A. C. Carr, D. Peretz, A. H. Kutscher, & I. K. Goldberg (Eds.), *Anticipatory grief*. New York: Columbia University Press, 1974.

Bolian, G. Psychiatric consultation within a community of sick children. *Journal of the American Academy of Child Psychiatry*, 1971, **10**, 293–307.

Bornstein, M. R., Bellack, A. S., & Hersen, M. Social skills training for unassertive children: A multiple baseline analysis. *Journal of Applied Behavior Analysis*, 1977, **10**, 183–195.

Braud, L. W. *The effects of EMG biofeedback and progressive relaxation upon hyperactivity and its behavioral concomitants*. Paper presented at the meeting of the Southwestern Psychological Association, Houston, 1974.

Brazelton, T. B. *Infants and mothers*. New York: Delacorte Press, 1969.

Brazelton, T. B. *Toddlers and parents*. New York: Delacorte Press, 1974.

Brewer, D. The role of the psychologist in a dialysis and transplantation unit. *Journal of Clinical Child Psychology*, 1978, **7**, 71–72.

Brick, H. J., & Scheiner, A. P. Education for handicapped children: A study of educational services in central Massachusetts. *Journal of Pediatric Psychology*, 1978, **3**, 77–80.

Brown, J., & Hepler, R. Stimulation—A corollary to physical care. *American Journal of Nursing*, 1976, **76**, 578–581.

Brown, R. A. Behavioral intervention with feeding problems. *Pediatric Psychology*, 1975, **3**, 11–12.

Bruch, H. Anorexia nervosa and its treatment. *Journal of Pediatric Psychology*, 1977, **2**, 110–112.

Butterfield, W. H., & Parson, R. Modeling and shaping by parents to develop chewing behavior in their retarded child. *Journal of Behavior Therapy and Experimental Psychiatry*, 1973, **4**, 285–287.

Camp, B. W. Verbal mediation in young aggressive boys. *Journal of Abnormal Psychology*, 1977, **86**, 145–153.

Cassell, S., & Paul, M. H. The role of puppet therapy on the emotional responses of children hospitalized for cardiac catheterization. *Journal of Pediatrics*, 1967, **71**, 233–239.

Chandler, M. J. Egocentrism and antisocial behavior: The assessment and training of social perspective-taking skills. *Developmental Psychology*, 1973, **9**, 326–332.

Chittenden, G. E. An experimental study in measuring and modifying assertive behavior in young children. *Monographs of the Society for Research in Child Development*, 1942.

Christ, A. E. Psychotherapy of the child with true brain damage. *American Journal of Orthopsychiatry*, 1978, **48**, 505–515.

Christophersen, E. R., & Rainey, S. K. Management of encopresis through a pediatric outpatient clinic. *Journal of Pediatric Psychology*, 1976, **1**, 38–41.

Clarke-Stewart, K. A. Popular primers for parents. *American Psychologist*, 1978, **33**, 359–369.

Cline, F. W., & Rothenberg, M. B. Preparation of a child for major surgery. *Journal of the American Academy of Child Psychiatry*, 1974, **13**, 78–94.

Collins, R. W. Importance of the bladder-cue buzzer contingency in the conditioning treatment for enuresis. *Journal of Abnormal Psychology*, 1973, **82**, 299–308.

Colman, M. D., Dougher, C. A., & Tanner, M. R. Group therapy for physically handicapped toddlers with delayed speech and language development. *Journal of the American Academy of Child Psychiatry*, 1976, **15**, 395–413.

Combs, M. L., & Slaby, D. A. Social-skills training with children. In B. B. Lahey & A. E. Kazdin (Eds.), *Advances in Clinical Child Psychology*, Vol. 1. New York: Plenum Press, 1977.

Cowen, E. L. Psychotherapy and play techniques with the exceptional child and youth. In W. M. Cruickshank (Ed.), *Psychology of exceptional children and youth*. New York: Prentice-Hall, 1955.

Craighead, W. E., Kazdin, A. E., & Mahoney, M. J. *Behavior modification: Principles, issues, and applications*. Boston: Houghton Mifflin, 1976.

Creer, T. L., & Christian, W. P. *Chronically ill and handicapped children: Their management and rehabilitation.* Champaign, IL: Research Press, 1976.

Creer, T. L., & Davis, M. H. Using a staggered-awakening procedure with enuretic children in an institutional setting. *Journal of Behavior Therapy and Experimental Psychiatry*, 1975, **6**, 23–25.

Cyphert, F. R. Back to school for the child with cancer. *Journal of School Health*, 1973, **43**, 215–217.

Dodge, M. R., & Harris, F. R. Use of reinforcement principles with autistic children. *Research Report*, 1969, **2**, 82–84.

Dodson, F. *How to parent.* New York: Signet, 1970.

Doleys, D. M., & Ciminero, A. R. Childhood enuresis: Considerations in treatment. *Journal of Pediatric Psychology*, 1976, **1**, 21–23.

Dollinger, S. J. *Family systems/behavioral treatment for psychogenic blackouts in an adolescent girl.* Paper presented at the meeting of the Southeastern Psychological Association, Washington, D.C., March 1980.

Dreikurs, R., & Grey, L. *A parents' guide to child discipline.* New York: Hawthorn, 1970.

Drotar, D. Death in the pediatric hospital: Psychological consultation with medical and nursing staff. *Journal of Clinical Child Psychology*, 1975, **4**, 33–35. (a)

Drotar, D. The treatment of a severe anxiety reaction in an adolescent boy following renal transplantation. *Journal of the American Academy of Child Psychiatry*, 1975, **14**, 451–462. (b)

Drotar, D. Psychological consultation in the pediatric hospital. *Professional Psychology*, 1976, **9**, 77–83.

Drotar, D. Family oriented intervention with the dying adolescent. *Journal of Pediatric Psychology*, 1977, **2**, 68–71.

Drotar, D. Adaptational problems of children and adolescents with cystic fibrosis. *Journal of pediatric Psychology*, 1978, **3**, 45–50.

Ellis, A. Rational-emotive guidance. In L. E. Arnold (Ed.), *Helping parents help their children.* New York: Brunner/Mazel, 1978.

Elmer, E., & Gregg, G. S. Developmental characteristics of abused children. *Pediatrics*, 1967, **40**, 596–602.

Epstein, L. H., Wing, R. R., Steranchak, L., Dickson, B., & Michelson, J. Comparison of family-based behavior modification and nutrition education for childhood obesity. *Journal of Pediatric Psychology*, 1980, **5**, 25–36.

Esperanca, M., & Gerrard, J. W. Nocturnal enuresis: Comparison of the effect of imipramine and dietary restriction on bladder capacity. *Canadian Medical Association Journal*, 1969, **101**, 721–724.

Evers, W., & Schwarz, J. Modifying social withdrawal in preschoolers: The effects of filmed modeling and teacher praise. *Journal of Abnormal Child Psychology*, 1973, **1**, 248–256.

Ferster, C. B. Positive reinforcement and behavioral deficits of autistic children. *Child Development*, 1961, **32**, 437–456.

Field, T. M. Maternal stimulation during infant feeding. *Developmental Psychology*, 1977, **13**, 539–540.

Forgatch, M. S., & Toobert, D. J. A cost-effective parent training program for use with normal preschool children. *Journal of Pediatric Psychology*, 1979, **4**, 129–145.

Foxx, R. M. Attention training: The use of overcorrection avoidance to increase eye contact of autistic and retarded children. *Journal of Applied Behavior Analysis*, 1977, **10**, 489–499.

Foxx, R. M. An overview of overcorrection. *Journal of Pediatric Psychology*, 1978, **3**, 97–101.

Foxx, R. M., & Azrin, N. H. Restitution: A method of eliminating aggressive-disruptive behavior of retarded and brain damaged patients. *Behavior Research and Therapy*, 1972, **10**, 15–27.

Foxx, R. M., & Martin, E. D. Treatment of scavenging behavior by overcorrection. *Behavior Research and Therapy*, 1975, **13**, 153–162.

Friedman, S. Self-control in the treatment of Gilles de la Tourette's syndrome: Case study with 18-month follow-up. *Journal of Consulting and Clinical Psychology*, 1980, **48**, 400–402.

Gardner, G. G. Adolescents with cancer: Current issues and a proposal. *Journal of Pediatric Psychology*, 1977, **2**, 132–134.

Gardner, J. E. Behavior therapy treatment approach to a psychogenic seizure case. *Journal of Consulting Psychology*, 1967, **31**, 209–212.

Gardner, R. A. *Therapeutic communication with children: The mutual storytelling technique*. New York: Science House, 1971.

Gardner, R. A. Psychogenic difficulties secondary to MBD. In J. D. Noshpitz (Ed.), *Basic handbook of child psychiatry*, Vol. 3. New York: Basic Books, 1979.

Garfinkel, P. E., Garner, D. M., & Moldofsky, H. The role of behavior modification in the treatment of anorexia nervosa. *Journal of Pediatric Psychology*, 1977, **2**, 113–121.

Geist, R. A. Consultation on a pediatric surgical ward: Creating an empathetic climate. *American Journal of Orthopsychiatry*, 1977, **47**, 432–444.

Geist, R. A. Onset of chronic illness in children and adolescents: Psychotherapeutic and consultative intervention. *American Journal of Orthopsychiatry*, 1979, **49**, 4–23.

Gesell, A., & Ilg, F. *Infant and child in the culture of today*. New York: Harper & Row, 1945.

Gil, D. G. Primary prevention of child abuse: A philosophical and political issue. *Journal of Pediatric Psychology*, 1976, **1**, 54–57.

Ginott, H. *Between parent and child*. New York: Avon Books, 1965.

Ginott, H. *Between parent and teenager*. New York: Avon Books, 1971.

Glynn, E. L., Thomas, J. D., & Shee, S. M. Behavioral self-control of on-task behavior in an elementary classroom. *Journal of Applied Behavior Analysis*, 1973, **6**, 105–113.

Gogan, J. L., O'Malley, J. E., & Foster, D. J. Treating the pediatric cancer patient: A review. *Journal of Pediatric Psychology*, 1977, **2**, 42–48.

Gordon, T. *Parent effectiveness training*. New York: Wyden, 1970.

Gottman, J. M., & McFall, R. M. Self-monitoring effects in a program for potential high school dropouts: A time-series analysis. *Journal of Consulting and Clinical Psychology*, 1972, **39**, 273–281.

Gratzick, E. W. Hospitalized children and young adults with cystic fibrosis. In P. Patterson, C. Denning, & A. Kutscher (Eds.), *Psychosocial aspects of cystic fibrosis*. New York: Foundation of Thanatology, 1973.

Groen, J. J., & Pelser, H. E. Experiences with and results of group psychotherapy in patients with bronchial asthma. *Journal of Psychosomatic Research*, 1960, **4**, 191–205.

Guerney, L. F. Play therapy with learning disabled children. *Journal of Clinical Child Psychology*, 1979, **8**, 242–244.

Heber, F. R. Sociocultural mental retardation: A longitudinal study. In D. G. Forgays (Ed.), *Primary prevention of psychopathology*, Vol. 2. *Environmental influences*. Hanover, NH: University Press of New England, 1978.

Heffron, W. A. Group therapy sessions as part of treatment of children with cancer. In C. Pockedly (Ed.), *Clinical management of children with cancer*. Aeta, MA: Sciences Group, 1975.

Heifeitz, L. J. Behavioral training for parents of retarded children: Alternative formats based on instructional manuals. *American Journal of Mental Deficiency*, 1977, **82**, 194–203.

Hoffman, I., & Futterman, E. H. Coping with waiting: Psychiatric intervention and study in the waiting room of a pediatric oncology clinic. *Comprehensive Psychiatry*, 1971, **12**, 67–81.

Horner, R. D., & Keilitz, I. Training mentally retarded adolescents to brush their teeth. *Journal of Applied Behavior Analysis*, 1975, **8**, 301–309.

Howarth, R. The psychiatric care of children with life threatening illness. In L. Burton, (Ed.), *Care of the child facing death*. Boston: Routledge & Kegan Paul, 1974.

Howell, S. E. Psychiatric aspects of habilitation. *Pediatric Clinics of North America*, 1973, **20**, 203–219.

Humphrey, G. B., & Vore, D. A. Psychology and the oncology team. *Journal of Clinical Psychology*, 1974, **3**, 27–29.

Hunter, S., Russell, H., Russell, E., & Zimmerman, R. L. Control of fingertip temperature increases via biofeedback in learning-disabled and normal children. *Perceptual and Motor Skills*, 1976, **43**, 743–755.

Irwin, E. C., & McWilliams, B. J. Play therapy for children with cleft palates. *Children Today*, 1974, **3**, 18–22.

Jackson, R. H., & Terdal, L. Parent education within a pediatric practice. *Journal of Pediatric Psychology*, 1978, **3**, 2–5.

Johnson, D. L. *A parent education program for Mexican-American families*. An unpublished manuscript, University of Houston, 1976.

Johnson, M. R. Mental health interventions with medically ill children: A review of the literature, 1970–77. *Journal of Pediatric Psychology*, 1979, **4**, 147–164.

Johnson, M. R., Martin, B., Whitt, J. K., & Weisz, J. *Anxiety reduction through fantasy in chronically ill and normal children*. Paper presented at the meeting of the American Psychological Association, Montreal, September 1980.

Johnstone, C. Parental stress service—How it all began. *Journal of Clinical Child Psychology*, 1973, **2**, 45.

Kagen, L. B. Use of denial in adolescents with bone cancer. *Health and Social Work*, 1976, **1**, 71–87.

Kaplan, D. M., Smith, A., & Grobstein, R. School management of the seriously ill child. *Journal of School Health*, 1974, **44**, 250–254.

Kaslow, F. W., & Abrams, J. C. Differential diagnosis and treatment of the learning disabled child and his/her family. *Journal of Pediatric Psychology*, 1979, **4**, 253–264.

Kaslow, F. W., & Cooper, B. Family therapy with the learning disabled child and his/her family. *Journal of Marriage and Family Counseling*, 1978, **4**, 41–49.

Katz, E. R., Kellerman, J., Rigler, D., Williams, K. O., & Siegel, S. E. School intervention with pediatric cancer patients. *Journal of Pediatric Psychology,* 1977, **2,** 72–76.

Kauffman, J. M., & Vicente, A. R. Bringing in the sheaves: Observations on harvesting behavioral change in the field. *Journal of School Psychology,* 1972, **10,** 263–268.

Kazdin, A. E. Issues in behavior modification with mentally retarded persons. *American Journal of Mental Deficiency,* 1973, **78,** 134–140.

Keller, M., & Carlson, P. The use of symbolic modeling to promote social skills in preschool children with low levels of social responsiveness. *Child Development,* 1974, **45,** 912–919.

Kellerman, J., Rigler, D., Siegel, S. G., & Katz, E. R. Disease related communication and depression in pediatric cancer patients. *Journal of Pediatric Psychology,* 1977, **2,** 52–53.

Kempe, R. S., & Kempe, C. H. *Child abuse.* Cambridge, MA: Harvard University Press, 1978.

Kent, M. W., & Rolf, J. E. (Eds.) *Primary prevention of psychopathology,* Vol. 3. *Social competence in children.* Hanover, NH: University Press of New England, 1979.

Kimmel, H. D., & Kimmel, E. C. An instrumental conditioning method for the treatment of enuresis. *Journal of Behavior Therapy and Experimental Psychiatry,* 1970, **1,** 121–123.

Kingsley, R. G., & Shapiro, J. A comparison of three behavioral programs for the control of obesity in children. *Behavior Therapy,* 1977, **8,** 30–36.

Klaus, M. H., & Kennell, J. K. *Maternal-infant bonding.* St. Louis: Mosby, 1976.

Kohlberg, I. J., & Rothenberg, M. B. Comprehensive care following multiple life-threatening injuries. *American Journal of Diseases of Children,* 1970, **119,** 449–451.

Koocher, G. P. Talking with children about death. *American Journal of Orthopsychiatry,* 1974, **44,** 404–441.

Koocher, G. P., & Sallan, S. E. Pediatric oncology. In P. R. Magrab (Ed.), *Psychological management of pediatric problems,* Vol. 1. Baltimore: University Park Press, 1978.

Korsch, B. M., Fine, R. N., Grushkin, C. M., & Negrete, V. F. Experiences with children and their families during extended hemodialysis and kidney transplantation. *Pediatric Clinics of North America,* 1971, **18,** 625–637.

Krumboltz, J. D., & Krumboltz, H. B. *Changing children's behavior.* Englewood Cliffs, NJ: Prentice-Hall, 1972.

Kubler-Ross, E. The languages of dying. *Journal of Clinical Child Psychology,* 1974, **3,** 22–24.

Kunzelman, H. D. (Ed.). *Precision teaching.* Seattle: Special Child Publications, 1970.

LaGreca, A. M., & Mesibov, G. B. Social skills intervention with learning disabled children: Selecting skills and implementing training. *Journal of Clinical Child Psychology,* 1979, **8,** 234–241.

LaGreca, A. M., & Ottinger, D. R. Self-monitoring and relaxation training in the treatment of medically ordered exercises in a 12-year-old female. *Journal of Pediatric Psychology,* 1979, **4,** 49–54.

LaGreca, A. M., & Santogrossi, D. A. Social skills training with elementary school students: A behavioral group approach. *Journal of Consulting and Clinical Psychology,* 1980, **48,** 220–227.

Lansky, S. B. Childhood leukemia: The child psychiatrist as a member of the oncology team. *Journal of the American Academy of Child Psychiatry*, 1974, **13**, 499–508.

Lansky, S. B., Lowman, J. T., Vats, T., & Gyulay, J. School phobia in children with malignant neoplasms. *American Journal of Diseases of Children*, 1975, **129**, 42–46.

Lask, B., & Kirk, M. Childhood asthma: Family therapy as an adjunct to routine management. *Journal of Family Therapy*, 1979, **1**, 33–49.

LaVietes, R. Mental retardation: Psychological treatment. In B. B. Walnar, J. Egan, & A. O. Ross (Eds.), *Handbook of treatment of mental disorders in childhood and adolescence*. Englewood Cliffs, NJ: Prentice-Hall, 1978.

Lewis, S. A comparison of behavior therapy techniques in the reduction of fearful avoidance behavior. *Behavior Therapy*, 1974, **5**, 648–655.

Lewis, S. Considerations in setting up psychological consultation to a pediatric hematology-oncology team. *Journal of Clinical Child Psychology*, 1978, **7**, 21–22.

Lindsley, O. Teaching parents to modify their children's behavior. In L. E. Arnold (Ed.), *Helping parents to help their children*. New York: Brunner/Mazel, 1978.

Linn, S. Puppets & hospitalized children: Talking about feelings. *Journal of the Association for the Care of Children in Hospitals*, 1977, **5**, 5–11.

Linscheid, T. R. Disturbances of eating and feeding. In P. R. Magrab (Ed.), *Psychological management of pediatric problems*. Baltimore: University Park Press, 1978.

Linscheid, T. R., Oliver, J., Blyler, E., & Palmer, S. Brief hospitalization for the behavioral treatment of feeding problems in the developmentally disabled. *Journal of Pediatric Psychology*, 1978, **3**, 72–76.

Lott, G. Psychotherapy of the mentally retarded: Values and cautions. In F. J. Menolascino (Ed.), *Psychiatric approaches to mental retardation*. New York: Basic Books, 1970.

Lovaas, O. I. Program for establishment of speech in schizophrenic and autistic children. In J. K. Wing (Ed.), *Early childhood autism: Clinical, educational, and social aspects*. London: Pergamon Press, 1966.

Lovaas, O. I., & Koegel, R. L. Behavior therapy with autistic children. *Seventy-second yearbook of the National Society for the Study of Education*. Chicago: University of Chicago Press, 1973.

Luber, J. F., & Shouse, M. N. Use of biofeedback in the treatment of seizure disorders and hyperactivity. In B. B. Lahey & A. E. Kazdin (Eds.), *Advances in clinical child psychology*, Vol. 1. New York: Plenum Press, 1977.

Magrab, P. R. Psychological management and renal dialysis. *Journal of Clinical Child Psychology*, 1975, **4**, 38–40.

Magrab, P. R. & Papadopoulou, Z. L. Renal disease. In P. R. Magrab (Ed.), *Psychological management of pediatric problems*, Vol. 1. Baltimore: University Park Press, 1978.

Mahoney, M., & Thoresen, C. E. *Self-control: Power to the person*. Monterey, CA: Brooks/Cole, 1974.

Maisto, A. A., & German, M. L. Variables related to progress in a parent infant training program for high-risk infants. *Journal of Pediatric Psychology*, 1979, **4**, 409–419.

Maletzky, B. M. Behavior recording as a treatment: A brief note. *Behavior Therapy*, 1974, **5**, 107–111.

Marshall, G. R. Toilet training of an autistic eight-year-old through operant conditioning therapy: A case report. *Behaviour Research and Therapy*, 1966, **4**, 242–245.

McDonnell, L. Paraverbal therapy in pediatric cases with emotional complications. *American Journal of Orthopsychiatry*, 1979, **49,** 44–52.

McGuiness, T., & Glasser, W. Reality guidance. In L. E. Arnold (Ed.), *Helping parents help their children*. New York: Brunner/Mazel, 1978.

McInnis, T. Training and maintaining staff behaviors in residential treatment programs. In R. L. Patterson (Ed.), *Maintaining effective token economies*. Springfield, IL: Charles C. Thomas, 1976.

Meichenbaum, D. H., & Goodman, J. Training impulsive children to talk to themselves: A means of developing self-control. *Journal of Abnormal Psychology,* 1971, **77,** 115–126.

Melamed, B. G., & Siegel, L. J. Reduction of anxiety in children facing hospitalization and surgery by use of filmed modeling. *Journal of Consulting and Clinical Psychology,* 1975, **43,** 511–521.

Melamed, B. G., Weinstein, D., Hawes, R., & Katin-Borland, M. Reduction of fear-related dental management problems with use of filmed modeling. *Journal of the American Dental Association,* 1975, **90,** 822–826.

Mesibov, G. B. *Effectiveness of several intervention strategies with some common childrearing problems.* Paper presented at the meeting of the American Psychological Association, San Francisco, August 1977.

Mesibov, G. B., & Fontaine, J. Use of token and response cost systems in sports activities with pre-adolescent boys. *Pediatric Psychology,* 1975, **3,** 26–27.

Mesibov, G. B., Schroeder, C. S., & Wesson, L. Parental concerns about their children. *Journal of Pediatric Psychology,* 1977, **2,** 13–17.

Minuchin, S. *Families and family therapy.* Cambridge, MA: Harvard University Press, 1974.

Minuchin, S., Rosman, B. L., & Baker, L. *Psychosomatic families: Anorexia nervosa in context.* Cambridge, MA: Harvard University Press, 1978.

Moustakas, C. E. *Psychotherapy with children: The living relationship.* New York: Ballentine Books, 1959.

Mowrer, O. H., & Mowrer, W. M. Enuresis—A method for its study and treatment. *American Journal of Orthopsychiatry,* 1938, **8,** 436–459.

Munson, S. W. Family structure and the family's general adaptation to loss: Helping families deal with the death of a child. In O. J. Sahler (Ed.), *The child and death.* St. Louis: Mosby, 1978.

Murphy, L. B., & Frank, C. Prevention: The clinical psychologist. *Annual Review of Psychoogy,* 1979, **30,** 173–207.

Nay, W. R. Intra-institutional "roadblocks" to behavior modification programming. In D. Marholin II (Ed.), *Child behavior therapy.* New York: Gardner Press, 1978.

Neisworth, J. T., & Smith, R. M. An analysis and redefinition of "developmental disabilities". *Exceptional Children,* 1974, **40,** 345–347.

O'Connor, R. D. Modification of social withdrawal through symbolic modeling. *Journal of Applied Behavior Analysis,* 1969, **2,** 15–22.

Oden, S., & Asher, S. R. Coaching children in social skills for friendship making. *Child Development,* 1977, **48,** 495–506.

O'Leary, K. D. Establishing token programs in schools: Issues and problems. In D. Meyers,

R. Martin, & I. Hyman (Eds.), *School consultation: Readings about preventative techniques for pupil personnel workers*. Springfield, IL: Charles C. Thomas, 1977.

O'Malley, J. E., & Koocher, G. P. Psychological consultation to a pediatric oncology unit: Obstacles to effective intervention. *Journal of Pediatric Psychology*, 1977, **2**, 54–57.

Oremland, E. K., & Oremland, J. D. (Eds.). *The effects of hospitalization on children: Models for their case*. Springfield, IL: Charles C. Thomas, 1973.

Patenaude, A. F., Szymanski, L., & Rappaport, J. Psychological costs of bone marrow transplantation in children. *American Journal of Orthopsychiatry*, 1979, **49**, 409–422.

Patterson, G. R., & Gullion, M. E. *Living with children*. Champaign, IL: Research Press, 1968.

Petrillo, M., & Sanger, S. *Emotional care of hospitalized children*. Philadelphia: Lippincott, 1980.

Pihl, R. O., Parkes, M., & Stevens, R. Nonspecific interventions with learning disabled individuals. In R. M. Knights & D. J. Bakker (Eds.), *Treatment of hyperactive and learning disordered children: Current research*. Baltimore: University Park Press, 1980.

Pike, E. L. C.A.L.M.—A timely experiment in the prevention of child abuse. *Journal of Clinical Child Psychology*, 1973, **2**, 43–45.

Plank, E. N., & Horwood, C. Leg amputation in a four-year-old: Reactions of the child, her family and the staff. In *An anthology of the psychoanalytic study of the child: Physical illness and handicap in childhood*. New Haven: Yale University Press, 1977.

Powell, L. The effect of extra stimulation and maternal involvement on the development of low-birth-weight infants and on maternal behavior. *Child Development*, 1974, **45**, 106–113.

Poznanski, E. O. The hospitalized child. In J. D. Noshpitz (Ed.), *Basic handbook of child psychiatry*, Vol. 3. New York: Basic Books, 1979.

Prugh, D. G., & Eckhardt, L. O. Psychophysiological disorders. In J. D. Noshpitz (Ed.), *Basic handbook of child psychiatry*, Vol. 3. New York: Basic Books, 1979.

Rae, W. A., & Stieber, D. A. Plant play therapy: Growth through growth. *Journal of Pediatric Psychology*, 1976, **1**, 18–20.

Ramey, C. T., Holmberg, M. C., Sparling, J. J., & Collier, A. M. An introduction to the Carolina Abecedarian project. In B. M. Caldwell & D. J. Stedman (Eds.), *Infant education for handicapped children*. New York: Walker, 1977.

Rathjen, D., Hiniker, A., & Rathjen, E. *Incorporation of behavioral techniques in a game format to teach children social skills*. Paper presented at the meeting of the Association for Advancement of Behavior Therapy. New York, December 1976.

Repp, A. C., & Deitz, D. E. Reducing inappropriate behaviors in classrooms and in individual sessions through DRO schedules of reinforcement. *Mental Retardation*, 1976, **14**, 11–15.

Rincover, A., & Koegel, R. L. Treatment of psychotic children in a classroom environment: II. Individualized instruction in a group. *Journal of Abnormal Child Psychology*, 1977, **5**, 123–136.

Ritter, B. Eliminating excessive fears of the environment through contact desensitization. In J. B. Krumboltz & C. E. Thoresen (Eds.), *Behavioral counseling: Cases and techniques*. New York: Holt, Rinehart & Winston, 1969.

Roberts, M. C., & Horner, M. M. A comprehensive intervention for failure-to-thrive. *Journal of Clinical Child Psychology,* 1979, **8,** 10–14.

Robertson, M., & Barford, F. Story making in psychotherapy with a chronically ill child. *Psychotherapy: Theory, Research, Practice,* 1970, **7,** 104–107.

Robinson, N. M., & Robinson, H. B. *The mentally retarded child.* New York: McGraw-Hill, 1976.

Rolf, J. E., & Hasazi, J. E. Identification of preschool children at risk and some guidelines for primary intervention. In G. W. Albee & J. M. Joffe (Eds.), *Primary prevention of psychopathology,* Vol. 1. Hanover, NH: University Press of New England, 1977.

Ross, D. M., & Ross, S. A. *Hyperactivity: Research, theory, and action.* New York: Wiley, 1976.

Ross, D. M., Ross, S. A., & Evans, T. A. The modification of extreme social withdrawal by modeling with guided practice. *Journal of Behavior Therapy and Experimental Psychiatry,* 1971, **2,** 273–279.

Rothenberg, M. B. The unholy trinity—Activity, authority and magic. *Clinical Pediatrics,* 1974, **13,** 870–874.

Routh, D. K. The short history of pediatric psychology. *Journal of Clinical Child Psychology,* 1975, **4,** 6–8.

Routh, D. K. Postdoctoral training in pediatric psychology. *Professional Psychology,* 1977, **8,** 245–250.

Russell, H. L., & Carter, J. L. Biofeedback training with children: Consultation, questions, applications and alternatives. *Journal of Clinical Child Psychology,* 1978, **7,** 23–25.

Safer, D. J., & Allen, R. P. *Hyperactive children: Diagnosis & management.* Baltimore: University Park Press, 1976.

Salhoot, J. T. The use of two group methods with severely disabled persons. In R. E. Hardy & J. G. Cull (Eds.), *Group counseling and therapy techniques in special settings.* Springfield, IL: Charles C. Thomas, 1974.

Salk, L. *What every child would like his parents to know.* New York: Warner, 1973.

Salk, L. Parenthood education: The responsibility of the pediatric psychologist. *Journal of Clinical Child Psychology,* 1975, **4,** 23–25.

Sarason, I. G., & Ganzer, V. J. Modeling and group discussion in the rehabilitation of juvenile delinquents. *Journal of Counseling Psychology,* 1973, **20,** 442–449.

Scarr-Salapatek, S., & Williams, M. L. The effects of early stimulation on low birth weight infants. *Child Development,* 1973, **44,** 94–101.

Schafer, D. S., & Maersh, M. S. (Eds.), *Developmental programming for infants and young children.* Ann Arbor: University of Michigan Press, 1977.

Schinke, S. P., & Wong, S. E. Evaluation of staff training in group homes for retarded persons. *American Journal of Mental Deficiency,* 1977, **82,** 130–136.

Schneider, M., & Robin, A. *Turtle Manual.* Unpublished manuscript, State University of New York at Stony Brook, 1975.

Schneider, S. F. Psychology and general health: Prospects and pitfalls. *Journal of Clinical Child Psychology,* 1978, **7,** 5–7.

Schowalter, J. E. The utilization of child psychiatry on a pediatric adolescent ward. *Journal of the American Academy of Child Psychiatry.* 1971, **10,** 684–699.

Schowalter, J. E. Hospital consultation as therapy. In J. D. Noshpitz (Ed.), *Basic handbook of child psychiatry,* Vol. 3. New York: Basic Books, 1979.

Schreibman, L., & Koegel, R. L. Autism: A defeatable horror. *Psychology Today,* 1975, **8,** 61–67.

Schroeder, C. S. *The psychologists' role in P.L. 94–142: Consultation strategies with peer groups of handicapped children.* Paper presented at the meeting of the American Psychological Association, Toronto, August 1978.

Schroeder, C. S. Psychologists in a private pediatric practice. *Journal of Pediatric Psychology,* 1979, **4,** 5–18.

Schroeder, C. S., & Schroeder, S. R. *A behavioral model to school consultation.* Paper presented at the meeting of the American Association on Mental Deficiency, Miami, May 1979.

Schroeder, S. R., Mulick, J. A., & Schroeder, C. S. Management of severe behavior problems of the retarded. In M. R. Ellis (Ed.), *Handbook of mental deficiency,* 2nd ed., New York: Erlbaum Associates, 1980.

Schroeder, S. R., Rojahn, J., & Mulick, J. A. Ecobehavioral organization of developmental day care for the chronically self-injurious. *Journal of Pediatric Psychology,* 1978, **3,** 81–88.

Seligman, R. A psychiatric classification system for burned children. *American Journal of Psychiatry,* 1974, **131,** 41–46.

Seligman, R. Emotional responses to burns in children. In J. G. Howells (Ed.), *Modern perspectives in the psychiatric aspects of surgery.* NewYork: Brunner/Mazel, 1976.

Shaw, W. J., & Walker, C. E. Use of relaxation in the short-term treatment of fetishistic behavior: An exploratory case study. *Journal of Pediatric Psychology,* 1979, **4,** 403–407.

Sheridan, M. S. Talk time for hospitalized children. *Social Work,* 1975, **20,** 40–44.

Slivkin, S. E., & Bernstein, N. R. Group approaches to treating retarded adolescents. In F. J. Menolascino (Ed.), *Psychiatric approaches to mental retardation.* New York: Basic Books, 1970.

Sourkes, B. Facilitating family coping with childhood cancer. *Journal of Pediatric Psychology,* 1977, **2,** 65–67.

Spinetta, J. J. The dying child's awareness of death: A review. *Psychological Bulletin,* 1974, **81,** 256–260.

Spinetta, J. J. Adjustment in children with cancer. *Journal of Pediatric Psychology,* 1977, **2,** 49–51.

Spivack, G., & Shure, M. B. *Social adjustment of young children.* San Francisco: Jossey-Bass, 1974.

Spock, B. *The common sense book of baby and child care.* New York: Duell, Sloane, & Pierce, 1946.

Stabler, B. Emerging models of psychologist-pediatrician liaison. *Journal of Pediatric Psychology,* 1979, **4,** 307–313.

Stacey, C. L., & DeMartino, M. F. (Eds.). *Counseling & Psychotherapy with the mentally retarded.* Glencoe, IL: Free Press, 1957.

Starfield B. Functional bladder capacity in enuretic and nonenuretic children. *Journal of Pediatrics,* 1967, **70,** 777–781.

Staub, E. The use of role playing and induction in children's learning of helping and sharing behavior. *Child Development*, 1971, **42**, 805–816.

Stephen, C., Stephano, S., & Talkington, L. Use of modeling in survival skill training with educable mentally retarded. *Training School Bulletin*, 1973, **70**, 63–68.

Sternlicht, M. Psychotherapy techniques useful with the mentally retarded. *Psychiatric Quarterly*, 1965, **39**, 84–90.

Tate, B. G., & Baroff, G. S. Aversive control of self-injurious behavior in a psychotic boy. *Behaviour Research and Therapy*, 1966, **4**, 281–287.

Thelen, M. H., Fry, R. A., Dollinger, S. J., & Paul, S. C. Use of videotaped models to improve the interpersonal adjustment of delinquents. *Journal of Consulting and Clinical Psychology*, 1976, **44**, 492.

Thomas, L. Patient groups for children who have cancer. In J. L. Schulman & M. J. Kupst (Eds.), *The child with cancer*. Springfield, IL: Charles C. Thomas, 1980.

Tjossem, T. D. (Ed.) *Intervention strategies for high risk infants and young children*. Baltimore: University Park Press, 1976.

Toker, E. Psychiatric aspects of cardiac surgery in a child. *Journal of the American Academy of Child Psychiatry*, 1971, 10, 156–186.

Vernick, J. Meaningful communication with the fatally ill child. In E. J. Anthony & C. Koupernick (Eds.), *The child in his family*, Vol. 2. *The impact of disease and death*. New York: Wiley, 1973.

Vernon, D. T. Use of modeling to modify children's responses to a natural, potentially stressful situation. *Journal of Applied Psychology*, 1973, **58**, 351–356.

Vore, D., & Wright, L. Psychological management of the family and the dying child. In R. E. Hardy & J. G. Gull (Eds.), *Therapeutic needs of the family: Problems, description and therapeutic approaches*. Springfield, IL: Charles C. Thomas, 1974.

Walker, C. E. Toilet training, enuresis, encopresis. In P. R. Magrab (Ed.), *Psychological management of pediatric problems*, Vol. 1. Baltimore: University Park Press, 1978.

Wallerstein, J. S., & Kelly, J. Divorce counseling: A community service for families in the midst of divorce. *American Journal of Orthopsychiatry*, 1977, **47**, 4–22.

Wheeler, M. E., & Hess, K. W. Treatment of juvenile obesity by successive approximation control of eating. *Journal of Behavior Therapy and Experimental Psychiatry*, 1976, **7**, 235–241.

White, B. L. *The first three years of life*. Englewood Cliffs, NJ: Prentice-Hall, 1975.

Williams, G. J. Child abuse. In P. R. Magrab (Ed.), *Psychological management of pediatric problems*, Vol. 2. Baltimore: University Park Press, 1978.

Willis, D. J. Preventive model for child abuse. *Journal of Pediatric Psychology*, 1976, **1**, 98.

Winder, A., & Medalie, M. Support for growth in cystic fibrosis teenagers. In P. Patterson, C. Denning, & A. Kutscher (Eds.), *Psychosocial aspects of cystic fibrosis*. New York: Foundation of Thanatology, 1973.

Wolf, M. M., Risley, T. R., & Mees, H. Application of operant conditioning procedures to the behavior problems of an autistic child. *Behaviour Research and Therapy*, 1964, **1**, 305–312.

Woods, T. L. Comments on the dynamics and treatment of disfigured children. *Clinical Social Work Journal*, 1975, **3**, 16–23.

Woodward, K. L., & Malamud, P. The parent gap. *Newsweek*, September 22, 1975, pp. 48–56.

Wright, L. Psychology as a health profession. *Clinical Psychologist,* 1976, **29,** 16−19.

Wright, L. Health care psychology: Prospects for the well-being of children. *American Psychologist,* 1979, **34,** 1001−1006. (a)

Wright, L. *Parent power.* New York: Psychological Dimensions, 1979. (b)

Wright, L., Schaefer, A. B., & Solomons, G. *Encyclopedia of pediatric psychology.* Baltimore: University Park Press, 1979.

Wright, L., & Walker, C. E. Behavioral treatment of encopresis. *Journal of Pediatric Psychology,* 1976, **1,** 35−37.

Zigler, E., & Hunsinger, S. Our neglected children. *Yale Alumni Magazine,* February 6, 1978, p. 41.

Zigler, E., & Muenchow, S. Mainstreaming: The proof is in the implementation. *American Psychologist,* 1979, **34,** 993−996.

Zlutnick, S., Mayville, W. J., & Moffat, S. Modification of seizure disorders: The interruption of behavioral chains. *Journal of Applied Behavior Analysis,* 1975, **8,** 1−12.

CHAPTER 5

The Pediatric Psychologist's Role in Catastrophic Illness: Research and Clinical Issues

JOHN J. SPINETTA
Elaine S. Elliott
James S. Hennessey
Vrinda S. Knapp
John P. Sheposh
Steven N. Sparta
Richard P. Sprigle

THE ROLE OF THE PEDIATRIC PSYCHOLOGIST[1]

The pediatric psychologist is in a unique position not shared by other health care professionals. While some physicians, nurses, social workers, and other allied health care professionals working with children with catastrophic illness are trained at the doctoral level in research methodology, and while it has become more common for doctoral level professionals in related disciplines to conduct psychosocial research in areas of behavioral pediatrics, the primary mandate of each of the other disciplines is not research, but service. Thus, while many doctoral level nurses have made excellent contributions to the field of catastrophic childhood illness (Martinson, 1976; Waechter, 1971), nurses by their profession are trained in service as their primary function. The same is true for social work. Outstanding contributions of a research nature have been made in the field of behavioral pediatrics by doctoral level social workers (Kaplan, Smith, Grobstein, & Fishman, 1973; Kaplan, Grobstein, & Smith, 1976). However, the primary function for which the social worker is trained is that of service. Similarly, while many of the early contributions to the field of behavioral pediatrics were made and continue to be made by research-oriented psychiatrists (Binger Ablin, Feuerstein, Kushner,

[1]This section was prepared by John J. Spinetta.

Zoger, & Mikkelsen, 1969; Friedman, Chodoff, Mason, & Hamburg, 1963; Schowalter, 1970), the primary function of the psychiatrist is service. The psychologist is the sole member of the pediatric health care team whose primary training, function, and professional role is research.

As a research clinician the pediatric psychologist has a unique role to play in a health care team's efforts to help children in the hospital—most notably those in critical life situations—to deal with their illnesses.

While this section will address certain catastrophic life situations (near-drowning, child abuse, neurological trauma, cancer, and cystic fibrosis), there are a myriad of other areas in child care in which a psychologist's research and clinical expertise can be helpful. These areas are discussed in detail in other sections of this book. An earlier two-volume series edited by one of the contributors to the present book, Phyllis Magrab (1978), covers such other areas as juvenile diabetes, renal disese, inherited disorders, birth traumas, toilet training, disturbances of eating and feeding, hyperactivity, seizure disorders, dyslexia, learning disabilities, hearing deficits, mental retardation, and the effects of divorce on a child.

It is not in consultation as an outsider, but in full working relationship on a health care team that psychologists can best bring to the fore their unique training and expertise, both as researchers and as clinicians. It is in this role that pediatric psychologists will be in a position to conduct rigorously designed research within the context of the health care unit which they serve.

Because it is so necessary for psychologists to become well trained in a particular medical area before they can conduct meaningful research and make relevant clinical judgments regarding a particular case, this chapter will treat only five areas of concern, and will do so in depth. Each section will model how a hospital-based pediatric psychologist can bring to bear both research and clinical training in dealing with a situation-specific and well-defined issue. This chapter of the book will detail specific applications of the psychologist's expertise and training in situations involving the emergency room (near-drowning and child abuse cases), the rehabilitation unit (cases of neurological trauma), and the outpatient setting (cases involving cancer and cystic fibrosis).

THE PEDIATRIC PSYCHOLOGIST AS ETHICIST-COUNSELOR: GUARDING PARENTAL AND CHILD RIGHTS IN CASES OF NEAR-DROWNING[2]

Recent Changes in Attitudes toward Life and Death Issues

In a 1975 volume entitled *The Sanctity of Social Life,* Crane observed that technology not only has had a pervasive effect on our daily lives but has also altered the process of dying. With the advent of new techniques which permit the physician

[2]This section was prepared by John J. Spinetta, John P. Sheposh, and Elaine S. Elliott.

to restore cardiac and respiratory functioning of patients and maintain these individuals for extended periods of time, the physician is increasingly faced with decisions involving ethical and moral considerations regarding sustaining the physical life functions of patients who have suffered brain death (Turbo, 1973).

Presently, there is no clear definition of death (Maguire, 1974). Beecher (1968) has proposed several criteria that define death: cellular criteria, physiological criteria (cessation of respiration and heartbeat), and social criteria (capacity to return to a reasonably normal life). A review of the studies that have attempted to identify the factors that affect physicians' decisions to sustain life suggests that consideration other than the physiological definition of death influence their decisions. Sudnow (1967) found that patients who were judged by medical personnel as greater contributors to society were more likely to receive heroic life-sustaining treatment. Crane's study (1975) of 3000 physicians revealed that a doctor's decision to actively treat a patient depended not only on physiological definitions of illness but also on the patient's capacity to interact with others. More intense treatment was recommended for some cases than others. The physically diagnosed salvageable patient was more likely to be actively treated than the severely brain damaged salvageable patient. The findings from Crane's study underscore the disparity between the traditional medical ethic concerning the treatment of such cases and the actual behavior of many physicians.

The influence of the values and attitudes of the patient's family on the physician's treatment decision obviously cannot be discounted. This is particularly true when the patient is a child. Crane (1975) acknowledged the importance of the attitude of the family in treatment decisions. In actual practice it is not always clear who makes the decision to use extraordinary measures. A pediatrician commented on Crane's questions concerning the role of physicians in such situations:

> [The] decision-making process may be so interwoven with the education of the parents and dealing with the parents' confused sense of responsibility for decision-making and underlying guilt that it is unclear exactly when and by whom the decisions were made, even though the physician then announced them as being his own.

Recently, there have also been increasing demands by patients and families to exercise their rights during treatment decisions. With growing public awareness of the issues surrounding death and dying, laypersons are unwilling to accept without question the doctor's judgment in such cases (Freidson, 1974; Reeder, 1972). Patients and families are beginning to demand a greater voice with doctors in life-sustaining decisions.

The extent to which physicians engage laypersons in the decisions to use life-sustaining extraordinary techniques further complicates a complex and most difficult decision. Cases involving children are especially difficult since others must obviously act on their behalf. In such cases, ethical and legal considerations dictate informed parental participation in the decision-making process. However, ethical concerns prevent the physician from overwhelming parents with information regarding the decision to use extraordinary means while they are emotionally shaken. It is in this context that the role of the pediatric psychologist becomes critical.

The case of near-drowning of children effectively demonstrates the complexities of the issues involved. Each year hundreds of children are pulled unconscious and not breathing from swimming pools. Paramedics are called, emergency resuscitation is applied, and the child is transferred to the emergency room still unconscious but with breathing restored. Critical decisions must be made by the physician and family at this point. Will this child ever regain full and effective use of his preincidence function? Will he remain in a comatose state for a period of time and then die?

How prepared are parents at the point of entry into the emergency room to make critical decisions regarding extraordinary efforts to be used in sustaining their child's life? Is informed consentient decision at all possible under such circumstances? It is at this critical point of entry of the child and parents into the emergency room that a pediatric psychologist, who is a full and functional member of the emergency medical team, can be of service to the child and family. This section summarizes two studies by the authors related to this issue, and draws conclusions relevant to pediatric psychologists who find themselves in such situations.

Two Studies

The following two studies by the authors of this section address the questions of the use of heroic life-sustaining measures in near-drowning cases, and in particular, the question of parental participation in such a decision. The first study is a series of interviews with parents whose children suffered extensive physiological insult from near-drowning, which necessitated the employment of life-sustaining measures. The second study is a survey of physicians' attitudes on this issue. Both studies are geared to understanding the pediatric psychologist's function, and the role he or she can play in increasing informed parental participation in decisions regarding the measures used to sustain their child's life. The data are intended primarily as illustrations of the problem, laying the groundwork for more extensive and controlled studies of the newly emerging social patterns on issues related to life and death. Broad social changes of the past decade (technological advances, informed consumerism regarding medical care, changing attitudes toward the sanctity of human life) require new approaches to the issue of the use of extraordinary life-sustaining measures. Because of the relative novelty of the circumstances, old norms need to be reworked and reapplied to the changing situations. Newly applied norms are required which would help both the physician and the parents make a more informed judgment regarding expected, appropriate, and ethical behavior in such circumstances.

In cases of near-drowning, parents are typically in such an emotional state upon their arrival at the emergency room that their ability to make a reasoned judgment is seriously in question. It is at this point that a pediatric psychologist assigned to the emergency room as a regular member of the medical emergency team, and who is experienced in such emergencies, is in a unique position to safeguard both the child's right to life and the parents' right to full participation in the decision of whether or not to sustain the life of their child.

The two studies reported in this chapter are geared to the development of viable hypotheses for future studies which would address the issue of the establishment of new norms. Given the present variability in both physician and parent responses in such life-and-death situations, parents need to become full participants in the decision of whether or not their child's life can be restored to full and effective functioning. If they determine that it cannot, then the parents need to know their moral, ethical, and legal rights and responsibilities regarding the termination of their child's life at that point in the emergency room. They need to know their rights and the child's rights regarding the decision not to resuscitate.

As a researcher-clinician, the pediatric psyhologist can play a vital role both in counseling that particular family and physician in the individual situation, and in conducting a highly reliable and well-designed study that would lead to a clarification of the issue in the broader psychosocial context of ethical norms regarding the sanctity of human life and the application of such norms in similar situations.

Study One: The Parents

The first phase of the study was undertaken to obtain insight into the experiences of 10 families whose children were near-drowning victims who, for a period of months, remained in a continual comatose state. The question asked of the parents was what they feel should be their role in the decision-making process, if and when the physicians in the emergency rooms and in the intensive care units feel medically certain that a decision becomes appropriate invoving a choice as to whether the life of the child should be prolonged by extraordinary means.

SUBJECTS AND METHOD

The subjects in the present study were parents whose children were near-drowning victims who after resuscitation were in a comatose state. The families were interviewed with an open-ended, semistructured interview schedule specifically designed for the study. Of the families who consented to informed participation in the study, five had children who were still alive, while five families had children who had died after a period of time in a comatose state. Of the former, two of the children recovered sufficiently from the coma to engage in some bodily activities. One of the two, though remaining functionally retarded, became ambulatory. Of the latter five, four of the children had been comatose less than one week prior to death; one had survived over three years prior to death.

After the initial contact by the hospital personnel, two interviewers, one male and one female, specifically trained for the task, made an appointment with the parents for the purpose of interviewing them. Medical records of each family were carefully reviewed prior to the contact. The interviewers spoke with physicians, nurses, and psychosocial personnel involved in each specific case. Both interviewers participated in each of the interview sessions. The interviews were tape-recorded with the permission of the parents, and later transcribed for content analysis.

RESULTS

Parental Involvement.   Table 1 presents responses of parents to three items regarding their involvement in the decision-making process. The first item asked what the parents would have decided had they been given a choice. Six families said that they would have chosen to sustain life by extraordinary efforts. Two of the sets of parents were ambivalent about whether they would have chosen to sustain their child in a probably comatose state as opposed to allowing nature to take its course, and the remaining two families would have opted for the removal of life support systems.

Quality of Life.   The second item concerned sustaining life regardless of the quality of that life. Four of the families felt that they would have opted for life even if there were little or no hope for eventual recovery.

Parent's Reasons for Parental Involvement.   The third item in the taped interview was the parents' views toward parental involvement and some of their conclusions regarding their role and that of the physician. One mother who was opposed to unilateral action, no resuscitation, on the part of the physicians stated:

> I think it would be very wrong for the doctors to decide to terminate a child instead of helping them. It is not meant for them to judge. I think their job is to help the child. They may be letting a child's life go who might pull out of it better than they think. It would be a very wrong, inhuman thing to do.

In a similar vein, another parent stated, "Nobody has more right to make a decision about your child than you do." In another interview, a father stated:

> The initial decision to revive the child is the doctors' decision. However, after parents know the child can go on his own or live with the help of the machine or whatever, at that point the parents should be consulted.

Another father responded:

> I think as far as we were concerned, the final decision is with us. All the doctor can do is give us his knowledge of what has transpired and the outlook. Then it should be

Table 1.   Parental Responses Regarding The Decision-Making Process[a]

	Child alive at time of interview				Child deceased at time of interview				
If you had been given a choice at the time would you have decided to sustain life?	A	Y	Y	Y	Y	Y	A	N	N	Y
Would you choose life, regardless of the quality?	N	Y	N	Y	N	Y	N	N	Y	N
Should the family be involved in the decision-making process?	A	Y	Y	Y_w	Y	Y	A	Y	Y	Y_w

[a]Y = yes; A = ambivalent; N = no; Y_w = weak.

strictly up to us. Hopefully, most parents can make the right decision for all parties concerned. They should rely heavily on what the doctor says, because he's the one who knows the medical implications, but the parents should be the ones to make the decision.

One of the parents who responded equivocally stated:

I think doctors should consult the family because the doctors don't have to live with the decision. The parents are thinking from the heart while the doctors are thinking from a practical standpoint of what's good for the general public.

Another parent stated:

I guess that parents are the only ones that can decide, but somehow it doesn't seem right to me that you can decide whether or not you just turn off somebody's life and that's all they have. I really don't think I could make that decision. I think I would know that's probably the best but I couldn't do it.

Another mother whose child was in a comatose state for an extended period of time, reflecting on the dilemma of the withdrawal of extraordinary life-sustaining measures, stated:

I never felt it would be better for him to die. He still had life. As long as he had life it was important to him.

One mother who expressed ambivalence with respect to parental involvement cited parents' lack of emotional readiness and competence:

At the time I don't think a parent is emotionally prepared to deal with that. They don't really know what is going on in the treatment room, and it's all happening so fast the doctors really don't have time to ask the parent's opinions. That's how it was for us. That's all I have to go on. I really don't think the parents could deal with that question. I think the doctors have more knowledge than any parent unless a parent has gone through med school or nursing or something. The little bit I knew really scared me. You know, I thought my son had died, which he had. The doctor came out and told me that he would live. He wouldn't be the same little boy that we had had, but I really didn't know what they meant.

A fourth family spoke of the reluctance of the parents to make such an irreversible decision as the withdrawal of extraordinary life-sustaining measures. The mother stated:

That's pretty hard. I probably would have rationalized that the best thing to do would be to take her off the supports, but I don't know if I could make the decision or not. I mean it's really hard to ask a mother to do so. There might be one chance in 10 million that if she stayed like that she would recover, but that's a chance your're pretty willing to take when it's your own child.

The following is the comment of a mother who had expressed reservations about involving parents in the decision:

I know I had it pounded into me that a doctor is trained to save lives and that is why they go through so much to resuscitate, but I have the feeling, too, that they know whose child is not going to have that much of a life. So somewhere along the line there's got to be a change. I don't see how it's going to just go on and on. When a child is born handicapped or whatever that's something that doctors and parents are more or less faced with from the very beginning. To resuscitate a child to just lay there for the rest of his life, I can't see any point in it.

Finally, one father expressed concern as to how the physicians themselves must react to the decision-making process:

I think that the doctor is probably more capable medically, but then I am worried that he becomes callous after the incident develops. I don't think you could find a person or doctor that is strong enough to make too many of these decisions and still be a doctor.

The interviews illustrate the ideosyncratic character of parents' views toward this dilemma and suggest that parents feel a human concern for difficulties faced by the physicians themselves in this life-and-death decision. None of the families suggested that physicians abrogate their role as the medical expert. On the contrary, the parents stated that the integrity of the physicians' role as medical expert must be maintained. While supporting the physicians in their medical role, the parents felt that such a broad human question demands the participation of the parents in a matter so much within their realm of responsibility and concern. The theme expressed throughout all of the interviews was that the parents have a compelling commitment to their particular child's life which is part and parcel of the parenting role itself and which is uniquely tied to the specific child in question. It must be stressed that the parents felt their input was necessary only after the physician had done all that she or he could do medically to resuscitate the child. Life itself is the primary issue for the parents. The quality of that life remains secondary.

The findings have implications for conclusions about the involvement of parents in cases which necessitate extraordinary life-sustaining measures. Although the number of families participating in the study was small, the information gathered can stimulate further dialogue and lead to future studies using a wider population base. It is clear from the responses to the questionnaires that the issue of parental participation in the decision-making process regarding the use of extraordinary life-sustaining efforts remains a controversial and most complex issue.

It is important to emphasize the fact that the parents interviewed were parents whose child at the time of the interview either had died or had undergone severe physiological damage because of the drowning incident. The parents' response to parental participation in the decision-making process was thoughtful and informed. Because they had direct experience, the parents recognized problems attendant to this situation. Despite these concerns and the pain involved in the parents' participation in the decision-making process, the majority felt that they should nevertheless be involved in such a situation. Whether their child had died or was still alive had no systematic effect on the parents' replies to this question.

Study Two: The Physician

The second phase of the study was a survey of physicians regarding the decision to use life-sustaining extraordinary means in the case of a child who was a near-drowning victim. All physicians contacted for the survey were living and practicing in San Diego County at the time of the study. Because of its temperate climate and large number of private swimming pools, this area is particularly prone to fresh-water-related accidents. One drawback with restricting the sample to this specific geographic area is that generalization of findings is constrained. However, the study is designed as exploratory, and results are offered as suggestive of areas for further, more detailed research.

METHOD

Instrument.   A 32-item questionnaire was devised to obtain systematic information about variables influencing physicians' attitudes toward parental involvement and toward the use of extraordinary means. The questionnaire included the following detailed case history of a child in a near-drowning incident.

> A three-year-old child with residuals of fresh water drowning is brought to the emergency room in an ambulance. Attempts made to resuscitate the child at the scene are unsuccessful. The father indicates that the child must have been in the water for approximately five minutes and that an estimated fifteen minutes have elapsed between time of discovery and time of arrival at the hospital. The heart is started in the emergency room and the child is placed on a respirator. The child is limp, cyanotic, and in a vigil state. His pupils are fixed and dilated. He is comatose with no response to deep pain. The electroencephalograph is diffusely abnormal with disturbed background. A decision as to whether or not to continue extraordinary measures to keep the child alive must be made.

The case was designed to include the specific medical information necessary for the physician's full understanding of the child's condition. The inclusion of an active but normal EEG was potentially more problematic for the physician since there are no clear guidelines for forming a decision in this case in contrast to that where the EEG is flat (Ad Hoc Committee of the Harvard Medical School, 1968). Professionals were asked to respond to questions regarding the case. Items in the questionnaire were devised in four clusters: (1) items assessing the physician's general attitude toward the use of extraordinary measures; (2) items assessing the role of parental needs, beliefs, and understanding in influencing the physician's attitude toward participative decision making; (3) items related to assessing the impersonal demands of the traditional medical norms, namely that the decision to use extraordinary means should be based solely on medical criteria; and (4) items assessing the physician's attitude toward parental involvement.

Subjects and Procedure.   The department heads of pediatrics and the heads of the emergency rooms in five San Diego County hospitals were contacted, given questionnaires, and asked to distribute these to physicians affiliated with the respective hospitals. Of the 180 questionnaires given out to physicians, a total of 101 were returned (58 from pediatricians, 19 from neurologists, and 24 from emergency room physicians). The majority of the respondents were married males, were at the time residents or full-time physicians on hospital staff, and had received their medical degrees after 1960.

RESULTS

Table 2 summarizes the physicians' responses to several of the questionnaire items. These data illustrate the absence of clear-cut expectations on the part of physicians in such instances. First, with reference to the use of extraordinary measures to sustain the lives of children in cases such as those described in the case study, it can be seen from Table 2 that physicians' opinions were split: 50% were in favor while 48% were opposed. Only 11% of the physicians reported that their hospitals have guidelines dealing with the use of life-sustaining measures. When asked if an ethics board was needed to deal with families in such situations, the physicians revealed a great deal of variability in the responses.

The fact that only 8% of the respondents expressed strong agreement with the statement that the decision to use extraordinary means should be based solely on medical criteria suggests that the physicians recognize that other factors must be taken into account in such decisions. A high proportion of the respondents (69%) regarded parental personal and religious beliefs as important to the decision. Regarding the question concerning the extent to which parents should be fully and actively involved in the decision to use extraordinary life-sustaining measures, 58% of the respondents indicated that parents should be accorded a high level of involvement.

Some differences were evident across specialties. One-way analyses of variance on the items revealed consistent differences between pediatricians and the other two specialties. Pediatricians saw a greater need for an ethics board $F(2,96) = 3.06, p < .01$; they placed greater importance on parents' personal and religious beliefs, $F(2,94) = 3.14, p < .05$; and they agreed to a lesser degree that the decision should be based solely on medical criteria, $F(2,96) = 6.05, p < .01$.

The findings of this study can be summarized as follows:

1. Physicians in our sample did not have a uniform view concerning the use of extraordinary measures in cases such as the one described above.
2. There was a difference of opinion as to whether such decisions should be based solely on medical criteria.
3. Differences were observed across specialties with pediatricians differing from the other two specialties regarding the entry of extramedical criteria into the decision-making process.

Physicians' Comments. Physicians were asked to write comments on their questionnaires. Some common themes emerged when these comments were reviewed.

THE CLINICAL MENTALITY.   One recurring theme which emerged was the physician's concern with the particular, individual case rather than with statistical units (Freidson, 1974). One physician wrote:

> Clear-cut cases are just that. As usual, the borderline cases require wisdom. This must, of course, be dependent on each individual case. This can't be taught or given through a knowledge of statistics, but must usually involve painful empathy on the physician's part to be effective.

Table 2.   Percentages and Frequencies[a] of General Attitude Responses

Item	Total percentage (n/101)
M.D.'s acceptance of extraordinary measures	
Pro	50 (51)
Con	48 (48)
NR[b]	2 (2)
Hospital in which M.D. practices has guidelines concerning extraordinary measures	
Yes	11 (11)
No	85 (86)
NR	4 (4)
Need for ethics board	
Strongly agree	9 (9)
Agree	23 (23)
Somewhat agree	27 (28)
Disagree	22 (22)
Strongly disagree	17 (17)
NR	2 (2)
Decision should be based solely on medical criteria	
Strongly agree	8 (8)
Agree	29 (30)
Somewhat agree	26 (26)
Disagree	25 (25)
Strongly disagree	10 (10)
NR	2 (2)
Importance of parental religious beliefs vis-à-vis parental participation	
Very much (utmost) importance	22 (22)
Much importance	47 (48)
Some importance	22 (22)
Little importance	0 (0)
No importance	5 (5)
NR	4 (4)
Extent to which parents should be involved	
Very much (utmost) involvement	17 (17)
Much involvement	41 (42)
Some involvement	26 (26)
Little involvement	10 (10)
No involvement	4 (4)
NR	2 (2)

[a]Frequencies, in parentheses, are similar to percentages, because of a subject population with an N of 101.
[b]NR = no response.

An emergency room physician commented:

> Because each family must be dealt with individually, development of a "protocol" or impersonal board of review seems unlikely to reduce their stress or help in their grief reaction.

Another physician, who disagreed with the notion of a formal educational program pertaining to these complex cases, commented:

We must treat patients as individuals and not as units in a protocol. The doctor-patient relationship should decide the course of events.

THE EXCEPTIONAL CASE.   Another theme which related to the physician's emphasis on idiosyncrasy was the physician's awareness of the exceptional case. Responses alluded to the physician's personal experience or a colleague's experience with a particular case which colored the doctor's attitude toward all similar cases. Usually it involved the remarkable recovery of a patient who had been considered past help. For example, one pediatrician wrote:

> It is difficult to decide what are extraordinary measures and in addition it is often difficult to predict prognosis. I have personally cared for 25−30 submersion patients [of] varying degrees of severity. I have seen one 13-year-old remain comatose and unresponsive for eight weeks who eventually made a full recovery.

And an emergency room physician commented:

> No effort should be spared to initially attempt to sustain any sign of life. Miraculous recoveries are rare but it does happen; it can and it will happen again.

THEMES WITHIN SPECIALTIES—EMERGENCY ROOM PHYSICIANS.   One point frequently voiced by the emergency room physicians was that everything that is medically possible should be done initially to sustain the life of the child, because of the physician's inadequate knowledge of the child's prior history at the time of admission. In general, these respondents felt that the decision to use extraordinary measures was not the responsibility of emergency room personnel. One of these respondents commented:

> I have been involved in several of these types of circumstances involving resuscitation of a child with the possibility of severe brain damage, some which later had essentially flat line EEGs. In each case where the result was unsatisfactory I have been subjected to criticisms for carrying out the resuscitation in the first place. I consider this criticism totally unfair and wrong. It may be an easy decision in retrospect . . . to say a child with total neurological catastrophe should not have been resuscitated, but I defy them to be the emergency physician on the scene with virtually no information as to the length of anoxic time interval faced with a child with no vital signs, and not attempt resuscitation. The place for the decision not to use extraordinary measures to sustain life is not in the emergency room except for rare and exceptional circumstances.

Another emergency room physician responded:

> I think initially all cases that are not "obviously" DOA in the ER should be resuscitated because (1) the initial history is obtainable only several minutes after arrival in the ER, (2) the initial appearance is not always reliable, and (3) the "medical-legal" aspects of not at least attempting resuscitation. However, even the initial efforts should not be very vigorous if there is no fairly strong response.

Another physician wrote:

> Some of the questions and simulations described are unrealistic and not applicable to the emergency department since they deal with problems and information occurring well after we must make a decision to act or not act. We usually get a body plus a

history of immersion; time estimates then are notoriously inaccurate and usually change several times before the facts are finalized. "Extraordinary measures" usually involve procedures and treatment in the following days—not an ER decision.

Similarly, another emergency room physician commented:

> Most often it is the emergency room physician who first encounters the decision to begin "extraordinary measures" in a given case. Termination then becomes the responsibility of the physician providing continuing care. In general; if in doubt, begin extraordinary measures.

THEMES WITHIN SPECIALTIES: THE FAMILY PEDIATRICIAN.   Whereas the majority of emergency room physicians' comments concerned employment of full medical resources for the sustainment of the child's life, pediatricians addressed their comments to the physician-family interaction. Most of these respondents expressed the attitude that once resuscitation had begun, the family should be actively involved in the decision if the physician perceived that they were able to handle it. For example, one pediatrician wrote:

> Parents should be told as much as they can understand, as often as necessary to help them understand the problem, and share in the decision as much as they are willing and able.

Similarly, another commented:

> I believe that parents can understand and participate to a meaningful degree in such decisions. They should not have to feel the full burden of responsibility nor should they have to order extraordinary measures stopped as in the Quinlan case.

And still another example of this concern with parental participation in the decision-making process:

> The question of how much to involve parents is very tricky. Certainly they should be advised early and repeatedly of the prognosis. Whether they can take part in making the decision to discontinue life support depends very much on the parents. Some are sure of what they wish done. Others are confused, unrealistic, denying—and I think likely to be themselves harmed by an attempt to involve them in the decision to discontinue life support. In those cases the physician must assume he burden of the responsibility rather than risk leaving the parents with lifelong guilt.

Although in general most of the comments concerning physician-family interaction were made by pediatricians, it should not be inferred that other specialties did not concern themselves with this problem. One emergency physician devoted much space to this topic. His comments are presented at length because they offer insight into the physician-family interaction and present a good overview of the basic issue.

> Although the medical situation and prognosis is usually readily appreciated in these cases, the emotional aspects for the family are sometimes prolonged and occasionally difficult to assess. The reaction of any one family member may influence all others. There is marked variability in our ability to cope with this type of stress and sudden grief. There is a definite tendency for parents to have latent guilt feelings about any catastrophic mishap to their child. In essence, the family often becomes the patient as the possible benefits to the injured family member become progressively limited.

CONCLUSIONS

It is clear from the two studies presented here that the issue of parental participation in the decision-making process regarding the use of extraordinary life-sustaining efforts remains a controversial and most complex issue. There is continuing disagreement as to whether it is a medical or extramedical problem. The majority felt that full information should be given to the parents, and that parents should be involved at east to some degree in the decision-making process. The fact that one-half of the respondents were opposed and the other half in favor of using such measures clearly indicates that the problem is not solely a medical one. A third of the physicians saw the need for a medical ethics board, and the written comments indicated an expressed desire for more formal and continuing education programs in the area of medical ethics. It was clear from the comments of the physicians that such guidelines should supplement but not replace individual professional judgments regarding the disposition of specific cases. Perhaps most important, the results demonstrate the sensitivity of physicians toward all aspects of this type of case.

Parental participation in the decision-making process was judged appropriate by the physicians only after the physician has done all that can be done from the medical point of view. The physicians felt that the integrity of the physician's role as medical expert must be maintained. The parents felt this, too. Both the physician and the parents felt that the parents' participation is called for when the decision of whether or not to continue extraordinary life-sustaining efforts reaches beyond the purely medical to broader human concerns, the answer to which must be based on a value system that goes beyond the medical. One concern expressed by both physicians and parents was that too hasty a decision might lead to failure to treat the treatable.

What emerged from our two studies was that, although there was no consensus on the decision of whether or not to sustain life, nor even a direction stated regarding this decision, there was agreement on the necessity of parental participation in the decision. Disagreement came as to the timing and amount of parental participation. Both the physicians and the parents emphasized that each case is and must remain specific and individual, and that no overall generalization would be appropriate in so delicate an area.

Relevant to the issue of lay participation in such decisions is the following quote from Crane (1975):

> Social and technological changes provide the context for the emergence of a loosely coordinated, norm-oriented social movement with two principal goals. The first goal appears to be improvement in the quality of interaction between dying persons and both professionals and nonprofessionals. . . . second goal of the movement is the enactment of legislation to strengthen the patient's right to refuse (Veatch, 1972) and to define death (Capron & Kass, 1972).

The explosion of literature on death and dying has caused a reevaluation of the place of death in our lives. Laypersons are becoming increasingly aware of the implications involved in complex medical decisions. As more openness takes place in our society regarding the complexities and available options in decisions such as life-and-death issues, it is expected that more parents will enter the crisis phase with a background of informed thought on such sensitive issues, and that the parents would thus be better prepared to enter into an informed-consentient participation in the resuscitation decision when the emergency arises.

The pediatric psychologist working as a fully functioning and regular member of the emergency room medical team is in a position to help both the physician and parents to come to terms with each of their roles, rights, and responsibilities in this complex area. Above all, the pediatric psychologist, as a trained researcher-clinician, is in a position to design and conduct rigorous studies of the basic question of parental informed consent in emergency-room situations, and from such well-designed studies to help develop updated norms based on important emerging social patterns. By placing into a research context the broad social processes which brought about the problematic situation and the emerging adaptive patterns used by both the physician and the parents to resolve the specific situation, the pediatric psychologist can help set higher-order standards that take into account the new technology without losing sight of the basic value of human life and the rights of the child to a full participation in that life.

THE PEDIATRIC PSYCHOLOGIST AS PARENTAL COUNSELOR IN CASES OF CHILD ABUSE: GUIDING THE PARENT TO THERAPY[3]

The pediatric psychologist in the emergency room is likely to run into near-drowning cases as a relatively rare event. However, the pediatric psychologist as a full, regular, and functional member of the emergency room health care team is likely to encounter cases of child abuse in increasing frequency as awareness of the phenomenon becomes more widespread. Because child abuse laws in most states are written to protect the child, the majority of the members of the health care team will be giving their attention to the child—and rightly so. The child must be cared for medically as well as psychologically and protected from further harm.

The parents are not neglected either, at least not by the protective forces: police and the legal establishment. After all, it is the parents or stepparents of the child who, in the majority of cases, are the perpetrators of the abuse, and the medical and legal community raises a rightful voice of anger at such abuse. Even though child abuse is increasing at an alarming rate, perhaps because of increased population, increased stress events within the family, such as unemployment, or perhaps merely because of greater public awareness and tighter reporting laws, it is still difficult for even the most seasoned of emergency room team members to understand how a parent could deliberately inflict harm on his or her own child. The medical emergency room health care team sees accidental trauma as a matter of course. For a person to deliberately inflict trauma on so helpless a victim as a young child, and

[3]This section was prepared by John J. Spinetta, Richard P. Sprigle, and James S. Hennessey.

for that person to be the child's own parent, runs counter both to the medical purpose of the medical team and to the feelings of each of its members.

It is because of this very difficulty in comprehending parental motives and the intense feelings against the abusing parent on the part of the medical emergency room health care team members that it is essential for the emergency room team to include as a full, functional, and regular team member a pediatric psychologist who can act as parental advocate. While the medical team members are attending to the child, and while the child-protective team members have as their obligation to bring the law to bear on the abusing parent, there is no one left to respond to the parent's very real cry for help. Is the abusing parent an overbearing child abuser of irreparable habit, or is the parent a weak and helpless human being who, after having abused the child, has sought medical care for the child and is sitting there begging to be stopped and helped? A pediatric psychologist as a regular and respected working team member, who has a good rapport with the other team members and who is well trained in sorting out the rare unconscionable abuser from the majority of low-self-esteem and weak parents crying for help, is in a unique position to become an advocate for the abusing parent at an emotional time when the parent seems least deserving of such an advocate.

Background for the Present Study

There was a time in child abuse work when efforts were placed totally on protecting the child and prosecuting the abusing parent (Helfer & Kempe, 1968). Then a period of awareness came when the parents themselves were seen as in need of help (Spinetta & Rigler, 1972). During the decade of the 1970s, a shift was made from an overly simplified view of causes of abuse (Helfer & Kempe, 1968) to an emphasis on the fact that the causes of child abuse are multiple and interactive (Belsky, 1980; Starr, 1979). In the middle of this decade, the parent was somehow lost as the controller of his or her own actions. With the growing emphasis in the literature on the fact that the causes of child abuse are multiple and interactive, many therapists who deal with parental personality and attitudinal variables were made to feel as if they were engaging in a futile effort (D'Agostino, 1975; Smith, 1975). Although many new and exciting identification and treatment programs for child abuse abounded throughout the country (National Center on Child Abuse and Neglect, 1975, 1976), very little encouragement was given to the therapist who did not have easy access to the new interdisciplinary treatment programs and who, in many instances, remained the sole therapeutic agent for a particular set of families (Steele, 1975). The problem was viewed as sufficiently complex that an individual therapist who deals solely with parental attitudes was often discouraged. In a study demonstrating that parental personality and attitude are important factors in the etiology of child abuse, Spinetta (1978) tried to give hope to the therapist that efforts in dealing with the parental personality are aimed in a profitable direction, and that it is possible to be effective in reducing potential for abuse.

It was not the intent of the 1978 study to suggest that factors of parental background or inadequacy are the sole determinants of child abuse. The fact is that the causes of child abuse are multiple and interactive; there is no single type of child abuser or single causative factor as sufficient explanation of abuse (Spinetta & Rigler, 1972). Emphasis on parental personality is in no way meant to detract from these other factors. Rather, it is suggested that helping the parent to develop the ability to maintain equanimity under stress is directly related to situational variables and can be of central value in the rehabilitative or preventive process.

It is in the broader context of situational variables that the question is raised: Why is it that the majority of parents do not abuse their children? Although in the socially and economically deprived segments of the population there is generally a higher degree of the kinds of stress factors found in abusing families, the great majority of deprived families do not abuse their children. Why is it that most deprived families do not engage in child abuse, though they are subject to the same economic and social stresses as those families who do abuse their children? Is there an actual difference between the types of stresses encountered by abusing parents and nonabusing parents within the same socioeconomic level (Gil, 1970, 1976), or is the difference due to the parents' manner of approaching the stress situation (Kent, 1976; Smith, 1975; Spinetta & Rigler, 1972; Young, 1976)? We hold the latter position. When one takes into account the fact that some well-to-do and middle-class families also engage in child abuse, then one must look for the causes of child abuse beyond mere socioeconomic stress. The problem of etiology remains insoluble at the demographic level alone. A brilliant theoretical formulation by Belsky (1980) and a masterful review by Starr (1979) underscore this point.

In 1978, we demonstrated that abusing mothers could be differentiated from nonabusing mothers on personality and attitudinal variables (Spinetta, 1978). A set of abuse-potential categories, independently derived from our own local sample's response to the Michigan Screening Profile on Parenting (Helfer, Schneider, & Hoffmeister, 1977), proved capable of differentiating significantly between abusing and nonabusing mothers within the same socioeconomic level. Our independently derived categories were subsequently analyzed by Schneider 1979), and found to correlate at a significant level with her own empirically derived categories. The empirically derived set of abuse-potential categories proved useful in significantly differentiating between abusing and nonabusing mothers within the same socioeconomic level in three areas: the tendency to become upset and angry, feelings of isolation and loneliness, and the fear of external threat and control. The abusing mothers differed significantly from nonabusing mothers in a middle socioeconomic level in the same categories; in their relationship to their own parents, both past and present; in having higher than normal expectations for their young children's performance; and in failing to separate their own feelings from those of their children. Although not at a significant level, abusing mothers differed from nonabusing mothers in the same socioeconomic level in the latter categories as well. Neglecting parents and spouses of abusers were also shown to be weak in the six abuse-potential categories.

We demonstrated that personality and attitudinal factors do make a difference. Abusing mothers differ from nonabusing mothers in areas of attitude and personality that have been clinically related to potential for abuse (Colman, 1975; Corey,

Miller, & Widlack, 1975; Kent, 1976; Paulson, Savino, Chaleff, Sanders, Frisch, & Dunn, 1974; Smith, 1975; Spinetta & Rigler, 1972; Steele, 1975; Tracy & Clark, 1974; Walters, 1975). The fact that neglecting mothers and spouses of abusers also scored high on the abuse-potential categories demonstrates the power of the test in pointing to weakness in parental personality and attitudes that can affect the parenting role itself, regardless of whether the results are actual physical abuse, neglect of the child, or passively allowing one's spouse to abuse the child. Intervention and direction is called for in each case.

As stated above, there was no suggestion made that factors of parental inadequacy and personality weakness are the sole determinants of child abuse. Certainly, those involved in the care of the abusing parent must continue to relieve the family as much as possible of overwhelming situational stresses. However, personality does play a role. The therapist who helps the parent develop the ability to maintain equanimity under stress can be of immense aid in the rehabilitative or preventive effort.

One must caution that the questionnaire cannot be used as a legally valid criterion for sorting out abusing from nonabusing parents, since false positives have been shown on occasion (Schneider, Hoffmeister, & Helfer, 1976; Schneider, 1970), and since false negatives can appear with those parents who refuse to answer the questions honestly. It is possible to fake answers by giving socially desirable responses. However, for those parents in a therapeutic situation who respond to the questionnaire with an honest desire to be helped, the responses can help point to weaknesses in areas that have been clinically shown to relate to potential for abuse. A therapist who directs interventional and preventive efforts toward the ameliora-tion of parental attitudes, attitudes toward both the self and the child, is not, as Alby (1975) suggested, misdirecting energies, but is rather helping reduce deviations from the norm in characteristics related to abuse potential and is ultimately helping reduce the actual abusive behavior.

Given that abusing parents differ from nonabusing parents in attitudinal and personality variables, are there differences among the abusing parents that might help explain why some profit from therapy while others do not (Helfer & Schmidt, 1976; Paulson et al., 1974; Tracy & Clark, 1974; Young, 1976)? The present study is an attempt to demonstrate that parents who refer themselves for help are at a greater level of readiness for therapy than those who remain under adjudication for child abuse within judicially mandated agencies.

Parental Readiness for Therapy: A Study

Using the Michigan Screening Profile on Parenting to differentiate between abusing and nonabusing mothers on personality and attitudinal variables, as shown above, we were able to derive empirically, through factor analysis, six clusters relating to high abuse potential: (1) a faulty relationship to one's own parents (= PARENTS), (2) the tendency to becoming easily upset and angry (= CONTROL), (3) the tendency for being lonely and isolated in social interactions (= AFFILIATIONS),

(4) a high expectation of one's own children at a level long preceding the child's developmental capacity to perform (= EXPECTATIONS), (5) the inability to separate one's feelings from those of the child (= SYMBIOSIS), and (6) the inordinate fear of external threat and control from authority figures (= THREAT). The parents who abused or neglected their children scored at levels of higher risk than did the nonabusing parents in all of the six categories, with abusing parents scoring at the highest-risk level throughout (Spinetta, 1978).

If it is true that the person who scores high in a particular category is indicating a weakness in an area showing high potential for abuse, then that person who answers honestly is also demonstrating awareness of the weakness, and thus readiness for therapy. Those who score at a low level on the categories, whether they are really low in abuse potential or merely faking an "expected social response," do not demonstrate the same need or readiness for therapy. For those parents in a therapeutic situation who respond to the questionnaire with an honest desire to be helped, the responses can help point to weaknesses in areas that have been clinically shown to relate to potential for abuse. Therapists who direct their interventive and preventive efforts toward the amelioration of parental attitudes, attitudes both toward the self and toward the child, are not misdirecting their energies but rather are helping reduce deviations from the norm in characteristics related to abuse potential, and are ultimately reducing actual abusive behavior (Derdeyn, 1977; Justice & Justice, 1976; Kempe, 1978; Spinetta, 1978). Since the Michigan Screening Profile on Parenting (Helfer et al., 1977) has already been shown to be powerful in pointing to weaknesses in parental personality and attitudes that can affect the very parenting role itself, and that therapeutic intervention is helpful in such cases, the present study was conducted to see if there were any differences among abusing parents between those who refer themselves for help and those who remain under adjudication within the judicial system.

Method

The six groups of subjects for the study came from two sources: (1) three groups were under adjudication within agencies mandated by the judicial system (neglect—$N = 68$; physical abuse—$N = 18$; and sexual abuse—$N = 6$), (2) three groups were voluntary referrals of differing natures (self-referred to nonpunitive, judicially mandated agency for neglect—$N = 135$; system-referred to a self-help group for abuse—$N = 20$; and self-referred to a self-help community-based treatment program for physical abuse—$N = 14$). There were 261 families participating in the study. Although more women than men have been found to abuse their children (Gelles, 1978; Gil, 1970; Helfer & Schmidt, 1976; Justice & Justice, 1976; Kent, 1976; Smith, 1975), child abuse is not an act solely of the mother. However, the questionnaire was administered only to women, to insure nonconfounding by differences in childrearing attitudes between men and women. Subjects were chosen in the following manner. The participating agencies agreed to administer the questionnaire to all of the mothers currently under their jurisdiction as active cases. The purpose of the study was explained in detail to the respective supervisors. Because of the sensitive nature of the accusation of child abuse and neglect, and to prevent socially desirable responses, parents were not told specifically that the survey's ultimate purpose was to differentiate abuse potential. Rather, parents were asked if they wished to take part in a survey on attitudes in bringing up children, conducted by the university to learn how parents viewed childrearing. In accord with the HEW guidelines, parents were promised that the results would remain anonymous, and that any parent who wished would be given the overall results upon completion of the study.

The instrument used for the study was the Michigan Screening Profile of Parenting (Helfer *et al.*, 1977) with the factor-analyzed categories of Spinetta (1978) as discussed above. The groups were analyzed by a 2 × 3 multivariate analysis of variance, voluntary-referrals versus system-mandated, in three groups: neglect, system-aware physical abuse, and self-aware abuse.

Results

Table 3 shows the means in scores for each of the groups in each of the six abuse-potential categories, and the results of the MANOVA analysis. The voluntary-referral groups demonstrated a greater readiness for therapy, scoring as more aware of weaknesses in each of the following areas: Overall ($p < .001$), Parents ($p < .001$), Feelings ($p < .01$), Affiliation ($p < .01$), and Threat ($p < .001$). Of the system-mandated, those parents who neglect their children as opposed to the other two groups demonstrated the greatest readiness for therapy. The neglect-population scored as most aware of weaknesses in the following areas: Overall ($p < .001$), Feelings ($p < .01$), Expectations ($p < .05$), and Threat ($p < .01$). Within the voluntary-referred group, the two self-referred (to system and to self-help) were highest, but not significantly so.

Discussion

It has been shown that the therapist who helps the parent to develop the ability to maintain equanimity under stress can be of immense aid in the rehabilitative or preventive effort (Spinetta, 1978). The present study attempted to differentiate readiness for therapy in several groups of abusing parents. The results indicated that parents who refer themselves to a community-based program that is geared to helping the parents, and is not punitive in nature are the most willing to admit weakness in areas related to high abuse potential. Whether the voluntary-referral parents score higher because they have a higher abuse potential than the others or merely because they are more honest in filling out the forms is not the critical issue. What is the critical issue is that the parents are not only aware of their areas of weakness but are willing to express that awareness. Such expression is a higher indicator of readiness to participate effectively and with motivation in proffered therapy sessions. Those parents who were system-referred to the self-help community based program also evidenced a high level of awareness of problem areas, more so than the system-based groups. It is clear from the data that it makes no significant difference whether the parents are self-referred or system-referred to the self-help programs as long as they willingly participate once they are there. The parents in the three voluntary-referred groups exhibited a sensitivity and self-

Table 3.   Mean Scores for Each of the Six Groups

	Parents	Feelings	Affiliation	Expectations	Symbiosis	Threat
Voluntary Referrals						
Self referred to system (CPPS, $N = 135$)	51.20	25.33	26.03	41.86	17.02	47.64
System-referred to self-help group (FSC, $N = 20$)	50.85	22.25	23.20	42.09	17.39	42.89
Self-referred to self-help group (FSC, $N = 14$)	55.14	25.43	25.79	38.36	15.71	44.64
System-Mandated						
Adjudicated neglect (DC, $N = 68$)	45.29	23.85	23.43	42.94	16.69	42.29
Adjudicated physical abuse (DC, $N = 18$)	45.17	18.72	22.61	32.33	16.22	36.06
Adjudicated sexual abuse (DC, $N = 6$)	36.00	20.33	21.67	41.83	18.50	33.67
Total mean score	49.08	24.15	24.79	41.31	16.87	44.60

Significant differences (df = 2254)

Voluntary referrals versus system mandated:
Overall:	$F = 4.92$, p < .001
Parents:	$F = 23.32$, p < .001
Feelings:	$F = 6.52$, p < .01
Affiliations:	$F = 9.94$, p < .01
Threat:	$F = 19.58$, p < .001

System mandated neglect versus system mandated abuse:
Overall:	$F = 1.79$, p < .001
Feelings:	$F = 4.97$, p < .01
Expectations:	$F = 3.51$, p < .05
Threat:	$F = 4.91$, p < .01

knowledge that demonstrate a higher potential for profiting from therapy than those in the system-mandated groups, who demonstrated either a lack of awareness of areas of weakness or a lack of willingness to share such awareness if present. The latter groups did not indicate the openness and sensitivity prerequisite to good therapy.

What the data point to are the differences between those programs that are primarily punitive in nature and those geared toward ameliorating the parents' attitudes and ability to become good parents. The researchers did not have any prior relationship with either set of respondents in the agencies. Even those parents referred to the self-help groups from the system demonstrated a willingness to share awareness of problem areas. The atmosphere of help rather than punishment appears to lend itself to this openness. Referrals to such community-based, nonpunitive self-help programs may provide the avenue for the parents to realize that they can be helped and that they can learn proper parenting skills based on a greater self-worth. Although there are some child-abusing parents who deliberately and intentionally set out to inflict harm on their children, these are typically few in number (Gil, 1970; National Center on Child Abuse and Neglect, 1975, 1976; Spinetta & Rigler, 1972; Walters, 1975). The majority of parents who admit to tendencies to abuse, given the supportive circumstances of a nonpunitive nature, have shown ability and willingness to profit from training in effective parenting. Self-awareness, training in greater self-worth, and reduction in areas of weakness demonstrated to be related to high abuse potential can be very effective in the ultimate reduction of the incidence of child abuse.

The pediatric psychologist, both as a specialist in the functioning of the human being as an individual member of society and as a scientist involved in research methodology, is in a unique position to best further the ability of the system, not only to protect the child from further abuse, but to help the parents regain their sense of self-worth and their ability to perform more adequately in their parenting role.

THE PEDIATRIC PSYCHOLOGIST IN THE REHABILITATION UNIT: LEARNED HELPLESSNESS AFTER TRAUMATICALLY INDUCED NEUROLOGICAL IMPAIRMENT[4]

When a child or young adult receives a neurological impairment from a motorcycle or automobile accident, or from an athletic accident, he or she may end up in a rehabilitation unit for a long period of time. While there, the child may find other children suffering similar neurological impairments from a variety of causes. Such children and young adults enter a phase of treatment which entails a serious interruption of their normal development. The psychological needs of such neurologically impaired victims are immense. What can the pediatric psychologist do to assist children and young adults in their emotional development?

To underscore the seriousness and extent of the problem, the rehabilitation unit of just one relatively small children's hospital (Children's Hospital and Health Center, San Diego) served 147 patients during the calendar year 1979. The breakdown is as follows: 65 girls and 82 boys with an average age of 5½ years. Some of the admitting diagnoses for these children were acute myelitis (e.g., Guillain-Barre,

[4]This section was prepared by Steven N. Sparta.

polio, and transverse myelitis); acute encephalopathies (e.g., those resulting from anoxia, hypoxia, meningitis, cerebritis, and encephalitis); trauma resulting in hemiplegia, paraplegia, or quadriplegia; metabolic and endocrine disorders (e.g., phenylketonuria and propionic acid); and neoplasms (e.g., brain tumors of various kinds). Still other patients of much fewer numbers were those receiving shunt revisions or experiencing complications of cleft lip and palate and multiple congenital anomalies.

Of the 147 patients admitted over the year, 47 were acute care cases. Eleven of the acute care patients were nonaccident related due to either parental neglect or intentional harm. Many of the accident-related cases resulted from vehicular or diving-related accidents.

While the pediatric psychologist who is a part-time consultant to the unit may attempt an effective but short-lived behavioral intervention, the pediatric psychologist who is a full, regular, and functional member of the rehabilitation unit's health care team will be more cautious to develop an intervention program which will be both successful in the specific situation and effective in the long-haul in the context of the child's normal out-of-hospital life. Even among children of the same sex, age, and diagnosis, the psychological significance of a disability will vary with the child's prior experience with illness, the personality of the child— particularly factors related to adaptive capacity patterns of familial interaction and social circumstances surrounding rehabilitation. Knowledge of these factors is critical to effective intervention.

With the intent of examining a small and carefully defined sample of neurologically impaired children, three children who had suffered significant neurological impairment were chosen for study. Some of their characteristics were described by staff who worked with these children as relative to "helplessness," and a comparison was made with the pattern of behavior described as "learned helplessness" (Seligman, 1975). The concept of "learned helplessness" seemed applicable to the observed lack of patient responses in a problem situation, and the sense that these children had overgeneralized their beliefs that one's actions were inconsequential toward desired outcomes.

Subjects were first screened on prehospitalization history, to rule out children with chronic disabilities. Of the children who had suffered dramatic neurological impairment—most typically reflected in spinal cord injury with quadriplegia or paraplegia—general descriptions were obtained of their hospital ward behavior, and ratings were completed on a scale intended to measure helplessness. To control for the effects of hospitalization per se, the same helplessness ratings were gathered on hospitalized children from rehabilitation and surgical wards who were expected to be discharged with a comparable level of prehospital functioning.

Descriptions of this kind were thought to provide an initial refinement of the rehabilitation population into clearer problem populations with greater amenability to understanding and treatment. This study is considered a pilot investigation into only one of presumably many kinds of emotional difficulties represented within the scope of rehabilitation. The study was conducted as a means of helping pinpoint more clearly the true nature of the psychological problems faced by children with neurological impairment, in a children's hospital rehabilitation unit. This section will also demonstrate clearly the role the pediatric psychologist plays as a researcher-clinician in the hospital setting. The pediatric psychologist cannot be merely a clinician. Research is a critical element that falls squarely within the scope and responsibility of the pediatric psychologist as a full, regular, and functioning member of a hospital unit's health care team.

Learned Helplessness: Laboratory and Naturalistic Studies

The term *helplessness,* while increasingly used in research on depression and underachievement, was originally used to denote an experimental state induced in infrahuman subjects (Seligman & Maier, 1967). Helplessness was described as the failure to take action which would terminate an aversive stimulus when the organism possessed the ability to do so. Thus dogs given helplessness training through trials of inescapable shock would not terminate a shock, even though they had previously been able to terminate shock within the same physical environment. In contrast to control animals whose behaviors following shock were characterized by intense activity, the helpless animals passively tolerated extreme amounts of shock. Although erroneous, the animals had acted as if events were uncontrollable—as if the outcome was independent of voluntary response. Few attempts were made to prevent its occurrence. The failure to act lent itself to the term *helplessness.*

The authors proposed that the animals exposed to inescapable shock learned that the probability of shock termination given a response was equal to the probability of shock termination given no response, or shock termination and responding were independent. Thus "in the same way that organisms can learn about contingencies, they can learn about the absence of contingencies" (Dweck & Goetz, 1977).

While helplessness has been operationalized in the laboratory with animals, the result can also be seen as a person's belief that one's actions are inconsequential. Moreover, this learning can generalize to similar situations, which seriously decreases the probability of attempting instrumental responses. The important feature is that it is not the physical world that engenders the psychological state of helplessness, but the organism's expectations about personal control. Thus with handicapped children it is not the handicap itself that would produce such a state but the child's evaluations about its significance in areas related to mastery.

The striking nature of such a finding has prompted much attention in related problems, such as depression (DeCharms, 1968, Seligman, 1975) and "attribution-ally related under achievement" (Dweck, 1975).

Some parallels can be drawn between the helplessness-related research and the passivity presumed with the study's sample. For purposes of discussion with children with significant neurological impairment, helplessness is defined by the low frequency of initiated activities; the lack of persistence at a task, or sustained attention; verbalizations reflecting hopelessness in being able to control encountered situations; and lack of carefulness or conscientiousness for those attempted tasks. These behaviors seem reasonably related to the definition of learned helplessness.

Learned helplessness has also been studied in children with severe and chronic learning problems (Dweck, 1975; Sparta, 1979). In achievement situations it "exists when an individual perceives the termination of failure to be independent of his responses" (Dweck & Goetz, 1977). The belief that one's actions do not matter may manifest itself in various classroom behaviors, including the student's deterioration of performance after failure; seldom raising his hand; initiation of work only on request; or not asking for help, but rather diverting attention to some nontask-related behavior. There is a familiarility of these classroom behaviors and later descriptions of the hospitalized children. It would seem that the radical changes in capability after trauma may well predispose one toward helplessness, which would extend to areas where exerted effort does make a difference. Helplessness in the suddenly incapacitated child may require clarification of the accurate limits of loss and, more important, the reestablishing of an attitude that effort and carefulness are genuinely productive.

The phenomenon of helplessness has also been investigated in mentally retarded adults. In these studies, helplessness was defined as the "inability to take effective action in a problem situation" (Floor & Rosen, 1975). Reports within this literature include the failure of such persons to take constructive actions for problems arising in their daily lives. For example, such persons might run completely out of funds before taking steps in obtaining a new job or applying for welfare (Cohen, 1960; Mattison, 1970).

Definitions of helplessness in these situations emphasized the motivational rather than the intellectual aspects of the person. Weight was given to personality factors consisting of a pattern of "inertia, passivity, or helplessness" (Floor & Rosen, 1975).

As with Seligman's laboratory definition, and Dweck's definition regarding underachievement, the literature on retardation also notes the person's lack of instrumental responses despite the ability to do so.

Method

Many diagnoses are represented on the rehabilitation ward, each type subject to the variabilities already mentioned. Before one would attempt to treat or study a "rehabilitation" patient, it would be necessary to specify the individual characteristics of this heterogeneous group. A first step toward problem definition is whether the disability represents a newly acquired set of problems, as in the acute cases, contrasted with chronic care cases whose hospitalization represents the latest manifestation of a continual adjustment since birth. It is assumed that the children in these two groups would differ in their behaviors shown in current hospitalization, given the radical shifts in body image, level of independence, sense of personal competence, and awareness of the daily living consequences. Examination was limited to cases representing sudden and significant shifts from pre-to-post injury functioning. More complex combinations of acute crisis in children with already existing chronic disabilities were omitted.

Subjects

Children from the Rehabilitation and Surgical wards of Children's Hospital and Health Center were selected according to the following considerations: excluded from consideration if younger than 3½ years of age, or older than 16 years; excluded if the child was from a different cultural background, which may have affected normal expectations of children's behavior regarding dependency or helplessness; excluded if the child's medical status precluded conscious awareness, normal intelligence or orientation; and holding constant the different levels of pre-and-post hospital functioning for each of the neurologically impaired and control groups. From this process, three subjects were obtained for each group.

The three patients that comprised the neurologically impaired sample were a 9½-year-old female with a spinal cord injury with asymetrical quadriplegia; a 3-year, 7-month-old female with a spinal cord injury with quadriplegia, and a 13-year, 1-month-old female with a cervical spine injury with quadriplegia. All three were on the rehabilitation ward and rated by a common set of raters. One control subject was also on the rehabilitation ward and rated by the same staff. This was an 11-year-old male with transverse myelitis, which was not chronic or incapacitating. Two other control subjects were chosen from the surgical ward of the hospital, and included a 7-year, 4-month-old arrhythmia patient discharged with full functioning, and a 6-year, 1-month-old male with an acute abdominal disorder, who was also discharged with full capabilities. Table 4 presents a summary of patient type, age, diagnosis, and number of raters that were knowledgeable of the patient's behavior.

The three control subjects were selected in order to rule out the effects of hospitalization per se and increase the likelihood that differences in helplessness among the neurologically impaired were a function of their sudden and pronounced loss of functioning. Results from all children were kept confidential and ratings were discussed anonymously.

Procedure

Information regarding the neurologically handicapped group consisted of (1) responses to an open-ended question regarding problem behaviors encountered by staff, and (2) ratings on a scale pertaining to helpless behaviors reflecting the hospital milieu. Responses to the open-ended question were gathered for the neurologically handicapped group only, while ratings were obtained for both groups.

To obtain an initial understanding of the extent of the neurologically handicapped children's needs, the daily nursing and support staff were asked to describe the three greatest problems in working with this type of patient. The question was open-ended to allow the maximum flexibility in choice of problem. The responses were given with the selected neurologically impaired individuals as a reference. All of the nursing staff familiar with these children completed descriptions, as did the physical therapists, occupational therapists, and speech, hearing, and language specialists involved.

Before proceeding with further study, these responses were reviewed to deter-

Table 4.   Subject Charasteristics by Diagnosis, Hospital Ward, and Age

Subject	Diagnosis	Ward	Raters	Age
Control				
1	Transverse myelitis: discharge with full functioning	Rehabil-itation	6	11 years
2[a]	Arrhythmia: discharge with full functioning	Surgical	1	7 years, 4 months
3[a]	Acute abdomen disorder: discharge with full functioning	Surgical	2	6 years, 1 month
Average age				8 years, 1 month
Neurologically impaired				
1	Spinal cord injury with asymetrical quadriplegia	Rehabil-itation	7	9 years, 6 months
2	Cervical spine injury with quadriplegia	Rehabil-itation	7	13 years, 1 month
3	Spinal cord injury with paraplegia	Rehabil-itation	8	3 years, 7 months
Average age				8 years, 6 months

[a]These patients were rated by different staff on the surgical ward.

mine whether there was any relevance to the helplessness construct. These behaviors were considered reflective and a measure was developed to assess helplessness behaviors within a hospital setting. The behavior rating scale used was adapted from one used to assess learned helplessness in a population of children experiencing extreme learning difficulties (Sparta, 1978). The adaptation of the items retained the characteristics of the helplessness definition, but the situations were transposed to reflect the appropriate hospital milieu. So, slight initiation of productive behavior could be reflected in rarely seen spontaneous practice of spoon-feeding behavior taught during occupational therapy. Carefulness, or consci-entiousness, could be reflected in how accurately a child performed an attempted task, as opposed to haphazardly responding and not utilizing the feedback from the unsuccessful trial. Persistence, the ability to sustain attention and effort over time, may be shown by the child who is trying to relearn feeding herself with a spoon in a slow and laborious manner, spills food onto her lap, yet repeats the trial as often as is necessary until she has eaten.

The nine-item scale was rated using a 5-point continuum of *never, seldom, sometimes, often,* and *always* with corresponding numerical values of 1 through 5. All items were not necessarily oriented in the same direction toward the helplessness definition, but the results were adjusted so that higher numerical values reflected greater helplessness. A description of the scale is contained in Table 5.

Table 5. Helplessness Rating Scale for Hospital Milieu

Patient Name: _____

Please rate the patient along the following scales, using a 1 to 5 point rating system.

1	2	3	4	5
Never	Seldom	Sometimes	Often	Always

Rating Scale

Patient asks questions about caring for self, for example, how to bathe self properly, how best to use a spoon while eating, etc.   _____

Patient verbalizes or shows positive mood when taking part in program, e.g., being asked to go to physical therapy   _____

Patient does only what is asked regarding program, rather than initiating tasks on own initiative   _____

Patient works with slight effort or carelessness for those tasks required by staff   _____

Patient will continue to work long periods of time after task started   _____

Patient will "come back stronger" after initially failing   _____

Patient waits in silence or refuses to comply with request when it is made   _____

Even though difficult, patient will keep trying or ask for help   _____

Patient asks about or performs something different than that assigned   _____

Descriptions and ratings were completed without rater knowledge of whether the subject was part of the hospital control group or the group under examination.

Results

The issue examined was whether neurologically impaired children show patterns of behavior related to a previously described state, termed helplessness, and whether these behaviors are not simply a function of a child being hospitalized.

Results of the open-ended questions were first examined in a content-validity fashion to determine whether the salient problem behaviors resembled the helplessness definitions. A representative sample of these responses were as follows:

The child is complaining about what is happening to him.

Frustration that patients don't express their concerns.

Setting limits on behavior.

The patient's motivation and willingness to try and practice different activities.

Although the patient is tired and depressed, how do I get him involved in therapy?

Waking her up in the morning for breakfast.

Having them involved in self-care activities.

Once rapport has been established, I find it difficult to cope with the moodiness and rejection that the kids push on you.

Lack of motivation.

The slow and difficult progress.

Frustration, depression, anger and refusal to accept their limitations.

Setting up a positive reinforcement system to motivate the kids in physical therapy.

[Child's name] won't try again if he doesn't get it the first time.

The commonalities seen in the foregoing were the negative affective expressions toward the child and staff, and insufficient motivation for the tasks demanded through the various rehabilitation activities. A fair number of these responses were directly related to similar themes described in the helplessness literature, regarding task initiation, persistence, and carefulness.

The results of the behavior ratings on both groups are presented in two ways, depicted in Figures 1 and 2. The first set of data represents an average helplessness rating for all nine questions on each child. Each average rating should be evaluated against the helplessness rating of the control subjects to rule out the effects of hospitalization per se. All three of the neurologically impaired patients showed more helplessness than all three of the control subjects, with an average for both groups equaling 3.4 and 2.0, respectively.

Figure 2 respresents the percentage of helplessness ratings for each child; in this case, a helpless rating was one of "often" or "always" to the helplessness question. The graphic differences are much greater for the neurologically impaired, consistently reflecting more helplessness than the control subjects. Average percentages for these groups were 50% helplessness behaviors for the neurologically impaired group versus 1.3% for the control group.

Discussion

The results show that there are different patterns of observed behavior with the traumatically impaired and hospitalized children on behaviors related to disturbances in initiation, carefulness, and persistence, a pattern termed *helplessness*. Before these general differences can be more adequately conceptualized within the helplessness theory, many conceptual and methodological refinements would be required.

The current definition was based on behavior observations of judged performance in a nonspecific situation. Multidetermined definitional criteria in situation-specific contexts would yield more accurate validity and reliability. Important potentially confounding variables that also have to be controlled include preaccident personality variables; the course of behavior change over time, from immediately following injury and beyond; degree of incapacitation; age must be controlled more carefully, as developmental stages will vary, for example, with initiative; raters should be trained along developed rating criteria and interrater reliability determined prior to

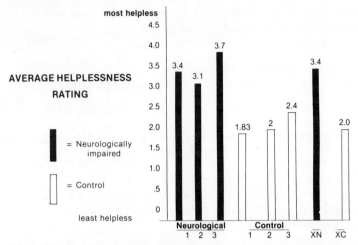

Figure 1. Average helplessness ratings among neurologically impaired and other hospitalized children.

observation; and the emphasis of the motivational aspects of behavior should cautiously address the possible behavioral effects of brain dysfunction (Reitan, 1974).

The foregoing descriptions of *helplessness* were intended to provide a framework from which to clarify and better plan for the treatment of one kind of pediatric patient. Helplessness does not describe the "psychological state" of the child; it does not "explain" aftereffects of trauma in an overly reductionistic manner; it does not ignore or contradict prior descriptions of stages involving loss of bodily function—and subsequent feelings or defenses such as depression, anger, identity

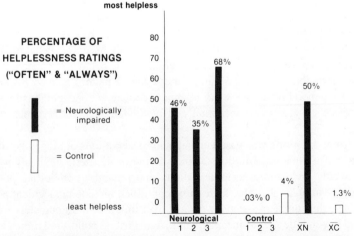

Figure 2. Percentage of helplessness ratings among neurologically impaired and hospital control subjects.

confusion, anxiety, isolation, and withdrawal or dependence (Dembo, Leviton, & Wright, 1956; Freud, 1917/1959; Grzesiak, 1979). The effects of helplessness can fit into these models.

These patterns, even when described in an exhaustive manner, are not considered fixed or universal among children. The child's personality prior to the illness or accident will significantly affect the adjustment to loss, and observable patterns of helplessness may vary accordingly. Additionally, the child's age during the adjustment will affect the nature of the meaningfulness of such issues. A framework for understanding this contribution is seen in Erikson's stages of psychosocial development, whereby patients who suddenly experience loss may experience a natural regression and an obligatory reworking of some previously surmounted developmental task (Erikson, 1968; Pepper, 1977). Thus older children may or may not rework a particular stage since chronological age itself does not insure that the developmental stage has been mastered.

The mechanisms underlying distortions in personal control involve an initial sense of mastery that is subsequently undermined after certain contingencies are perceived by the subject. Helplessness is the psychological state that frequently results when events are uncontrollable. "A person or animal is helpless with respect to some outcome when the outcome occurs independently of all voluntary responses" (Seligman, 1975). It would not be difficult to generalize this conception to these children's experiences of trauma following their previous mastery in a variety of situations. The effects of helplessness have not only included motivational consequences, pimarily that involving initiation of voluntary responses (Seligman & Maier, 1967), but disruptions of learning (Hiroto, 1972) and emotionality are heightened (Seligman, 1975). In the case of these hospitalized children, these effects would interact with each other, and possibly further its continuance. This is thought to exist in observations of these children during physical or occupational therapy. During these times they attempt few activities, express hopeless beliefs about the limits of their perceived ability or inability to control, and when they manage to attempt some task, they are subject to additional learning difficulties that increase the likelihood of failure.

The implications for such benign terms as "initiation, conscientiousness, and persistence" of tasks can be quite significantly related to direct health status as well as emotional well-being. One example is provided by Anderson and Andberg's (1979) examination of recovery rates of paraplegics suffering decubitus ulcers. In most previous investigations focused on physiologic and mechanical mechanisms underlying tissue ischemia, it was found that quadriplegics as a group (rather than paraplegics) had a history of fewer pressure sores. However, in Anderson's study, psychosocial factors of high responsibility in skin care and satisfaction with the activities of life were significantly associated with the decreased incidence of decubitus ulcers. The use of select psychological treatments with carefully chosen rehabilitation patients—each treatment different and logically derived from the needs of the child—should hold promise for the total health of the child.

The problems of initiation, carefulness, and persistence have been outlined in the context of the Children's Hospital environment. How do these problems manifest themselves over time especially in specific contexts of school and at home? What are the characteristics and attitudes of children with similar personality and neurological disability that have accomplished a successful adaptation? How might these differences in the successful group suggest treatment? What are the parallels of helplessness-related research with this population of children? These are all issues that can be resolved only by further study.

As stated in the introduction of this section of the book, it is pediatric psychologists, by their unique training both as researchers and as clinicians, who are in the position of conducting such research within the context of the health care unit which they serve. It is this unique combination of the research and clinical role in which pediatric psychologists are trained that form the unique function that pediatric psychologists can serve within the hospital structure. For the pediatric psychologist to opt for one role or the other, be it research or be it clinical application, is for the pediatric psychologist to give up what makes him or her a unique professional and defines his or her role within the health care system.

THE PEDIATRIC PSYCHOLOGIST AS CHILD ADVOCATE IN LIFE-THREATENING ILLNESS: HELPING THE CHILD LIVE WITH CANCER[5]

As a regular member of the pediatric hematology-oncology health care team, the pediatric psychologist is in a unique position to make a critical contribution of a research and service nature to the betterment of a child's life. The emphasis in this section, as throughout this chapter, is on the necessity for the pediatric psychologist dealing with catastrophic illness and trauma to be a full, regular, and functional member of the pediatric health care team. Any attempt to fulfill the role on a part-time or consultative fashion, in this author's opinion, will be futile, and worse, may even be misleading. A thorough knowledge of the illness, an ongoing rapport with the other team members, and a shared knowledge of family history and family functioning, over time, are elements critical to an ethically sound and long-term-effective intervention. A brief, behaviorally oriented encounter between a psychologist or psychiatrist as a one-time consultant and the family and/or child undergoing a long-standing chronic illness may prove initially effective in the immediate situation. However, in this author's experience, the long-term interests of the child and family are best served by an intervention program which encompasses the family's long-range needs as well as the specific situation calling for immediate resolution. It is to the pediatric psychologist who plans to become a

[5]This section was prepared by John J. Spinetta. During the preparation of this section, the author wa supported in part by Grant Number CA 21254, awarded by the National Cancer Institute, Department of Health and Human Services. The author wishes to thank Faith Kung, MD, of the University of California, San Diego School of Medicine; Donald Schwartz, MD, and Gary Hartman, MD, of Children's Hospital and Health Center, San Diego, and their staffs for their continued support and encouragement.

full, regular, and functional member of a pediatric hematology-oncology team to whom this section is addressed.

Psychosocial Issues in Childhood Cancer[6]

Some chronic diseases of childhood, while debilitating, follow a known course. Because the course is predictable, parents and patients alike can learn to cope well, given sufficient time, energy, and assistance. The uncertain and the unpredictable make it more difficult to cope well. The varieties of childhood cancer fall into the category of the uncertain.

Less than 20 years ago, childhood cancer was considered invariably fatal. The general course of each type of cancer was fairly predictable, and parents were counseled in ways of preparing for the death of the child. The time lag between diagnosis and death was brief. Today, the outlook for the survival of the child with cancer has improved dramatically. Many children live five years and more beyond the point of diagnosis. Many are considered cured. This increased chance for survival of the child with cancer has changed the psychosocial needs of caregivers and families. While medical advances have bettered the survival rates, the psychosocial problems faced by the children and their families have multiplied. Even when the child achieves a five-year or longer survival, uncertainty remains (Koocher & O'Malley, 1980). The cancer can recur.

How do parents live with this uncertainty? How do the children adapt to living with a life-threatening illness? What happens to the siblings? Are there ways that professionals can help facilitate the coping and adaptation of patient and family? Can we be satisfied with merely helping the patient and family adapt, or can we help the child continue to grow and develop, despite the illness? The literature on the psychosocial repercussions of childhood cancer ranges from the pessimistc tones of a decade ago, when it was believed that the majority of children suffer psychological damage, to the more optimistic tones of recent years. Much has been written about the child, the child's family, and those who treat the child. This section will deal with these issues, as well as with the child's attempts to return to a normal school life. It is the theme of helping the child live with the cancer that will be the primary focus of the present section.

History of the Research

There is no doubt that the extension of the life of pediatric cancer patients through medical developments has had a profound impact on the interests and the approach of mental health professionals and researchers working in pediatric oncology since 1960. A masterful literature review by Slavin (1980) highlights the trends over the past 20 years, with careful attention given to the way that the cancer experience has

---

[6]The remainder of this section appears, with minor changes, as "Psychosocial issues in childhood cancer: How the professional can help." In D. K. Routh & M. L. Wolraich (Eds.), *The Advances in Behavioral Pediatrics,* Vol. 3. Greenwich, CT: Jai Press, in press.

changed as a result of the evolving medical outlook for these patients, and to the new issues which are emerging as childhood cancer is increasingly viewed as a chronic disease. A comparison of newer volumes (such as those by Adams, 1980; Kellerman, 1980; Koocher & O'Malley, 1980; Schulman & Kupst, 1980; and Spinetta & Deasy-Spinetta, 1981a) with the classic volumes and papers of a decade ago (Binger *et al.*, 1969; Bozeman, Orbach, & Sutherland, 1955; Easson, 1970; Friedman, Chodoff, Mason, & Hamburg, 1963) points to the change in emphasis from one of preparing for death to one of preparing for life.

THE CHILD'S KNOWLEDGE OF MEDICAL IMPLICATIONS

When the early work on psychosocial aspects of childhood cancer was undertaken, most children died shortly after diagnosis. Psychosocial concern was aimed at helping the parents prepare the child for death and prepare themselves for life without the child. A major question for parents, clinicians, and mental psychosocial personnel was whether or not to tell the child about the impending death, and at what age. In our early work (Spinetta, 1974; Spinetta & Maloney, 1975; Spinetta, Rigler, & Karon, 1973, 1974), we demonstrated that children as young as 5 years of age became aware that theirs was no ordinary illness, even when no one had told them. At a level often preceding their ability to conceptualize their awareness in adult terms, the children were very aware that theirs was a very serious illness. Eventually, they came to know that they too might die from the illness. Our advice to the adults dealing in the children's lives was to allow the children to speak openly about their concerns so that they could receive support in their struggles.

As the current medical treatments succeed in prolonging the lives of many children and curing some, it is easier to discuss the illness and its prognosis, because the future can be discussed with a great deal more optimism than previously. It has also become clear in recent years that children's coping skills are much more adequate and mature than had been previously thought (Spinetta, 1977). In addition, there is growing evidence that talking about one's fears and fantasies relative to the cancer can be supportive and reassuring and can lessen levels of anxiety (Slavin, 1980).

COMMUNICATION AS A SUPPORT MECHANISM

Concern has shifted from the issue of telling or not telling to one of communication as an effective support mechanism. Research has centered on how to effectively maintain open levels of communication within a family, allowing the parents to remain in their role as support network for the child. It was shown that as a child who knows little about his illness nears death, he tends to separate from those around him, and exhibits increased feelings of isolation and loneliness (Spinetta *et al.*, 1974). In contrast, children whose families maintained an open level of communication throughout the course of the illness not only demonstrated a higher level of self-regard but were closer to family members than children whose families did not maintain an open level of communication Spinetta & Maloney, 1978; Spinetta, Swarner, & Sheposh, 1980).

Even now, with all of the medical advances, some children do die of cancer, and they must be prepared for that death. Parents and caregivers must also be prepared.

However, the children typically live longer before their death than in years past. Even those children who will die can live fully until the moment of their death (Martinson, 1976). Allowing the children to attend school and have a positive outlook toward a productive and fulfilled future can be as helpful to those who will eventually die as to those who will become long-term survivors (Clapp, 1976; Deasy-Spinetta & Spinetta, 1980, 1981; Greene, 1976; Kaplan *et al.*, 1973; Katz, Kellerman, Rigler, Williams, & Siegel, 1977; Lansky, Lowman, Vats, & Gyulay, 1975; van Eys, 1977). Kagen-Goodheart (1977) wrote of helping the children with cancer continue in their forward growth and commitment to life by helping them to reenter their normal world as soon as possible after initial cancer treatment. This "reentry" often involves having the child go to school despite outward signs of sickness such as hair loss or excessive weight, or despite negative effects of medication on ordinary bodily functioning. Regular school attendance is considered vital, not only to foster normal development, but to prevent isolation from peers and social regression. A positive school experience can provide the child with a sense of accomplishment and social acceptance, strengthening his faltering self-esteem and lessening maladaptive emotional responses to the illness (Slavin, 1980). The theme of the child's reentry into a normal world will be addressed in detail throughout this section.

Coping with Diagnosis and Treatment

The childhood cancers are a group of diseases. Each disease has its own natural history, a relatively predictable course from the time that it first becomes apparent, through a period of spreading, to death. The goal of treatment is to interrupt or alter the natural history of the disease. The psychological impact of the cancer is complex.

The time of diagnosis and initial treatment is the first of a series of events with which the child and family must cope. In fact, many families have pointed to the event of diagnosis as the most serious of the entire disease course. When a child is diagnosed with cancer, each family member is affected. Parents and siblings must develop methods of dealing with the child's cancer. They must also adjust to the practical limitations placed on their lives by the child's illness. Basically sound families are confronting an inordinate amount of stress and need help to begin to master at least some of the day-to-day elements of the task. Families must live with the uncertainty of the illness. They hope for a susained remission, while at the same time prepare for the possible loss of the child.

AGGRESSIVE TREATMENT

Therapeutic programs in the past were aimed at keeping the child comfortable. Today, treatment is undertaken with the hope of cure. Such therapy is often aggressive to the point that the effects of the treatment are as painful as the effects of the disease (Koocher Sallan, 1978). Not only are the chemotherapies tolerated differently by each child, but wide variations occur within the same individual at various times. Parents and children must accept and incorporate this aggressive treatment in the hope of a greater good, the child's ultimate cure.

As issues relative to diagnosis become less immediate, the issues that come to the fore for the children center on coping with the cancer treatments. Recently, we set forth a series of tasks, originally described by Lazarus (1976), as helpful in evaluating the adaptational efforts of children with cancer (Spinetta, 1977). These coping tasks are (1) tolerating or relieving distress associated with the illness; (2) maintaining a sense of personal worth; (3) maintaining positive personal relationships with parents, peers, and caregivers; and (4) meeting the specific requirements of particularly stressful situations, utilizing the resources available. Researchers recently have spoken to each of these issues (Adams, 1980; Kellerman, 1980; Schulman & Kupst, 1980; Spinetta & Deasy-Spinetta, 1981a). The increased use of self-relaxation or hypnosis techniques for relieving distress associated with the treatments has resulted in less pain for the children (Dash, 1980; Hartman, 1980; Zeltner, 1980). The area of preparation for untoward events has received much emphasis in recent literature (Slavin, 1980).

The treatments can result in a variety of side effects. Hair loss can be an emotionally trying experience for all of the children, teenagers as well as younger children. Although family and friends become accustomed to the children's appearance and the hair does grow back eventually, the hair loss can be very embarrassing for most of the children. Other problems include dramatic weight gain or loss, mouth ulcers, muscle spasms, skin rashes, skin discolorations, scars, organ losses, and amputations (Koocher & Sallan, 1978). Preparation for these can be helpful, but the problems are not resolved at a single intervention. Problems in adaptation continue throughout the disease course. As old problems are resolved, new ones appear. Chronic vomiting is a virtually inescapable part of chemotherapy. Some children may even become so conditioned to expect the side effect of vomiting that they begin to vomit hours before the medication is given, in anticipation of receiving it.

Depression of a child's immune responses presents a constant concern because of the child's increased susceptibility to all manner of infection (Koocher & Sallan, 1978). When a child with cancer develops infections during the course of treatment, the infections are considerably more dangerous than in the normal child. The frequency of these interruptions in daily living adds considerably to the family's level of stress. Other frequently voiced concerns of the children include forced dependence on others and loss of bodily control, both coming at a time when they have begun to mature. The painful muscle spasms, nausea, and disorientation as a function of chemotherapy causes the child concerns.

The age and level of development of the child makes a difference in how the child responds to the illness and treatments. A brief review of a child's age-related responses and concerns will follow.

The Child's Age, Experience, and Level of Development

A prerequisite to a meaningful communication with a child about his illness and treatment is a basic understanding of developmental levels in the growth of the child's thought processes, notably those surrounding the concepts of life and death. There are many books and articles which speak to this issue (Esson, 1970; Grollman, 1967; Hostler, 1978; Jackson, 1965; Koocher, 1973; Spinetta, Spinetta, Kung, & Schwartz, 1976; Spinetta & Deasy-Spinetta, 1981b). Although it is difficult to do justice to so complex a topic in so brief a space, the issue will be addressed at this point in an overview fashion, so that it can be placed in proper perspective. The topic will be addressed in two phases: (1) the child's concept of death, and (2) the seriously ill child's concept (or understanding) of death.

THE CHILD'S CONCEPT OF DEATH

Concepts of death are age-related in children and differ with intellectual ability and development (Anthony, 1940; Hostler, 1978; Koocher, 1973; Nagy, 1948; White, Elsom, & Prawat, 1978). It is generally believed that during the first two years of life there is no understanding of death as such, but fear of separation from protecting, comforting persons is present in its most terrifying intensity. While death is not yet a fact of life for the child going on 3, anxiety about separation remains all pervasive. Some time between the ages of 3 and 5, most children first comprehend the fact of death as something that happens to others. At this time, the concept of death is still vague. It is associated with sleep, and the absence of light or movement, and is not yet thought of as permanent. In contrast to toddlers, most children of this age are able to withstand and understand short separations. They often respond more spontaneously and with less anxiety to questions about death than do older children. They are also curious about dead animals and flowers. However, children between 3 and 5 typically deny death as a final reality. They believe death is accidental and they themselves will not die.

Attitudes and concepts of children do not change abruptly at any given age but evolve gradually and with wide individual variation. This is true whether one is talking about the concept of time, the concept of space, or the concept of death. From approximately the age of 6, the child seems gradually to be accommodating himself or herself to the proposition that death is final, inevitable, universal, and personal. Many 6- and 7-year-olds suspect that their parents will die someday, and that they too may die, but only in the very distant future. Children in these early school years show a strong tendency to personify death. Many children at their initial awareness and discovery of death are horrified, confused, and angered. Although some authors feel that because of exposure a child in the present day and age is coming to grips with the concept of death at a young age (Hansen, 1973), most still agree that the child under 10 has not yet attained a well-developed understanding of death (White et al., 1978). As children approach adolescence, they are equipped with the intellectual tools necessary to understand time, space, life, and death in a logical manner. At about the age of 10 or 11 the fact of the universality and the permanence of death becomes understandable.

What we have discussed to this point is the normal development of the ability to conceptualize death in children. A speeding up of the process occurs when the child is faced with death at an early age, often at a level preceding the child's ability to conceptualize it (Bluebond-Langner, 1974, 1977; Spinetta, 1974; Waechter, 1971).

THE SERIOUSLY ILL CHILD'S CONCEPT OF DEATH

It is important when speaking to children with a life-threatening illness about the concept of death to understand differences in ability to conceptualize because of the child's age and level of development. At the same time, it must be remembered that a child who is experiencing the day-to-day effects of a life-threatening illness, and the often drastic changes in the emotional climate that accompany this disease, may become aware of his own impending demise at a much younger age than his healthy peers (Spinetta, 1974). As shown above, recent studies of 6- to 10-year-old children with life-threatening illnesses reveal that, despite efforts by parents and medical personnel to keep the child from becoming aware of the prognosis, he somehow picks up a sense that the illness is no ordinary illness. The fear of abandonment and separation, characteristic of the younger child, has added to it a fear of bodily harm and injury and possible awareness of his own impending death, or, at the very least, the awareness at a level preceding his ability to conceptualize it, that something very serious is happening. The awareness of his own impending death becomes stronger as the child nears death (Bluebond-Langner, 1977; Spinetta et al., 1973, 1974).

The Adolescent.   Adolescence brings with it additional problems and concerns. There are changes and conflicts that accompany ordinary adolescence; the addition to these of the diagnosis of cancer makes it traumatic (Adams, 1980; Clapp, 1976; Drotar, 1977; Easson, 1970; Katz et al., 1977; Plumb & Holland, 1974). There are basic developmental tasks the adolescent must accomplish, whether he has cancer or not: achieving a sense of who he is; establishing independence from parents; adjusting to sexuality; forming mature relationships with peers of both sexes; and planning for a future in terms of job and marriage. Adolescents have a need to assert their independence at the same time that their illness forces dependence on physician, hospital staff, and parents. Anything that can be done to help them retain a sense of decision and independence while under treatment is most helpful. Rebellion is a common teenage trait. Building up trust and rapport will help allay some of the rebellious nature of teenagers. Communicating directly with them will help them maintain a level of maturity and independence that will help them sustain self-esteem.

Adolescents normally look forward to what their lives will be like in the future. Most begin thinking about careers and marriage. The adolescent with cancer may be concerned about whether his disease will limit the possibilities open to him (National Cancer Institute, 1979). Sterility may be a possible side-effect of some treatments. They may see their friends getting married and having children and wonder if they will be able to do so as well. Yet, in spite of the uncertainty about the future, the adolescent cancer patient must be encouraged to make realistic plans. Parents and caregivers must provide the emotional support for them to do so. Psychological support for adolescent cancer patients must take into account their developmental needs. Peer support groups are good ways to help them talk about the illness with someone who will understand. Often adolescents have a difficult time talking to adults. Forming a group of adolescents with cancer allows them to talk openly with peers about common disease-related and nondisease-related problems. An ongoing adolescent support group has been an integral part of our own intervention program (Deasy-Spinetta, 1981; Spinetta, Deasy-Spinetta, Milaren, Kung, Schwartz, & Hartman, 1981).

How does a health care professional begin to help a child and family deal with the cancer diagnosis, aggressive treatment regime, and life-threatening prognosis? It is essential that the health care professional understand the family's role as support system for the child and establish from the beginning an open level of communication. This issue will be addressed at this point.

Communication with Family Members

While the health care professional must attempt to understand the particular family structure and environment under which an individual child must live and grow, and while each family's adaptive capabilities and coping styles may differ, there are common patterns of communication among family members that are peculiar to the families of children with a life-threatening illness. It is these common elements which will be addressed here.

If it is true that children as young as 4 or 5 are aware of the serious nature of their illness, what do they do with this knowledge and awareness? Do they talk openly with their families about the prognosis, or do they live in silence with the knowledge? What roles do the families play in interaction with children wishing to talk or not to talk about their illness? Studies of family communication patterns about the issue of serious illness in children show that the level of family communication about the illness, as expressed in the mother's judgment of communication, relates to coping strategies in the child (Spinetta & Maloney, 1978). Families in which levels of communication about the illness are high are those families in which the children exhibit a nondefensive personal posture, express a consistently close relationship with the parents, and express a basic satisfaction with self. The parental level of willingness to discuss the illness is most important in the child's decision about what to do with the knowledge. Children who have the personal desire and parental permission to discuss their illness openly within the family structure are in the best position to receive the type of support they need (Spinetta, 1978).

Circumstances of pain, reactions to medication and treatment, and the death of older children from the illness all play a role in children's increasing awareness of the severity of their illnesses. Some professionals encourage denial in order for the children to maintain mental as well as physical comfort, and to a point, some brief denial may appear helpful (Alby & Alby, 1973; Howarth, 1974; Lazarus, 1980). However, children, siblings, and parents are best served in the long run by being encouraged to bring into the open their anxieties about the illness and its possible consequences (Alby & Alby, 1973; Futterman & Hoffman, 1973; Spinetta et al., 1976).

In a series of interviews conducted with families whose children had died from a life-threatening illness after the age of 6, the most frequently discussed issue was the extent to which the family had communicated with the child about the possible terminal effects of the illness (Spinetta et al., 1980). About half of the families interviewed felt they had talked freely and openly with their children about their impending deaths. None of the parents who had spoken openly with their child felt that too much had been said; on the contrary, these parents felt that a higher level of closeness was achieved with the child than might have occurred otherwise. The memory of the open discussions and exchange of family values before the child's death had sustained the families during the mourning process. The siblings in the open group reported having had time to say goodbye to their dying brother or sister, to resolve old quarrels, and to help their dying sibling in efforts to say goodbye as well.

The families whose children had died without open discussion of the illness or of the imminent death usually wished they had spoken more openly with their child. These parents reported feelings of incompleteness and nonresolution. Those siblings who reported unresolved feelings regretted not having been forewarned or not having had time to say goodbye and settle differences before the child's death.

Further studies are needed as to what to say and when, taking into consideration the severity of the illness, parental and sibling readiness, and age levels of the children. Nevertheless, studies to date point to the fact that children understand that their illnesses are serious, and encouraging children to talk about the illness usually has beneficial short- and long-term effects on all family members, including the life-threatened child.

Though desirable, open communication in all families in all circumstances is not always possible. Although open communication is generally of supportive value to the sick child, a forced openness too soon can be destructive for some specific families. Some parents are initially unable to communicate openly under the stress of a seriously ill child and exhibit maladaptive behavior, being inaccessible, withdrawn, and remote. The goal in working with these parents should be to help them become aware of the false sense of equilibrium that comes from excessive denial of the problem and the harm such denial can cause the sick child. Temporary use of denial of a serious illness can allow the family time to pull together adaptive resources. However, in dealing with such a family, care should be taken to prevent the "temporary" state of denial from becoming self-perpetuating.

We have found that the life-threatened child chooses whether or not to talk about his illness based on his experiences within the family regarding openness of communication about illness. A child may choose silence because he senses that his family forbids discussion of the illness, or the child may communicate openly because the family reinforces openness. Either choice represents a different style of coping. The choice of silence can lead to excessive denial and avoidance and a feeling of rejection and isolation. The child may feel that he has been left alone to work out his problems. In contrast, open discussion, stemming from the sincere attempts of family members to communicate concern and support, encourages expression of feelings. Open expressions of the child's fears relative to the illness can lead to mutual support among family members, helping the child achieve a balanced adaptive equilibrium.

THE FAMILY AS A SUPPORT SYSTEM

When open communication begins in a family, complex sets of feelings emerge. Openness increases expressed levels of anxiety within the family and commits family members, as well as others who must deal with the family members, to a confrontation with the severity of the illness. The open family may be torn apart by the confrontation or it may come through the adaptive struggle with members having grown closer together, having gained an ability to struggle valiantly in future life conflicts, and having achieved a level of confidence, strength, and reevaluation of basic life commitments that will make for a more effective and fulfilled life.

People use coping mechanisms to deal with crisis (Lazarus, 1980). In families coping with a life-threatening illness, it is important to place the coping patterns of each member within the context of the family's primary role as support environment for its members. If a family loses its common objectives, reduces cooperation among members, if members do not reciprocate services (most notably in the sexual roles of the spouses), or fail to coordinate functions, or lack consensus of emotional attitudes, then, no matter how well an individual member adapts to a life-threatening diagnosis, the family itself has failed in its primary function of social support of its members. The result is family disorganization and possible disintegration if the situation continues for long. While individual family members may cope effectively and well without family support, effective coping is the exception in families in which communication is minimal and disorganization is high.

In the family of a child with a life-threatening illness, parents are often so overwhelmed by the illness that they do not prepare for ordinary events; for example, a child diagnosed with a life-threatening illness at 2 years of age can at 5 begin to have problems in school simply because his mother did not engage in the ordinary preparatory steps for school. If the child had not developed a life-threatening illness some time earlier, the mother would have placed into perspective the child's needs for preparation for school, with its accompanying social demands from the child's school-aged peers. What happens is a basic failure in family coping and adaptation: the mother's attempts at coping with her child's illness, though successful regarding the illness, leave the mother with little energy to deal with the child's new problem, entry into school. The mother, while coping with the illness, is not giving her child the type of support needed to cope with a nondisease task. Similarly, other ordinary life transitions of children, such as entry into junior high school, pubescence, or transfer to a new city, can become crises because the family, overwhelmed by a life-threatening diagnosis in the child, has frozen efforts at growth. It is as if the family unit were saying to itself: "If only we can hold it all together and keep from falling apart, we'll make it." Such a mode of coping with the illness precludes the type of openness to growth and change that is necessary as the children move through various developmental crises on their way to adulthood. Such a family fails to devote the necessary energy to help the child in a time of greatest nondisease need.

SIBLINGS

What has been stated about the child with a life-threatening illness also holds for the siblings. The siblings of a child with a life-threatening illness are often neglected by the parents, not because sibling needs are not important, but because their needs take on a lesser importance relative to the diagnosis of a life-threatening illness. Siblings in the families of children with a life-threatening illness often face alone the developmental tasks necessary to achieve adulthood. Attempts by the siblings to seek help from parents often meet with a plea to be mature and generous, and to respect the needs of the ill child. Even the mentally strong and healthy sibling cannot be expected to go through life's transitional stages without support, from parents who have "burned-out" from strategies used in coping with their ill child's diagnosis (Cairns, Clark, Smith, & Lansky, 1979; Johnson, Rudolph, & Hartman, 1979; Kagen-Goodheart, 1977; Kaplan et al., 1976; Lavigne & Ryan, 1979; Slavin, 1980; Sourkes, 1977, 1980; Spinetta, 1981b).

SPOUSES

What has been said about the child with a life-threatening illness and his siblings also holds for the parents. The parents, occasionally in unison but more often in their own separate ways, expend their energies dealing with the illness. Often, remaining life tasks, such as career, finances, and sexual life, take on a lowered significance (Stehbens & Lascari, 1974). When a parent's needs are not met within the family unit, the parent may turn outside the family to fulfill the needs. Sometimes separation and divorce can result from this activity. However, with proper and continued counseling support, spouses may be drawn closer together because of their shared experiences. Divorce is not inevitable (Lansky, Cairns, Hassanein, Wehr, & Lowman, 1978; Spinetta et al., 1980).

In summary, a family spends a large amount of energy in attempting to keep itself from becoming disorganized and disintegrated under the overwhelming threat to the life of one of its members. In the process of dealing with a life-threatening illness, the family finds itself with little energy left to fulfill its primary function as a support team to each of its members. Individual members may find their own special needs unmet. What must occur is that family members communicate their needs at a level that can be effectively understood by others in the family. Unless this communication occurs and individual family members are able to continue to receive support for their own needs from the family system, those individuals will be forced to look elsewhere for the support the family no longer gives.

SOURCES OF SUPPORT

As parents prepare to meet the new demands imposed on them by their child's illness, it is wise for them to take an inventory of what individuals or systems of belief they can rely on as a source of support in this time of stress (Spinetta et al., 1976). It might be good to look back and analyze who or what helped during previous stressful times.

A group of parents who had lost their child to cancer was asked to list the sources of support they depended upon during the duration of their child's illness (Spinetta, 1981a). Not all indicated the same sources, but the list included: spouse, friends, relatives, hospital staff, religious beliefs, clergy, professional counselors, the sick child himself, and other parents of sick children.

The spouse was a supportive factor in many but not all of the marriages. Some people turned to friends because they accepted the fact that they could not communicate with their partner. The hospital staff was of assistance to many families. Parents as a whole had great respect for the medical competence of their physician and appreciated the doctor's and nurses' understanding and sensitive care of their child. Religion was a powerful factor in the lives of many parents who had a strong religious belief prior to the diagnosis. By far the strongest source of support was the presence of an understanding spouse or close friend to whom the parent could turn as problems arose. It was not unusual for parents to derive strength from their own child. Finally, parents have found other parents of children with cancer a source of support. Parents of children with cancer share common concerns, fears, and problems. They are able to establish supportive bonds with one another that cut across social, economic, and racial barriers.

In many hospitals, parents have organized parents groups which meet on a regular weekly or monthly basis to share common problems and concerns (Adams, 1980; Heffron, Bommelaere, & Masters, 1973; Knapp & Hansen, 1973). These parental groups serve a healthy function in helping parents attain a feeling of mastery in coping with some of the more difficult aspects of the illness and diagnosis.

The goal of working with the families of children with a life-threatening illness is to help them strengthen their own adaptive capabilities and coping styles. The health care professional treating the child must take into account the family structure and environment (van Eys, 1977). To help family members use the support systems they will need during the remaining months or years of their child's life, and after the child's death, is the goal for which the professional dedicated to the care of the total child must strive.

Returning to School

A major part of normal growth and development for all children involves school. For a child with a life-threatening illness, a return to school represents a continuation of life, hope for the future, and an attempt to reestablish equilibrium—an equilibrium that does not deny the fact of the illness but encompasses the new reality base of a potential threat to life (Greene, 1975; Kagen-Goodheart, 1977; Kaplan et al., 1973; Katz & Kellerman, 1977; Kirten & Liverman, 1977; Lansky et al., 1975; Zwartjes & Zwartjes, 1980). School personnel play a crucial role in determining whether or not the child with a potentially life-threatening illness can live a normal life, since so much of the child's day is centered on school. Teachers, counselors, school nurses, and administrators must be prepared to deal with this added responsibility (Deasy-Spinetta & Spinetta, 1980a, 1980b).

The physician, either directly or through a school-trained educational liaison who is an integral member of the health care team, can best help the child by opening and keeping open lines of communication with the school.

A return to school for a child with a life-threatening illness involves personal interaction, typically with one teacher at the elementary school level, five or more at the secondary level, plus school nurses, counselors, administrators, and peers. Each of these individuals brings to the child their own philosophy of life, attitudes toward death, and understanding of the illness. Furthermore, each school often has an identifiable attitude toward working with any child with a medical problem in the regular classroom. It is, therefore, imperative to prepare significant school personnel for the reentry of the patient-student. The school needs: first, accurate medical information specific to the particular student/patient; second, an understanding of the psychosocial implications of the illness as it relates to the child and his family, and finally, a referral source, someone who is part of the health care team, who can answer questions as they arise. When this is done, the school, the environment in which the child spends many hours each day, will promote rather than interfere with the child's efforts to cope with his school life within the context of the illness. If the school is not adequately prepared, the environment in which the child spends many hours each day may interfere with the child's efforts to cope with his school life within the context of the illness.

PREPARING THE TEACHER

Health care professionals associated with the medical management of potentially life-threatening illnesses in children realize that the children are living longer than in the past. However, professionals outside the medical environment, such as school teachers, frequently equate life-threatening illnesses with death. Since such illnesses no longer always result in death, this attitude must be addressed if teachers are to be adequately prepared to handle children with life-threatening illnesses in the classroom. Just as each member of the medical staff has his or her own philosophical position on death, so too does each member of the school staff. A specific teacher's philosophy of death may differ from that of colleagues and from that of the parents of the child. The presence of a possibly life-threatened child in the classroom causes reflection and concern among the school staff. For some teachers this may be a personally unsettling experience. It is necessary to assist teachers in understanding their own attitudes and emotional responses toward the concept of death. The teacher must also gain an appreciation of the child's understanding of death and realize that each family has its own manner of dealing with such a crisis. It is important to help teachers realize that all children are very sensitive to nonverbal cues in their environment. If the teacher is uneasy about having a child with a potentially life-threatening illness in the classroom, the child will sense this at a nonverbal level and there may be negative consequences in his academic and social performance. The child will also sense a warm, caring supportive attitude on the part of the teacher. The teacher must realize that she or he is working not only with a child but also with a family in crisis.

It is also important to help teachers understand that a child with a serious illness can continue to achieve and develop, and may have years of valuable life ahead. Hope is essential in dealing with these students. Unlike denial, hope does not interfere with healthy adjustment and is entirely compatible with an acceptance of reality (Lazarus, 1980). When caregivers lose the hope for cure, development can be hampered. Some caregivers may expect a child to die and therefore not do what is needed to help the child develop. This attitude, termed "psychological euthanasia" (van Eys, 1977), may serve to protect caregivers but is devastating to the child in the classroom. It is imperative, then, that teachers be helped to understand that a child with a life-threatening illness is a living, growing, developing child valiantly trying to learn in spite of a difficult situation.

SPECIFIC ISSUES RELATIVE TO SCHOOL

Many children with a potentially life-threatening illness have difficulties in school for a variety of reasons. Hair loss, weight loss or gain, and reduced stamina are the most obvious and most frequently discussed. Yet many children who have an understanding of the reasons for these obvious physical changes and have been well prepared by both the medical staff and their parents can explain to their classmates the reasons for the physical changes, and thereby gain the understanding and support of their peers. The more directly school-related problems can be more devastating than the disease-related problems, simply because the former are more subtle and easily overlooked; for example, a child with a serious illness may either have or develop a reading problem. Teachers who view the child as living despite the illness see the need for referring the child for appropriate diagnostic evaluation and remediation. Teachers who view the child as dying do not refer, and the child goes from grade to grade carrying the burden, not only of the illness, but also of a worsening reading difficulty.

Attendance at school may be a problem because of frequent clinic visits and occasional hospitalizations. Many teachers are very cooperative and flexible and allow the child to make up work. Others, especially at the secondary level, do not. The adolescent's need for privacy, coupled with a teacher's need for an excuse for absence, can often conflict. This especially becomes a problem when the child's teachers do not accept the fact of the illness, or the adolescent refuses to tell the teacher what he or she really has. Bridging this communication gap is critical and can best be done by a professional trained both in the school and in the hospital environments.

A well-prepared teacher is a valuable link in the total care of the child. A teacher who is prepared to deal with the family in crisis, as well as with the child, is in a position to communicate with parents in a way health care professionals might not be. For example, many children are found to have the illness before entering school. Beginning school is a significant step for all children and their parents. If the child is successful in entering school, the parents feel rewarded in their efforts to promote normal growth and development. If a child has problems in school, parents may link the problems to some other cause. If the child has an illness, they may blame the illness for nonillness-related difficulties. A well-prepared teacher will point out to these parents that many other children have difficulties at the beginning of school as well, and that the difficulties are not those only of children with a serious illness. This support of the parents at a critical transition time by a competent teacher helps the child.

The transition from elementary to junior high school is stressful for all students, not merely for the student with a life-threatening illness. School-related activities are particularly significant for the adolescent patient. Diseases and their treatment may prevent or impede successful development of autonomy, acquisition of consistent body image and sex roles, establishment of peer relations, and the adoption of future-oriented social and intellectual preparation. It is important to allow an adolescent to maximize her or his sense of control, and the school is one area where the adolescent patient can do this. It is essential that school personnel understand the particular illness and its related consequences as they apply to the adolescent.

Since children with life-threatening illnessess are living longer and seeking a normal life by attending school, communication with the school becomes not a luxury, but a vital and essential element in the total care of the child. Everyone involved benefits from expanded communication with the child's school. The child is happier in school; teachers are more comfortable in their roles; the parents are content that the child is safe, productive, and functioning like other children his age; and the physician obtains a more complete picture of the child. Teachers and other school personnel play a significant role in the life of the child. Given adequate preparation, information, and support, they are an essential and valuable link in the total care of the child.

Conclusion

The major dilemma facing parents of a child with cancer is between the amount of time and mental effort to be devoted to concern for the cancer and its treatment, and the amount of time to be devoted to the continuation of a normal living pattern, both for the child with cancer and for the remaining family members. Work, the home, the siblings, the schools, the normal life of the patient—all of these must continue. The critical factor is at what level these will continue. Does coping merely mean getting on with the task of life, or can it include a healthy growth which includes the joy of living? Parents need help to keep their lives moving forward. Our research has demonstrated that the parental self-image does not change because of the illness (Spinetta *et al.*, 1980). What does change is the parent's ability to handle day-to-day kinds of problems (Kalnins, 1980). These are problems that come to the fore during the course of remission. During ordinary clinic visits for treatments, it is the day-to-day issues that become important; issues that may have been readily resolvable prior to the illness now take on a different challenge. Many parents feel unable to make the needed decisions alone without the help, understanding, support, and input of an understanding team member.

NEED FOR A PSYCHOSOCIAL TEAM MEMBER

What the parents need is a professional who is both trained in counseling and therapy, and who is up-to-date on psychosocial research findings regarding responses of parents who are struggling with the continual task of maintaining normalcy in the light of having a child with cancer who is undergoing treatment. It is during times of relapse recurrence when the strain becomes great, and the parents feel especially overwhelmed by the tasks, when life in effect does stop while the child becomes the central and sole focus for a while, that they turn to the professional for help. It is critical to have such a professional assigned to the team whose primary task is dealing with these psychosocial concerns of the family (Koocher & Sallan, 1978). This will give the family members a pivotal person on whom they can depend, even though they may also turn to the nurse or physician for counsel.

The availability of psychological consultation services in pediatric oncology cannot be considered a luxury. The ever-increasing complexity and variables in the treatment programs demand a relatively sophisticated consultant who can function smoothly as a member of an oncology treatment team (Koocher & Sallan, 1978). Issues about side-effects of treatment, troublesome symptoms, relations with staff members, and a hundred other potential concerns cannot be met effectively by a therapist at the local mental health center, a school counselor, or a private practitioner away from the clinic. The other members of the oncology treatment team must have consultants they know, whose judgment they trust, and with whom they can relate on a regular basis.

It is therapy in the broadest sense which is being addressed here. Often parents are reluctant to talk to an assigned therapist directly about a problem, for fear of being labeled abnormal or pathological. What is critical is that the parent, sibling, and child realize that talking about day-to-day concerns is not only appropriate and acceptable, but that the need to do so is normal. While parental concerns from the outset may be existential, and very much related to the potentially life-threatening nature of the illness, what will emerge after a time will be first medical and treatment-related concerns, and then nonmedical family concerns. When the initial shock has worn off, the family members need to know that there is someone on the team to whom they can turn to have their questions resolved, both medical and nonmedical. This rapport must be established from the outset; the parents will fare best when they are able to return to the business of living as soon as possible after the diagnosis and initiation of treatment.

CONTINUED HOPE, EVEN TO THE END

Lazarus (1980) talks about the aspects of denial. One must maintain hope at all costs, hope that this particular child will be the one to make it. Use of the best medical treatment will be one step toward that goal. A second and equally important step is the psychological commitment toward life on the part of spouses, siblings, and patient. A child who is going to live will need to continue to develop and grow, and to continue to pursue schooling with the objective of full adult participation in life. If the child does make it as a survivor of the cancer experience, the patient should not have fallen so far behind that catching up to normal living becomes an additional burden.

If the child relapses, hope can still be kept alive, though it becomes more difficult to do so. It is not uncommon for family members to be committed to growth and development, and, at point of relapse or recurrence, to give up hope. When a child does achieve a remission again, the family members then bear the additional burden of having to regroup forces and continue moving forward, with diminished hope. The parents need help to pull them through these phases of relapse/remission to keep their commitment to life fully functional.

If the child does eventually become terminal, as a large number of children do, then a point comes when the parents must face the fact of the child's death and make difficult decisions about cessation of treatment, recessation procedures, home care during the final phase. Even at this point, a family must continue its commitment to the value of life for each of its members. The patient will have been well served by having tried as much as possible to live a fulfilled life, despite the cancer. At the point of death, such a child will die with the memory of having lived fully at least for a while. Such a child may continue to fight the death, but at least when death comes will have felt that life was not set aside because of the cancer. A continued commitment of the family to schooling and family activities during the course of the child's disease will be a memory the child can cherish at the end. It is very important for the children and adolescents to achieve as much as possible during the time they have left. Keeping up physical appearance, keeping up with schoolwork, most especially during the final phases of the illness, are critical to the self-worth of the patient. For adolescents, love, security, and freedom from pain are equally important as for younger children. The more their parents can be with them and communicate with them with openness and honesty, the more adolescents can be helped to resolve their feelings at the time of death (Adams, 1980).

Parents who have given this commitment to continued life and living, who have not spoiled their sick child, who have allowed the siblings to live their lives as well, and who have continued their own spouse relationships will find their strength to accept the death of the child when it comes. While the sadness and grieving will not be diminished after the death of the child, the ability to return to a full and functioning life after the death will be greatly enhanced for those who were able to go on with the business of living during the life of the child (Spinetta et al., 1980).

CAREGIVERS

There are effects on caregivers as well. It is difficult to see so many children die without being saddened and hurt when the deaths occur. The emotional costs are high, but the rewards are even higher. There is the opportunity to work with highly motivated family members and to see significant beneficial progress in short periods of time. There is the continuous reward of playing an important role, helping at a crucial time in the life of a family. Some patients die. The caretaker who periodically has sad feelings, and can reasonably accept them, will remain in the field, and be productive (Koocher & Sallan, 1978; Koocher, 1979).

NO SINGLE ANSWER

While a family's responses at point of diagnosis may be so exceptional as to point out that family as low risk, most families are in need of care throughout. Some families ebb and flow in their abilities to handle issues; some do well at the beginning but grow progressively in need of help. There is no single pattern.

There is no single prescription for dealing with childhood cancer. There are many variables: the type of cancer, the severity of the illness, the prognosis, the age of the child, the family history of coping, the present family support system, as well as economic and other factors that may impinge in an ongoing manner on the course of the treatment and response to the treatment.

One of the pioneers in this work expressed the problem exceptionally well:

Each parent and sibling reacts to a fatal illness individually, in a manner consistent with his own personality structure, past experience, current crises, and the particular meaning or special circumstances associated with the loss threatening him. To help them, one must know each one and his relations to his or her friends, how they react to the initial diagnosis, how their grief process begins, and how they cope. One should know, too, something of their beliefs about life, death, and religion, their response to previous crises, and their current burdens and sources of support. (Binger *et al.*, 1969, p. 418)

This is a large task, but then, the life of a child is not a small responsibility. Will we meet the task of helping the child with cancer live a full and happy life, even if that life will be foreshortened?

THE PEDIATRIC PSYCHOLOGIST AS FAMILY ADVOCATE IN LIFE-THREATENING ILLNESS: HELPING THE FAMILY SUSTAIN A CHILD WITH CYSTIC FIBROSIS[7]

As with the child with cancer, so too has much been done in recent years to prolong the life of a child with cystic fibrosis. What was once inevitably and too quickly fatal has become a chronic illness, with a shortened life span. And with the chronicity has come its inseparable psychosocial concomitants. The individual's chance of survival with cystic fibrosis well beyond the childhood and adolescent years, enhanced by recent medical advances, has brought with a lengthened life span, an increase in problems in normal living, and a prolongation of emotional complications among the patients, their parents, and siblings.

A unique feature of the medical care of the child and young adult with cystic fibrosis is the presence of cystic fibrosis centers carefully placed geographically in population areas throughout the United States, to give the best of medical and psychosocial care to every patient in each catchment area. While other catastrophic childhood illnesses share the concept of a center, few others have so fully, extensively, and carefully mapped out centers throughout the country, such that each major population center has a medical facility specifically staffed by a combined medical and psychosocial team. Cystic fibrosis is an illness so intrusive in nature, both physically and psychologically, on the functioning of the family and of each of its members, that a health care team at a Cystic Fibrosis Center can readily use two psychosocial members: a social worker, to deal directly with psychological needs, and a pediatric psychologist, to study family needs in detail and to research the effectiveness of differing modes of intervention. As the patient is living longer, such combined interdisciplinary clinical and research efforts become critical to the future well-being of the patient. The presence of Cystic Fibrosis Centers throughout the country makes it possible to conduct research efforts in a highly controlled and geographically adaptive manner.

---

[7]This section was prepared by John J. Spinetta and Vrinda S. Knapp.

What Is Cystic Fibrosis?

When one mentions the word *cancer,* the general public response is one of recognition, perhaps with overly negative connotations, of an illness that is potentially life-threatening. When one mentions the words *cystic fibrosis,* the ordinary layperson's response is: "What is that?" What many people do not realize is that cystic fibrosis is not only invariably fatal—even though the patient is now living longer—but is so intrusive as to render a "normal" family life achieveable only through intense and determined efforts on the part of all family members.

What is cystic fibrosis? Cystic fibrosis quite simply is an inherited and currently incurable disease that attacks the lungs and the digestive system, an effect of insufficiency of secretion of pancreatic digestive enzymes. In most visible terms, it is accompanied by a chronic coughing to expel excessive sputum, by intestinal and bowel difficulties, and by embarrassing flatulence and offensive stools. Secondary effects include retarded physical development, with small stature and delayed sexual characteristics, sterility in the male, and potential health dangers in childbearing for the female. A shortened life span now is inevitable, with death occurring most commonly in the early adult years.

The commonest inherited condition in populations of Caucasian origin, cystic fibrosis is inherited as an autosomal recessive gene. When both parents are carriers, each child in the family has a one in four chance of acquiring the condition at conception. Although non-Caucasians also can be carriers, the incidence in blacks is only 1 in 1700 live births, while for Asians, the incidence is 1 in 100,000 live births.

Management of the patient diagnosed as having CF is complex and varied because secondary consequences of the basic underlying disorder are widespread. In their *Manual of Diagnosis and Management,* Anderson and Goodchild (1976) list several factors that play an important part in successful management: early diagnosis; control of progression of chest infection by inhalation therapy and drugs; maintenance of adequate nutrition with pancreatic enzyme replacement and dietary management; the treatment and control of other complications such as diabetes mellitus and meconium ileus equivalent; and, more important, the acceptance, both by the patient and by the family, of limitations in normal living which the condition imposes.

Recent literature on the subject reveals the growing concern of professionals over the psychological complications accompanying the prolongation of the child's life. This section summarizes the issue, surveying the types of difficulties faced by patients at various ages, the effects of the illness on parents and siblings, and the growing need for ongoing research and service on helping families in the management of the emotional and psychosocial problems associated with the illness.

Effects on the Child

When the disease is first recognized, the family typically is overwhelmed by the thought of its fatality. But as the patient begins involvement in a lifetime program of intensive treatment, concerns shift to anxiety about the restrictions associated with the illness, both social and physical. The primary anxieties and conflicts of the patient relative to the illness contain some of the elements of a fatal illness, but most closely resemble those of a chronic illness (Patterson, Denning, & Kutscher, 1973).

THE CHILD UNDER 10

The problems for the young child, though not often openly discussed by the child, are nonetheless real and intense. Researchers claim that many more than expected of the ill children under 10 are already emotionally vulnerable, in danger either of disorganization under stress or, more commonly, of becoming unduly rigid and constricted with a resulting impoverishment of personality and disability to function (Falkman, 1977; Kulczycki, Robinson, & Berg, 1969; Mattsson, 1972; Turk, 1964). The young child with cystic fibrosis experiences physical limitation and distress, internalized fears, and excessive dependence. Inability to compete in physical activity and considerable absence from school, together with excessive shame and name calling by peer groups, may contribute to a lowered self-esteem and to a sense of personal failure (Gratzick, 1973; McCrae, 1975; Meyerowitz & Kaplan, 1973).

Although the girls under 10, as a group, seem to have a more adequate view of themselves than boys, they, too, suffer from the consequences of a restricting and energy-depleting illness. Both the boys and the girls fail to be as aggressive and self-assured as others their age; many see themselves as younger than they really are, and as dependent and inadequate. The children complain about the interruption of play, dietary deprivations, and physical limitations which prevent them from keeping up with others. The chances for enjoying the meaningful and pleasure-giving experiences of normal youth were limited in the past. Most recently, there have been attempts made to have the children with cystic fibrosis share such experiences as slumber parties and camp outings (Docter, 1973; Selden, 1973).

Afraid that other children will be uncomfortable with peers that are different, the children often try to conceal the condition in order to facilitate peer relationships, sometimes even escaping into fantasy life as a respite from the problems of reality (Lawler, Nakielny, & Wright, 1966; Leiken & Hassakis, 1973; Tropauer, Franz, & Dilgard, 1970) thus increasing even further their psychosocial distance from peers. Even children in the preschool years exhibit severe problems, reverting to primitive behavior patterns or becoming restricted in the range of their activities, interests, and interpersonal relationships. Withdrawal and avoidance are common. Given the tendency in our culture to praise the aggressive, healthy, and socially active child, with little room for the child who does not fit in, it is no wonder that the child with cystic fibrosis tries to deny the illness. This denial can be costly, in terms of emotional health (Cytryn, Moore, & Robinson, 1973).

Coupled with the many problems associated with the chronicity of the illness is the inevitable probability of an early death. Although in most of the studies of children in this age group there is a general absence of overt depression, this does not necessarily mean that the children are free from preoccupation with their disease. Children are acutely attuned to nonverbal signals, and can readily pick up signals at variance with expressed adult communication (Reeves, 1973; Spinetta & Deasy-Spinetta, 1980). At some level of awareness the child gets the message: you have a very serious illness, and eventually you are going to die from it. A child is likely to handle such awareness in the manner that least threatens his dependency, by going along with whatever story his parents give (Spinetta, 1978). It does not take long for professionals working with severely ill children to come to the realization that awareness of death for a child can be engraved at some level that precedes the child's ability to talk about it. A child might well know that he has an ultimately fatal illness long before he can say so (Spinetta, 1974).

Faced with a reality which neither the child or parents can change, the child tries to live with it. The defenses employed are not always effective.

THE ADOLESCENT

For the older child, the conflicts are more readily visible and the conditions better understood (Boyle, di Sant'Agnese, Sack, Millican, & Kulczycki, 1976; Davies & Addington, 1973; Drotar, 1977; McCollum & Gibson, 1970). Although the emerging adolescent may not willingly participate in group discussions, he or she spends a good deal of time gaining intellectual mastery of the illness, achieving hope from the older youngsters who have the same illness but who, in many cases, seem to be adapting. As the child reaches adolescence, the prolonged child-parent dependency intensifies the feelings of being different from peers. Adolescence brings with it increased concerns about physical stature, bodily functioning, and thin, frail appearance.

Added to the adolescent's anxiety about the restrictions the disease imposes on a growing desire to socialize with and be accepted by peers is a gnawing preoccupation with ultimate disability and eventual death (Tropauer et al., 1970). In contrast to the younger child who often fools parents concerning knowledge of impending death, the adolescent has an intense need to communicate preoccupations, anxieties, and fears. When there is no one around who will listen or understand, or most especially when the adolescent receives negative reinforcement for expressing socially unacceptable thoughts, she or he becomes very depressed. There are striking parallels between the depressions experienced by the adolescent with cystic fibrosis, and the emotional and psychosocial ingredients of suicide (Sibinga, Friedman, & Huang, 1973). Disease-related adolescent deaths may as often be the result of deliberate as of accidental failure to comply with medical management (Meyers, Dolan, & Mueller, 1975).

It is difficult to be an adolescent. When one adds to the normal problems of growing into adulthood the added problems associated with a life-threatening illness, it is no wonder that suicide is often a basic motive in the adolescent's refusal to receive or help maintain the necessary therapy (Meyers et al., 1975; Winder & Nedalie, 1973). Death by a fatal illness is tragic; the loss of one's desire to live is equally tragic.

THE YOUNG ADULT

As the patient reaches adulthood, interest in heterosexual relationships activates questions about marriage and childbearing. The young adult becomes "cautiously future oriented'' (Gratzick, 1973), making career and family plans with the knowledge that one's adult life span will very likely be short, and that the disease itself may well limit and in some cases, especially with males, even remove entirely one's ability to have children (Meyerowitz & Kaplan, 1973). Thoughts of marriage and a normal adult life bring with them increased concern over making realistic vocational choices that take into account a basic lack of energy and vitality, periods of hospitalization, and disease-related financial burdens (Boyle *et al.* 1976; Spinetta, Deasy-Spinetta, McLaren, Kung, Schwartz, & Hartman, 1981).

Faced with an inevitable and harsh reality, the patient with cystic fibrosis needs help to cope. Where does he or she turn? The patient, especially the younger child, looks inevitably to the family.

Effects on the Family

When individuals belong to families, they do not suffer their problems of stress independently. The disease affects the family as well as the child. Families may begin to fall apart. There is a reduction in occupational and social mobility, with increased social isolation. The family pattern may become one of continual stress. Serious financial burden, depletion of savings, foregoing of luxuries, resentments against the ill child are all part and parcel of the illness (Farkas & Schnell, 1973; Lawler, *et al.*, 1966)

Sometimes parents harbor wishes to desert their children and be free of the burden they must bear (Burton, 1975; Gayton, Friedman, Tavormina, & Tucker, 1977). These ambivalent feelings not only add to their guilt about having given birth to the child but often add to the burden of the child, who cannot help but pick up these feelings of resentment. In many cases, hospitalization may be dictated by the parents rather than by the patient's medical needs. The parents often become confused as to how they should behave exhibiting frequent dilemmas of how solicitous they should be or how much expectation they can place on their child. An entire life-style develops over the years based on cycles of treatments and visits to the doctor, all occurring at the expense of personal needs and the loss of the simplest amenities of daily life (Barbero, 1973).

Siblings are by no means free of the burdens of the illness. They, too, must defer their own needs and desires as the patient becomes the focus of attention. Siblings complain of deprivation and sacrifice: they begin to demand more of their parents' time, develop somatic complaints of their own, and sometimes even pretend that they, too, have some serious illness (Gayton *et al.*, 1977; Tropauer *et al.*, 1970). Excessive guilt often accompanies their wish for the ill child to become really sick or to die. Their school work begins to suffer, and the strain often results in poor school adjustment and even delinquency.

Mothers not only have the sick child and siblings to contend with, but often have the added burden of a father's lack of participation in the administration of therapy, his disinclination to discuss his feelings and get involved, and increased sexual tension (Burton, 1975; Lawler *et al.*, 1966). Talk of separation and divorce is common among the parents. As if this were not enough, above all stands the thought that, despite the most adequate of care and despite all of the sacrifices involved, death will someday intervene, for some earlier, for others later.

It is the rare patient and family that does not incur some psychological complications and problems in adapting to such an illness. These psychological and emotional complications may intensify the stress for everyone, especially the sick child, and eventually create additional difficulties for the physician in the total management of the case. In some instances, disturbance may be so severe as to interfere directly with the medical treatment. The famly needs help to cope.

FAMILY COPING

Cystic fibrosis poses serious problems for the coping ability of the family as a unit. If stress is great enough and sufficiently prolonged, the role of the family as a buffer for its members and aid for the ill child can be impaired or even destroyed. It seems clear that the family unit is a critical factor in the adaptation of a child to illness (Spinetta, 1978, 1980).The extent and severity of emotional and psychosocial effects of the illness on the child depend not merely on the child's own emotional reserves and coping mechanisms, but on the degree of support the child sustains from the immediate environment (Burton, 1975; Meyerowitz & Kaplan, 1973). Prior interaction and experience of the child and family, various factors such as age, degree, and duration of handicap, qualities and duress of prior treatment and hospitalization, temperament, social, cultural, and emotional environment are among the facets that determine the pattern of reaction to the illness (Barbero, 1973). A healthy family will have a greater chance to cope properly with the illness than will a family that is marginal in terms of psychological health.

But even in stable, well-adjusted families, parents have marked difficulty in talking to their child about the condition. They are often too involved in coping with their own very real problems (Spinetta & Deasy-Spinetta, 1981). Many parents do not have the personal resources to give the child both an intellectual understanding of the disease, at the child's own level, and, much more important, emotional support and an opportunity to communicate and share his personal anxieties. Even with healthy parents, there can be a tendency to cope with one's own problems, avoiding the child and his or her questions, or answering the questions in a superficial manner (Gayton et al., 1977; Lawler et al., 1966). This may lead the child to mistrust the parents, and can leave him or her increasingly anxious, fearful, and confused. The parents need help both in giving the emotional support the child needs and in facing their own anxieties relative to the illness.

The Role of the Pediatric Psychologist

The most logical place for the family to seek aid is the medical facility which is already dealing with the physical aspects of the problem. A pediatric psychologist or social worker who is a hospital CF team member can be very helpful in anticipating and in meeting the situation in a constructive manner (Drotar, 1977). The less communicative and the less emotionally supportive the members of the family are to each other, the more likely it will be that difficulties in adjustment to the illness will occur (Spinetta & Maloney, 1978), and the greater the need for outside sources of psychological help. A readily available team member who has experience with psychosocial adjustment is an indispensable aid to health family coping.

As stated above, CF is so intrusive a disease, both physically and psychologically, on the functioning of the family and of each of its members, that a health care team at a CF Center can readily use two psychosocial team members: a social worker, to deal directly with psychological needs, and a pediatric psychologist, to study family needs in detail and to research the effectiveness of differing modes of intervention. As the patients with CF are living longer, into adult years, such combined interdisciplinary clinical and research efforts become critical to the future well being of the CF patient.

Significant advances have been made in improving the chances of a longer life for a child with CF, shifting the focus of the illness gradually from fatality to chronicity. But it is not enough merely to keep the patient alive longer. Much more needs to be accomplished toward a unified and effective approach to the psychosocial and emotional care of the child, the adolescent, and the young adult striving toward adulthood. In helping the CF patient live longer, health care professionals must also help the patient live as full a life as possible, administering to emotional as well as to physical needs. Otherwise, CF will become an illness in which the patient is kept medically alive, but left psychologically dead (van Eys, 1977). A well-trained and alert social worker can help alleviate some of the difficulties, help the family strengthen its own coping resources, and, ultimately, help the child and young adult lead a happier as well as a longer life. Taking a cue from work in other childhood catastrophic illnesses (Spinetta & Deasy-Spinetta, 1981, in press), a well-trained research psychologist, as an equally active member of the CF Center's health care team, can research both the needs and the effectiveness of intervention methods to give direction to this field in its increasing awareness of psychosocial issues.

On a more global level, well-conducted research on the psychosocial concomitants of CF has as its ultimate goal the recognition by health care policymakers of the necessary role of psychosocial support systems in the treatment of catastrophic and chronic childhood illness. The implication of such recognition on financing the development of a true model and system of health care delivery is obvious.

OVERVIEW

A single theme has dominated this chapter: the role of the pediatric psychologist as a researcher-clinician in the hospital setting. Each section has been a detailed attempt at understanding how a pediatric psychologist might function with a particular disease entity in a particular situation. As stated more than once above, well-conducted and rigorous research on the psychosocial concomitants of catastrophic childhood illness has as its primary goal the well-being, both present and future, of the child-patient and the family. A vital step in the achievement of this goal is to conduct research that is so well designed and relevant to the child's psychosocial health care needs that health care policymakers at the national level will recognize the necessary role of psychosocial support systems in the treatment of catastrophic illness and will, accordingly, finance the development of a true model and system of health care delivery that will encompass the critical psychosocial needs of the children. Any help which the pediatric psychologist as researcher-clinician can give in furthering this goal will be a large step toward the care of the child with a catastrophic illness.

REFERENCES

Adams, D. W. *Childhood malignancy: The psychosocial care of the child and his family.* Springfield, IL: Charles C. Thomas, 1980.

Ad Hoc Committee of Harvard Medical School. A definition of irreversible coma: Report of the Ad Hoc Committee of the Harvard Medical School to examine the definition of brain death. *Journal of the American Medical Association,* 1968, **205,** 337–340.

Alby, K. T. Preventing child abuse. *American Psychologist,* 1975, **30,** 921–928.

Alby, N., & Alby, J. M. The doctor and the dying child. In E. J. Anthony & C. Koupernik (Eds.), *The child in his family,* Vol. 2. *The impact of disease and death.* New York: Wiley, 1973.

American Psychiatric Association. *Diagnostic and Statistical Manual* (Proposed draft of revision). Washington, D.C.: American Psychiatric Association, 1979.

Anderson, C., & Goodchild, M. *Cystic Fibrosis: Manual of diagnosis and management.* Oxford: Blackwell Scientific Publications, 1976.

Anderson, T., and Andberg, M. Psychosocial factors associated with pressure sores. *Archives of Physical Medicine and Rehabilitation,* 1979, **60,** 341–346.

Anthony S. *The child's discovery of death.* New York: Harcourt Brace, 1940.

Barbero, G. J. The child, parents and doctor in death from chronic disease. In P. R. Patterson, C. R. Denning, & A. H. Kutscher (Eds.), *Psychosocial aspects of Cystic Fibrosis.* New York: Columbia University Press, 1973.

Beecher, K. Ethical problems created by the hopelessly unconscious patient. *New England Journal of Medicine,* 1968, **278,** 1425–1430.

Belsky, J. Child maltreatment: An ecological integration, *American Psychologist,* 1980, **35,** 320–335.

Binger, C. M., Ablin, A. R., Feuerstein, R. C., Kushner, J. H., Zoger, S., & Mikkelsen, C. Childhood leukemia: Emotional impact on patient and family. *New England Journal of Medicine,* 1969, **280,** 414–418.

Bluebond-Langner, M. I know, do you?: Awareness and communication in terminally ill children. In B. Schoenberg, A. Carr, D. Peretz, & A. Kutscher (Eds.), *Anticipatory grief.* New York: Columbia University Press, 1974.

Bluebond-Langner, M. Meanings of death to children. In H. Feifel (Ed.), *New meanings of death.* New York: McGraw-Hill, 1977.

Boyle, I., di Sant'Agnese, P., Sack, S., Millican, F., & Kulczycki, L. Emotional adjustment of adolescents and young adults with Cystic Fibrosis. *Journal of Pediatrics,* 1976, **88,** 318–326.

Bozeman, M. F., Orbach, C. E., & Sutherland, A. M. Psychological impact of cancer and its treatment: The adaptation of mothers to the threatened loss of their children through leukemia. *Cancer,* 1955, **8,** 1–33.

Burton, L. Tolerating the intolerable: The problems facing parents and children following diagnosis. In L. Burton (Ed.), *Care of the child facing death*. Boston: Routledge & Kegan Paul, 1974.

Cairns, N. U., Clark, G. M., Smith, S. D., & Lansky, S. B. Adaptation of siblings to childhood malignancy. *Journal of Pediatrics*, 1979, **95**, 484 – N487.

Capron, A. M., & Kass, L. R. A statutory definition of the standards for determining human death: An appraisal on proposals. *University of Pennsylvania Law Review*, 1972, **121**, 87 – 117.

Clapp, M. J. Psychosocial reactions of children with cancer. *Nursing Clinics of North America*, 1976, **11**, 73 – 82.

Cohen, J. An analysis of vocational failure of mentally retarded people placed in the community after a period of institutionalization. *American Journal of Mental Deficiency*, 1960, **65**, 371 – 375.

Colman, W. Occupational therapy and child abuse. *American Journal of Occupational Therapy*, 1975, **29**, 412 – 417.

Corey, E. J., Miller, C. L., & Widlack, F. W. Factors contributing to child abuse. *Nursing Research*, 1975, **24**, 293 – 295.

Crane, D. *The sanctity of social life: Physicians' treatment of critically ill patients*, New York: Russell Sage Foundation, 1975.

Cytryn, L., Moore, P. V. P., & Robinson, M. E. Psychological adjustment of children with Cystic Fibrosis. In E. J. Anthony & C. Koupernik (Eds.), *The child in his family*, Vol. 2. *The impact of disease and death*. New York: Wiley, 1973.

D'Agostino, P. Strains and stresses in protective services. In N. B. Ebeling & D. A. Hill (Eds.), *Child abuse: Intervention and treatment*. Acton, MA: Publishing Sciences Group, 1975.

Dash, J. Hypnosis with pediatric cancer patients. In J. Kellerman (Ed.), *Psychological aspects of childhood cancer*. Springfield, IL: Charles C. Thomas, 1980.

Davies, M., & Addington, W. Psychosocial aspects of Cystic Fibrosis family life as they affect medical management. In P. R. Patterson, C. R. Denning, & A. H. Kutscher (Eds.), *Psychosocial aspects of Cystic Fibrosis*. New York: Columbia University Press, 1973.

Deasy-Spinetta, P. The adolescent with cancer: A view from the inside. In J. J. Spinetta & P. Deasy-Spinetta (Eds.), *Living with childhood cancer*. St. Louis: Mosby, 1981.

Deasy-Spinetta, P., & Spinetta, J. J. The child with cancer in school: Teachers' appraisal. *American Journal of Pediatric Hematology/Oncology*, 1980, **2**, 89 – 94.

Deasy-Spinetta, P., & Spinetta, J. J. The school and the child with cancer. In J. J. Spinetta & P. Deasy-Spinetta (Eds.), *Living with childhood cancer*. St. Louis: Mosby, 1981.

DeCharms, R. *Personal causation*. New York: Academic Press, 1968.

Dembo, T., Leviton, G., & Wright, B. Adjustment to misfortune—A problem of social psychological rehabilitation. *Artificial Limbs*, 1956, **3**, 4 – 62.

Derdeyn, A. P. Child abuse and neglect: The rights of parents and the needs of their children. *American Journal of Orthopsychiatry*, 1977, **47**, 377 – 387.

Docter, J. The chronically ill child: Soma and psyche. In P. R. Patterson, C. R. Denning, & A. H. Kutscher (Eds.), *Psychosocial aspects of Cystic Fibrosis*. New York: Columbia University Press, 1973.

Drotar, D. Family oriented intervention with the dying adolescent. *Journal of Pediatric Psychology,* 1977, **2,** 68–71.

Dweck, C. The role of expectations and attributions in the elevation of learned helplessness. *Journal of Personality and Social Psychology,* 1975, **31,** 674–685.

Dweck, C., & Goetz, T. Attributions and learned helplessness. In J. Harvey, W. Ickes, & R. Kidd (Eds.), *New directions in attribution research,* Vol. 2. Hillside, NJ: Lawrence Erlbaum Associates, 1977.

Easson, W. M. *The dying child.* Springfield, IL: Charles C. Thomas, 1970.

Erikson, E. *Identity: Youth and crisis.* New York: Norton, 1968.

Falkman, C. Cystic fibrosis: A psychological study of 52 children and their families. *Acta Paediatrica Scandinavica,* 1977, 269.

Farkas, A. & Schnell, R. A psychological study of family adjustment to Cystic Fibrosis. In P. R. Patterson, C. R. Denning, & A. H. Kutscher (Eds.), *Psychosocial aspects of Cystic Fibrosis.* New York: Columbia University Press, 1973.

Floor, L., & Rosen, M. Investigation of helplessness in mentally retarded adults. *American Journal of Mental Deficiency,* 1975, **79,** 565–572.

Freidson, E. *Profession of medicine.* New York: Dodd, Mead, 1974.

Freud, S. Mourning and melancholia. In J. Riviere (trans.), *Collected papers,* Vol. 4. New York: Basic Books, 1979. (Originally published 1917)

Friedman, S., Chodoff, P., Mason, J., & Hamburg, D. Behavioral observations of parents anticipating the death of a child. *Pediatrics,* 1963, **32,** 610–625.

Futterman, E., & Hoffman, I. Crisis and adaptation in the families of fatally ill children. In E. J. Anthony & C. Koupernik (Eds.), *The child and his family,* Vol. 2. *The impact of disease and death.* New York: Wiley, 1973.

Gayton, W. F., Friedman, S. B., Tavormina, J. F., & Tucker, F. Children with Cystic Fibrosis: I. Psychological test findings of patients, siblings, and parents. *Pediatrics,* 1977, **59,** 888–894.

Gelles, R. Violence toward children in the United States. *American Journal of Orthopsychiatry,* 1978, **48,** 580–592.

Gil, D. G. *Violence against children: Physical abuse in the United States.* Cambridge, MA: Harvard University Press, 1970.

Gil, D. G. Primary prevention of child abuse: A philosophical and political issue. *Journal of Pediatric Psychology,* 1976, **1**(2), 54–57.

Gratzik, H. W. Hospitalized children and young adults with Cystic Fibrosis. In P. R. Patterson, C. R. Denning, & A. H. Kutscher (Eds.), *Psychosocial aspects of Cystic Fibrosis.* New York: Columbia University Press, 1973.

Greene, P. The child with leukemia in the classroom. *American Journal of Nursing,* 1975, **75,** 86–87.

Grollman, E. A. (Ed.) *Explaining death to children.* Boston: Beacon Press, 1967.

Grzesiak, R. Psychological services in rehabilitation medicine: Clinical aspects of rehabilitation psychology. *Professional Psychology,* 1979, **11,** 511–N520.

Hansen, Y. *Development of the concept of death: Cognitive aspects.* Doctoral dissertation, California School of Professional Psychology. Ann Arbor, MI: University Microfilms, 1973, **640,** 73–19.

Hartman, G. Hypnosis as an adjuvant in the treatment of childhood cancer. In J. J. Spinetta & P. Deasy-Spinetta (Eds.), *Living with childhood cancer.* St. Louis: Mosby, 1980.

Heffron, W. A., Bommelaere, K., & Masters, R. Group discussions with the parents of leukemic children. *Pediatrics,* 1973, **52,** 831–840.

Helfer, R. E., & Kempe, C. H. (Eds.) *The battered child.* Chicago: University of Chicago Press, 1968.

Helfer, R. E., & Schmidt, R. The community-based child abuse and neglect program. In R. E. Helfer & C. H. Kempe (Eds.), *Child abuse and neglect: The family and the community.* Cambridge, MA: Ballinger, 1976.

Helfer, R. E., Schneider, C., & Hoffmeister, J. K. *Manual for use of the Michigan Screening Profile of Parenting.* East Lansing: Michigan State University Press, 1977.

Hiroto, D. Focus of control and learned helplessness. *Journal of Experimental Psychology,* 1972, **102,** 187–193.

Hostler, S. I. The development of the child's concept of death. In O. J. Z. Sahler (Ed.), *The child and death.* St. Louis: Mosby, 1978.

Howarth, R. The psychiatric care of children with life-threatening illnesses. In L. Burton (Ed.), *Care of the child facing death.* Boston: Routledge & Kegan Paul, 1974.

Jackson, E. N. *Telling a child about death.* New York: Hawthorn Books, 1965.

Johnson, F. L., Rudolph, L., & Hartman, J. Helping the family cope with childhood cancer. *Psychosomatics,* 1979, **20,** 241–251.

Justice, B., & Justice, R. *The abusing family.* New York: Human Sciences Press, 1976.

Kagen-Goodheart, L. Re-entry: Living with childhood cancer. *American Journal of Orthopsychiatry,* 1977, **47,** 651–658.

Kalnins, I. V., Churchill, M. P., & Terry, G. E. Concurrent stresses in families with a leukemic child. *Journal of Pediatric Psychology,* 1980, **5,** 81–92.

Kaplan, D. M., Smith, A., Grobstein, R., & Fishman, S. Family mediation of stress. *Social Work,* 1973, **18**(4), 60–69.

Kaplan, D. M, Grobstein, R., & Smith, A. Predicting the impact of severe illness in families. *Health and Social Work,* 1976, **1**(3), 72–81.

Katz, E. R., Kellerman, J., Rigler, D., Williams, K. O., & Siegel, S. E. School intervention with pediatric cancer patients. *Journal of Pediatric Psychology,* 1977, **2**(2), 72–76.

Kellerman, J. (Ed.) *Psychological aspects of cancer in children.* Springfield, IL: Charles C. Thomas, 1980.

Kempe, C. H. Child abuse: The pediatrician's role in child advocacy and preventive pediatrics. *American Journal of the Diseases of Children,* 1978, **132,** 255–260.

Kent, J. T. A follow-up study of abused children. *Journal of Pediatric Psychology,* 1976, **1**(2), 25–1.

Kirten, C., & Liverman, M. Special educational needs of the child with cancer. *Journal of School Health,* 1977, 170–173.

Knapp, V., & Hansen, H. Helping the parents of children with leukemia. *Social Work,* 1973, **18,** 70–75.

Koocher, G. P. Childhood, death, and cognitive development. *Developmental Psychology,* 1973, **9,** 369–375.

Koocher, G. P. *Pediatric cancer: Psychological problems and the high costs of helping.* Presidential Address, Division 12, Section 1, at the 87th Annual Convention of the American Psychological Association, New York, 1979.

Koocher, G. P., & O'Malley, J. E. (Eds.) *The Damocles syndrome: Psychosocial consequences of surviving childhood cancer.* New York: McGraw-Hill, 1980.

Koocher, G. P., & Sallan, S. E. Pediatric oncology. In P. R. Magrab (Ed.), *Psychological management of pediatric problems,* Vol. 1. *Early life conditions and chronic diseases.* Baltimore: University Park Press, 1978.

Kulczycki, L., Robinson, M., & Berg, C. Somatic and psychosocial factors relative to management of patients with Cystic Fibrosis. *Clinical Proceedings of the Childrens Hospital of Washington, D.C.,* 1969, **25**, 320–324.

Lansky, S. B., Cairns, N. U., Hassanein, R., Wehr, J., & Lowman, J. T. Childhood cancer: Parental discord and divorce. *Pediatrics,* 1978, **62**, 184–188.

Lansky, S., Lowman, J. T., Vats, T., & Gyulay, J. School phobia in children with malignant neoplasms. *American Journal of Diseases in Children,* 1975, **129**, 42–46.

Lavigne, J. V., & Ryan, M. Psychological adjustment of siblings of children with chronic illness. *Pediatrics,* 1979, **63**, 616–627.

Lawler, R. H., Nakielny, N., & Wright, N. A. Psychological implications of Cystic Fibrosis. *Canadian Medical Association Journal,* 1966, **94**, 1043–046.

Lazarus, R. S. *Patterns of adjustment.* New York: McGraw-Hill, 1976.

Lazarus, R. S. The costs and benefits of denial. In J. J. Spinetta & P. Deasy-Spinetta (Eds.), *Living with childhood cancer.* St. Louis: Mosby, 1980.

Leiken, S. J., & Hassakis, P. Psychological study of parents of children with Cystic Fibrosis. In E. J. Anthony & C. Koupernik (Eds.), *The child in his family,* Vol. 2. *The impact of disease and death.* New York: Wiley, 1973.

Magrab, P. R. (Ed.) *Psychological management of pediatric problems,* 2 vols. Baltimore: University Park Press, 1978.

Maguire, D. C. *Death by choice.* Garden City, NY: Doubleday, 1974.

Martinson, I. M. (Ed.) *Home care for the dying child: Professional and family perspectives.* New York: Appleton-Century-Crofts, 1976.

Mattison, J. *Marriage and mental handicaps.* Pittsburgh: University of Pittsburgh Press, 1970.

Mattsson, A. Long-term physical illness in childhood: A challenge to psychosocial adaptation. *Pediatrics,* 1972, **50**, 801–811.

McCollum, A., & Gibson, L. Family adaptation to the child with Cystic Fibrosis. *Journal of Pediatrics,* 1970, **77**, 571–578.

McCrae, W. Emotional problems in Cystic Fibrosis. *Physiotherapy,* 1975, **61**, 252–254.

Meyerowitz, J. H., & Kaplan, H. B. Cystic Fibrosis and family functioning. In P. R. Patterson, C. R. Denning, & A. H. Kutscher (Eds.), *Psychosocial aspects of Cystic Fibrosis.* New York: Columbia University Press, 1973.

Meyers, A., Dolan, T., & Mueller, D. Compliance and self-medication in Cystic Fibrosis. *American Journal of the Diseases of Children,* 1975, **129**, 1011–1013.

Nagy, M. The child's theories concerning death. *Journal of Genetic Psychology,* 1948, **73**, 3–27.

National Cancer Institute. *Coping with childhood cancer: A resource for the health professional.* Bethesda, MD: U.S. Department of Health and Human Services, 1979.

National Center on Child Abuse and Neglect. *Child abuse and neglect: The problem and its management,* 3 vols. (DHEW Publ. OHD 75–30073). Washington, DC: U.S. Government Printing Office, 1975.

National Center on Child Abuse and Neglect. *Federally funded child abuse and neglect projects 1975.* (DHEW Publ. OHD 76-0076). Washington, DC: U.S. Government Printing Office, 1976.

Patterson, P. R., Denning, C. R., & Kutscher, A. H. (Eds.) *Psychosocial aspects of Cystic Fibrosis.* New York: Columbia University Press, 1973.

Paulson, M. J., Savino, A. B., Chaleff, A. B., Sanders, R. W., Frisch F., & Dunn, R. Parents of the battered child: A multidisciplinary group therapy approach to life-threatening behavior. *Life Threatening Behavior,* 1974, **4**, 18-31.

Pepper, G. The person with a spinal cord injury: Psychological care. *American Journal of Nursing,* 1977, **77**, 1330-1336.

Plumb, M. M., & Holland, J. Cancer in adolescents: The symptom is the thing. In B. Schoenberg, A. C. Carr, A. H. Kutscher, D. Peretz, & I. Goldberg (Eds.), *Anticipatory grief.* New York: Columbia University Press, 1974.

Reeder, L. G. The patient-client as a consumer: Some observations on the changing professional-client relationship. *Journal of Health and Social Behavior,* 1972, **13**, 406-412.

Reeves, R. B. Pastoral care of Cystic Fibrosis patients and their families. In P. R. Patterson, C. R. Denning, & A. H. Kutscher (Eds.), *Psychosocial aspects of Cystic Fibrosis.* New York: Columbia University Press, 1973.

Reitan, R. Psychological effects of cerebral lesions in children of early school age. In R. Reitan & L. Davison (Eds.), *Clinical neuropsychology: Current status and applications.* Washington, DC: V. H. Winston & Sons, 1974.

Schneider, C. Prediction of child abuse potential. Invited address presented at the 59th Annual Convention of the Western Psychological Association San Diego, CA, April 7, 1979.

Schneider, C., Hoffmeister, J. K., & Helfer, R. E. A predictive screening questionnaire for potential problems in mother-child interaction. In R. E. Helfer & C. H. Kempe (Eds.), *Child abuse and neglect: The family and the community.* Cambridge, MA: Ballinger, 1976.

Schowalter, J. E. The child's reaction to his own terminal illness. In B. Schoenberg, A. Carr, D. Peretz, & A. Kutscher (Eds.), *Loss and grief: Psychological management in medical practice.* New York: Columbia University Press, 1970.

Schulman, J. L., & Kupst, M. J. (Eds.). *The child with cancer: Clinical approaches to psychosocial care—Research in psychological aspects.* Springfield, IL: Charles C. Thomas, 1980.

Selden, R. F. Improvement of self-image in the dying child. In P. R. Patterson, C. R. Denning, & A. H. Kutscher (Eds.), *Psychosocial aspects of Cystic Fibrosis.* New York: Columbia University Press, 1973.

Seligman, M. *Helplessness.* New York: Freeman, 1975.

Seligman, M., & Maier, S. Failure to escape traumatic shock. *Journal of Experimental Psychology,* 1967, **74**, 1-9.

Sibinga, N. S., Friedman, C. J., & Huang, N N. The family of the Cystic Fibrosis patient. In P. R. Patterson, C. R. Denning, & A. H. Kutscher (Eds.), *Psychosocial aspects of Cystic Fibrosis.* New York: Columbia University Press, 1973.

Slavin, L. S. Evolving psychosocial issues in the treatment of childhood cancer: A review. In G. P. Koocher & J. E. O'Malley (Eds.), *The Damocles syndrome: Psychosocial consequences of surviving childhood cancer.* New York: McGraw-Hill, 1980.

Smith, S. M. *The battered child syndrome*. London: Butterworths, 1975.

Sourkes, B. Facilitating family coping with childhood cancer. *Journal of Pediatric Psychology*, 1977, **2**(2), 65–67.

Sourkes, B. Siblings of the pediatric cancer patient. In J. Kellerman (Ed.), *Psychological aspects of childhood cancer*. Springfield, IL: Charles C. Thomas, 1980.

Sparta, S. Treatment of helpless children through cognitive interpretations of failure: An examination of some therapeutic influences. Unpublished doctoral dissertation, University of California, 1978.

Sparta, S. Treatment of helpless children: An examination of some potentially therapeutic influences. Presented at the annual meeting of the American Psychological Association, New York City, September 1979.

Spinetta, J. J. The dying child's awareness of death: A review. *Psychological Bulletin*, 1974, **81**, 256–260.

Spinetta, J. J. Adjustment in children with cancer. *Journal of Pediatric Psychology*, 1977, **22**, 49–51.

Spinetta, J. J. Communication patterns in families dealing with life-threatening illness. In O. J. Z. Sahler (Ed.), *The child and death*. St. Louis: Mosby, 1978. (a)

Spinetta, J. J. Parental personality factors in child abuse. *Journal of Consulting and Clinical Psychology*, 1978, **46**, 1409–1414. (b)

Spinetta, J. J. Disease-related communication: How to tell. In J. Kellerman (Ed.), *Psychological aspects of childhood cancer*. Springfield, IL: Charles C. Thomas, 1980.

Spinett, J. J. Adjustment and adaptation in children with cancer: A three-year study. In J. J. Spinetta & P. Deasy-Spinetta (Eds.), *Living with childhood cancer*. St. Louis: Mosby, 1981. (a)

Spinetta, J. J. The sibling of the child with cancer. In J. J. Spinetta & P. Deasy-Spinetta (Eds.), *Living with childhood cancer*. St. Louis: Mosby, 1981. (b)

Spinetta, J. J., & Deasy-Spinetta, P. Coping with childhood cancer: Professional and family communication patterns. In M. G. Eisenberg, J. Falconer, & L. C Sutkin (Eds.), *Communications in a health care setting*. Springfield, IL: Charles C. Thomas, 1980.

Spinetta, J. J., & Deasy-Spinetta, P. (Eds.) *Living with childhood cancer*. St. Louis: Mosby, 1981. (a)

Spinetta, J. J., & Deasy-Spinetta, P. Talking about death with children with a life-threatening illness. In J. J. Spinetta & P. Deasy-Spinetta (Eds.), *Living with childhood cancer*. St. Louis: Mosby, 1981. (b)

Spinetta, J. J., Deasy-Spinetta, P., McCaren, H. H., Kung, F. H., Schwartz, D. B., & Hartman, G. A. The adolescent with cancer. *Seminars in Oncology*, 1981. (In press.)

Spinetta, J. J., Deasy-Spinetta, P. M., McLaren, H. H., Kung, F. H., Schwartz, D. B., & Hartman, G. A. The adolescent's psychosocial response to cancer: A literature review and critique. *Seminars in Oncology*, 1981 (In press).

Spinetta, J. J., & Maloney, L. J. Death anxiety in the outpatient leukemic child. *Pediatrics*, 1975, **65**, 1034–1037.

Spinetta, J. J., & Maloney, L. J. The child with cancer: Patterns of communication and denial. *Journal of Consulting and Clinical Psychology*, 1978, **48**, 1540–1541.

Spinetta, J. J., & Rigler, D. The child-abusing parent: A psychological review. *Psychological Bulletin*, 1972, **77**, 296–304.

Spinetta, J. J., Rigler, D., & Karon, M. Anxiety in the dying child. *Pediatrics,* 1973, **52,** 841–845.

Spinetta, J. J., Rigler, D., & Karon, M. Personal space as a measure of the dying child's sense of isolation. *Journal of Consulting and Clinical Psychology,* 1974, **42,**751–756.

Spinetta, J. J., Spinetta, P. D., Kung, F., & Schwartz, D. B. *Emotional aspects of childhood cancer and leukemia: A handbook for parents.* San Diego: Leukemia Society of America, 1976.

Starr, R. H. Child Abuse. *American Psychologist,* 1979, **34,** 872–878.

Steele, B. F. Working with abusive parents from a psychiatric point of view. *Child abuse and neglect: The problem and its management.* National Center on Child Abuse and Neglect, Vol. 3, (DHEW Publ. OHD, 75–30073). Washington: U. S. Government Printing Office, 1975, pp. 65–114.

Stehbens, J. A., & Lascari, A. D. Psychological follow-up of families with childhood leukemia. *Journal of Clinical Psychology,* 1974, **30,** 394–397.

Sudnow, D. *Passing on.* Englewood Cliffs, NJ: Prentice-Hall, 1967.

Tracy, J. J., & Clark, E. J. Treatment for child abusers. *Social Work,* 1974, **19,** 338–342.

Tropauer, A., Franz, M. N., & Dilgard, V. W. Psychological aspects of the care of children with Cystic Fibrosis. *American Journal of Diseases of Children,* 1970, **119,** 424–432.

Turk, J. Impact of Cystic Fibrosis on family functioning. *Pediatrics,* 1964, **34,** 67–71.

Van Eys, J. (Ed.) *The truly cured child: The new challenge in pediatric cancer care.* Baltimore: University Park Press, 1977.

Veatch, R. M. *Allowing the dying patient to die: An ethical analysis of New policy proposals.* Hastings-on-Hudson, NY: Institute of Society, Ethics, and the Life Sciences, 1972.

Waechter, E. H. Children's awareness of ftal illness. *American Journal of Nursing,* 1971, **7,** 1168–1172.

Walters, D. B. *Physical and sexual abuse of children: Causes and treatment.* Bloomington: Indiana University Press, 1975.

White, E., Elsom, B., & Prawat, R. Children's conceptions of death. *Child Development,* 1978, **49,** 307–310.

Winder, A. H., & Medalie, M. Support for growth in Cystic Fibrosis teenagers. In P. R. Patterson, C. R. Denning, & A. H. Kutscher (Eds.), *Psychosocial aspects of Cystic Fibrosis.* New York: Columbia University Press, 1973.

Young, M. Multiple correlates of abuse: A systems approach to the etiology of child abuse. *Journal of Pediatric Psychology,* 1976, **1**(2) 57–61.

Zeltzer, L. The adolescent with cancer. In J. Kellerman (Ed.), *Psychological aspects of childhood cancer.* Springfield, IL: Charles C. Thomas, 1980.

Zwartjes, W. J., & Zwartzes, G. School problems of children with cancer. In J. L. Schulman & M. J. Kupst (Eds.), *The child with cancer: Clinical approaches to psychosocial care—Resarch in psychological aspects.* 82 Springfield, IL: Charles C. Thomas, 1980.

CHAPTER 6

The Role of the Psychologist in Pediatric Outpatient and Inpatient Settings

Dennis Drotar
Pauline Benjamin
Robert Chwast
Carole Litt
Paul Vajner

Pediatric psychology has undergone extraordinary professional growth since 1965. The number of psychologists in medical settings has increased rapidly, and the scope of their activities has widened enormously. This growth has been accomplished without an explicit definition of the roles and functions of pediatric psychologists and without a clear understanding of the impact of the hospital setting on their professional functioning.

Much of the literature germane to the practice of pediatric psychology has dealt with new settings and programs and with the early stages of consultation with pediatricians. While such reports have certainly helped to clarify professional identity and role definition, the profession of pediatric psychology is now at the stage where it becomes increasingly important to grapple with issues relevant to the middle and ongoing stages of the consultation process. What follows will describe clinical practice and consultation from the perspective of psychologists who have worked together within a pediatric hospital and have developed a service that has been in existence for more than a decade.

We will critically discuss the roles and functions of the pediatric psychologist in inpatient and outpatient medical milieus with particular emphasis on how the structural and organizational aspects of the hospital shape consultation and clinical care activites. We begin with an overview of psychologists' experiences in a variety of pediatric placements and a description of the evolution of our own service in a large, university-based pediatric hospital. Methods of consultation and clinical intervention which have proved successful in accommodating to the structure of our setting will be presented. The impact of the unique aspects of hospital culture and organization on clinical practice will be described in detail. Finally, the problems and prospects that characterize evolving psychologist-pediatrician collaborations will be noted.

The authors of this chapter, a group of five pediatric psychologists, form a Division of Psychology within a large, highly specialized pediatric department. All psychologists hold joint appointments in the Departments of Psychiatry and Pediatrics of the School of Medicine, Case Western Reserve University. The division is physically housed within a large pediatric teaching hospital, Rainbow Babies and Childrens Hospital, which is a referral center for northeastern Ohio and an integral part of a large university-based hospital complex. Rainbow Babies and Childrens Hospital contains a 220-bed inpatient service and an outpatient division consisting of approximately 15 specialty and primary care clinics. The hospital provides primary care for both middle-class and inner city families and is a tertiary care center serving patients from a large geographic area. Although this hospital is larger and more complex than many facilities in which pediatric psychologists now practice, the consultation and patient care issues which have emerged here are nonetheless relevant to a variety of pediatric environments.

VARIETIES OF PEDIATRIC SETTINGS

The physical and organizational characteristics of pediatric facilities play an extremely important role in determining the activities of the psychologists who work in them. Indeed, the "setting" has been designated the principal factor in distinguishing the role of the pediatric psychologist from that of the clinical child psychologist (Tuma, 1975).

Basically, there are three types of pediatric settings: the hospital inpatient unit, the ambulatory care facility (outpatient clinic or private pediatric office), and the comprehensive care center for chronic illness which may offer a combination of outpatient and inpatient care. At first glance these locations may appear to be very different from one another. For example, a hospital ward for surgical patients may seem different physically from an outpatient clinic or a private pediatric office. However, they share the common characteristic of having been created primarily to provide physical care to those in need of medical attention. It is this fact that determines the nature of the physical environment in which the pediatric psychologist must work. Such an environment frequently is antithetical to the milieu traditionally thought most conducive to good psychotherapeutic work.

Within outpatient facilities, pediatric psychologists have consulted in smaller pediatric practices as well as larger ambulatory care centers. Schroeder (1979) has described an innovative consultation program involving work with pediatricians in a private practice. Services included brief telephone consultation with patients, office visits, and educational group meetings for parents. The parent groups addressed topics pertinent to children including aspects of normal development (toilet training, sibling rivalry) as well as special problems in childrearing (divorce, foster care).

Phone consultations were brief, approximately 15 minutes each, and office visits were used for diagnostic screening or treatment by providing advice or education. Similarly, Smith, Rome, & Freedheim (1967) have reported another example of a psychologist functioning in a private pediatric practice involving one-half day per week of consultation. Screening and brief intervention were important components of service. Two-thirds of the families referred to the psychologist were seen only three or four times. In each of these private practice settings, children from infancy through adolescence were seen for referral questions ranging in content from normative aspects of child development to more severe behavioral disorders.

Pediatric psychologists often provide outpatient services within ambulatory programs located in large hospitals in order to reduce patient waiting time frequently imposed by outpatient mental health facilities (Botinelli, 1975). Such psychological services may overlap with those offered by traditional child guidance centers but they provide more rapid service and afford more comprehensive educational and consultative resources for pediatricians. Toback, Russo, & Gururaj (1975) have described a diagnostic service offered to children with concomitant medical problems and to younger preschoolers in a large ambulatory pediatric clinic at an inner city teaching hospital. School-age children who had access to other sources of psychological health care were generally not seen. The majority of children had diagnoses of lead poisoning, brain damage, and mental retardation while a lesser number had psychiatric disorders or emotional problems secondary to chronic illness.

Pediatric psychologists also practice in general and community-based hospitals. Pitcher (1978) delineated a program within a rural community hospital in which the psychologist was requested to see adults and children on both inpatient and outpatient services. Her program emphasized immediate short-term services to patients referred by general practitioners and subspecialists. Within this rural setting, the psychologist was also available for consultation to the community's Head Start program, the state rehabilitation service, and the local center for the developmentally disabled.

Pediatric subspecialty groups provide opportunities for consultation which may encompass activities on either an inpatient or outpatient basis. Johnson's (1979) review of mental health interventions with medically ill children outlines programs of psychological consultation to a variety of subspecialties including nephrology, cardiology, oncology, hematology, and surgery. Psychologists' activities with subspecialty groups may include only direct service, or they may encompass consultative attempts to foster an holistic, comprehensive-care treatment milieu for the chronically ill child and family.

Pediatric psychologists in large, multispecialty hospitals are involved in planning hospital organization and structure. Ack (1974) has discussed his role as Director of Mental Health within a large pediatric hospital. In addition to the familiar psychological services, a primary responsibility of his group was to address the overall "ecology" of the hospital, which included grappling with policies regarding admission procedures, parent visitation rules, and so on.

Finally, the educational role of pediatric psychologists in pediatric placements has become increasingly important. Recent recommendations by the Task Force on Pediatric Education (1978) and the U.S. Public Health Service (1978) place an increasing emphasis on behavioral pediatrics and psychosocial education in pediatric training. Psychologists in these settings teach pediatricians and other health care providers via informal and formal consultations, regular medical ward and psychosocial rounds, pediatric teaching conferences and more specialized child development seminars. The psychologist who works with pediatric trainees must make accommodations in approach and style which take into account the schedules, interests, and fatigue of house staff who are overstressed and often have little energy for formal didactic activities.

DEVELOPMENT OF THE AUTHORS' SERVICE

Our clinical activities take place in a large multispecialty hospital in which pediatric psychology has grown considerably over an 11-year period. Our early clinical activities were initially dominated by referrals from the inpatient service. In line with Wright's (1967) description of pediatric psychology activities, nearly half of the consultations involved intellectual or developmental problems associated with a large variety of disorders including language disabilities, chronic illness, psychosocial deprivation, and congenital anomalies. Approximately 30% of all referrals were concerned with management of patients with chronic illness and related adjustment problems, or with acute medical psychosocial crises such as abuse, accidents, burns, and so on. Less than 10% of referrals concerned children referred for primary behavior or psychiatric disorders (Drotar, 1977a).

In our setting, one finds the typical and remarkably varied problems of the pediatric patient population: attachment disorders, failure-to-thrive and feeding problems of infancy, developmental disabilities and neurological disorders, mild and reactive behavior problems, learning disabilities, psychosomatic illnesses, emotional concomitants of acute and chronic illness, child abuse and neglect, pediatric emergencies, suicidal behavior, and issues of patient compliance. This range of problems has required our group to develop sophisticated skills in intervention, consultation, and specialized assessment. The large number of referrals which occur in the context of brief hospitalizations or in periods of medical and family crisis has required that we develop skills in short-term intervention. Ongoing psychotherapeutic treatment of medically ill children has necessitated our flexibility with respect to theoretical orientation, timing of treatment, and our facility with various treatment modalities, including psychodynamic psychotherapy, parent guidance, and family therapy.

Consultation and educational activities have been part and parcel of our service from the outset. We have combined both didactic and case-oriented approaches to reach pediatric house staff in a number of settings, which have included informal case consultations and weekly psychosocial rounds. These activities serve a variety of functions such as screening of referrals, problemsolving concerning psychosocial management problems, and ventilation of feelings (Drotar, 1976b, 1977b). The following case vignette describes the multiple needs which a single consultation can fulfill.

> The psychologist consulting to the inpatient division serving young children was contacted with regard to a situation of suspected child abuse. The family and child involved presented difficulties for everyone. The foreign-born mother, who felt isolated and distraught, was able to respond well to one house officer. Through direct supervision, the psychologist helped this resident to more fully evaluate the problems of this mother and child, and to support the mother through the embarrassing exposure to which she was subjected. The psychologist carried out a formal developmental evaluation of the child which had been appropriately requested by the house staff. That same week, he presided over psychosocial ward rounds at which this case served as a springboard for discussion of child abuse, cross-cultural observation, and interviewing techniques. In a separate meeting with nursing personnel, this family was again discussed. There, the focus was on the difficulties mother posed for nursing staff. The recurrent feelings of anger and sadness that child abuse cases trigger in health care workers were also addressed.

Over the course of time, the Division of Psychology has geared its activities to cover discrete and manageable hospital units which demand varying styles of consultation. We currently organize weekly psychosocial rounds on four of our eight inpatient divisions. Our consultative strategies for these meetings vary with the specific needs and characteristics of the divisions on which they occur and the individual styles of the psychologists who assume responsibility for them. On our infant and toddler unit, weekly psychosocial rounds include nursing and house staff and blend didactic and case-centered approaches in order to focus on a particular patient or problem. Frequently, the infant under consideration is brought to the rounds so that participants may observe firsthand the particular symptoms or developmental issues to be discussed. Children observed by the group might include those with failure-to-thrive, congenital anomalies, or feeding disorders.

On the division which houses young school-age children, the psychologist has had to gear his meetings to the needs of a staff who work with many chronically or terminally ill children. On this floor, deaths occur frequently, and the consultant must be ready to help the staff grapple with the feelings of loss, grief, frustration, and anger engendered by the demise of patients in their care. Here, rounds often focus less on the psychosocal management of specific patients and more on the ongoing issues of loss and grief resolution.

A different model for psychosocial rounds has evolved on our children's orthopedic division. On this unit, psychosocial rounds have evolved from a single weekly meeting at which one child was discussed to a system of "work rounds" at which treatment plans for all children on the division are discussed. This change became necessary because of the particular characteristics of the orthopedic service. At our institution, orthopedic surgeons care for adults as well as for children. The time pressures inherent in providing surgical care have limited the surgeons' presence on the pediatric ward. In addition, occupational and physical therapy, social service, and other disciplines crucial to rehabilitative efforts with orthopedic patients are housed off the division and are neither highly visible nor available for regular informal exchanges regarding patient care. This lack of direct availability of key staff had contributed to poor interdisciplinary collaboration and to morale problems among all staff. Many staff members voiced a wish for stronger physician leadership in comprehensive planning efforts on behalf of their patients. When this was not forthcoming, the psychologist initiated weekly work rounds at which interdisciplinary planning could be carried out for every patient on the division. The organization of these work rounds was not easily accomplished because of longstanding patterns of mistrust among the various medical and nonmedical disciplines. There were many weeks when few people attended or when certain groups of professionals refused to attend. Initially, staff viewed the rounds as the "psychologist's meeting" rather than a process in which they could be collaborators. However, in time, these meetings have become an integral part of the ward's culture. They now have their own impetus and continue regularly even during those weeks when the psychologist is unable to attend.

The rounds conducted by the psychologist on the unit serving adolescents and young adults at times incorporate all the techniques described above. The majority of the patients cared for on this unit suffer from long-term chronic illnesses such as cystic fibrosis or have severe, life-threatening diseases such as cancer. Many of these patients undergo repeated lengthy hospitalizations, and the hospital staff grows to know them well. As on other wards emotions run high when these patients experience medical crises or when they die. However, the fact that the patients here are very close in age to the nurses and house officers charged with their care adds a dimension of anxiety not necessarily experienced on other wards. Finding a suitable time to hold psychosocial rounds has been a problem. Work loads for every discipline are heavy, and there is always a crisis or an influx of new admissions that requires attention. We have settled on a mid-week meeting time when at least some representatives of each discipline are available. The current patient census is reviewed, medical plans are discussed, and staff are encouraged to share observations which bear on the patients' psychological functioning and adjustment to their medical problems. This format serves the multiple needs of case planning, interstaff communication, education regarding specific emotional problems of adolescence, and ventilation and resolution of energy-sapping emotions produced by such a high-pressured milieu.

Our ambulatory clinics provide pediatric residents with their only opportunity to follow a group of children and their families for the full three years of the residency program. Within this continuity care experience, we are participants in didactic meetings, teachers of basic interviewing skills, case consultants, and collaborator-teachers working with selected patients conjointly with house staff, as in the following example:

A 2-year-old girl with delayed and atypical development was referred to us for developmental assessment by a third year resident who was about to complete his residency. We found the child to be emotionally disturbed, developmentally delayed, and clinically hyperactive. The mother was a seriously depressed woman who had borne this girl, her only child, late in life. She saw the girl as "normal" and was very threatened by the consultation request. The pediatrician, anxious that the mother "accept" a diagnosis of retardation, caused her to flee the clinic for a period of several months. When she finally returned some months after the original resident had left, we arranged to precept a new trainee on the case. This resident had already expressed an interest in child development and had a good working relationship with the consultant. He had arranged to start an elective rotation suggested by the consultant at a diagnostic preschool for retarded and disturbed children. With help, he was able to feel less pressured that the mother accept a diagnosis and was able to help her enroll the child in a diagnostic preschool. For the next three years, this resident followed the child, working with the psychologist to coordinate a program of comprehensive medical care and to respond with sensitivity to the mother's needs. At the end of three years the child had improved markedly. Although still mildly retarded, she no longer manifested serious emotional problems nor was she hyperactive. Her mother was now able to view her daughter's limitations more realistically and was much less depressed.

Such clinical experiences help pediatric residents appreciate varying modes of family adaptation to stress over time and recognize the importance of the physician-patient relationship in the management of psychosocial problems. All too frequently, many similar cases are turned over to psychologists when residents do not have continuing support to maintain their involvement.

UNIQUE CHARACTERISTICS OF PEDIATRIC SETTINGS

Limitations on Physical Space and Time

The requirements of medical practice present the psychologist with unfamiliar physical and philosophical terrain. Typically, medical care is dispensed in physical surroundings which tend to diminish the patient's sense of autonomy and individuality. Physical space is at a premium in most pediatric hospitals. Children and their families spend time on crowded wards or in congested, noisy clinics. In these settings, the patient's body is exposed and invaded not only by the doctor but by technicians, laboratory personnel, and nursing staff. Close proximity of rooms, lack of soundproofing, and frequent interruptions deprive child and family of the privacy necessary to introduce and explore sensitive psychological issues. Although their emotional difficulties may be manifest, they are often denied or dismissed by patients because of the feelings engendered by the lack of privacy and autonomy.

Medical activity takes place within a severely compressed time span. Physicians see large numbers of patients each day and therefore must try to solve each problem as rapidly as possible. Where many patients vie for the attention of few health care providers, the likelihood of discerning significant emotional problems can be markedly reduced. The physician's attention to any one patient is diffused and often primarily allocated to medical problems. Diagnoses are made quickly and treatment carried out with dispatch. Physicians strive for, and patients are oriented to expect, rapid resolutions of their complaints. Both may be sorely disappointed when their efforts fail to produce quick results. Unfortunately, the strenuous tme pressures inherent in the setting often serve to inhibit patients' expression of their emotional concerns. These pressures affect the physician's perceptions of the psychologist. Physicians who work with many patients at one time frequently do not realize that psychologists see children or families individually in contacts that require considerable interview time, and that psychological intervention takes place in a series of contacts rather than in discrete units. On an inpatient unit, time pressures are compounded by a constantly shifting cadre of professionals and nonprofessionals. In this atmosphere, interaction between hospital personnel and patients can become brief, mechanical, and impersonal. The necessity to fit into this booming, buzzing environment frequently comes as a shock to the traditionally trained psychologist accustomed to working in refined privacy seeing one patient an hour for as long as is necessary to bring about results.

Medical Authority

Even more important than the unfamiliar and often inhospitable physical characteristics of pediatric settings is the traditional "medical model" or philosophy which governs the functioning of physicians and affects their relations with psychologists. Central to this medical philosophy is the concept of medical responsibility. This concept underlies the highly regimented hierarchy of authority in which the individual physician assumes total control over patient care. "Other health care providers are expected to implement treatment plans within their designated role or area of expertise and are accorded responsibility and prestige commensurate with how closely their skills approximate those of a physician" (Tefft & Simeonsson, 1979).

The traditional medical hierarchy system is supported by a number of operations which are quite foreign to psychological practice. For example, the method by which medical practitioners typically communicate is of major significance. Pressured by large patient loads and the complexity of hospital care, physicians have developed the problem-oriented chart method of communicating with their medical colleagues. Pertinent information regarding the diagnosis and treatment of patients (often organized according to a "problem list") is written in hospital charts and order books where those charged with carrying out the care may read their instructions. Other professionals are expected to record their activities and observations of patients for the doctor's enlightenment. Although this system is highly practical for assuring that necessary information gets passed on from one shift of workers to another, it underscores the impersonal nature of medical care. A psychologist who is accustomed to sharing his thoughts and impressions in person may find it difficult to convey the subtleties of psychological concepts within the terse style dictated by the medical chart format. This format of communication further precludes the "give and take" personal dialogue often necessary to formulate effective plans for follow-up care and collaborative treatment.

Another aspect of the medical hierarchy which psychologists find awkward is the tendency for role and status to be signified through style of dress. Each medical discipline has adopted a system of uniforms which clearly identify the wearer and his position. Physicians wear white coats, nurses white uniforms, and in a teaching hospital, trainees at different levels wear uniforms which more closely approximate that of senior staff with each step up the ladder of training. Psychologists must decide whether to adopt the physician's white coat, and perhaps gain some of the functional status attached to it, or to shun the uniform and struggle to establish visibility and professional identity through their activities.

In their role of ultimate authority, physicians have developed a traditional style of practice governed by what Rothenberg (1974) has described as an "unholy trinity of activity, authority, and magic." Under pressure to "do" something quickly to help reduce pain and cure illness, physicians tend to perpetuate patients' belief in the magic of medicine by dispensing orders for treatment with an air of authority, assuring patients that all will be well if they comply. Such an approach may prevent the pediatrician from learning psychosocial information which may be crucial for the successful outcome of treatment. If physicians leap into activity without taking the time to consider patients in the context of their stages of psychosocial development, cultural background, and family situations, they may actually cause psychological harm while performing miracles for the body.

Interdisciplinary Nature of the Setting

By virtue of the care they must provide, pediatric medical facilities require the close cooperative interaction of a number of disciplines. This is especially true of a hospital inpatient service which must provide not only for children's medical needs but also for their daily needs of food, clothing, shelter, emotional nurturance, and education. Doctors, nurses, dietitians, laboratory technicians, physical and occupational therapists, social workers, teachers, and child life workers all may need to contribute directly to a child's hospital care. With so many people involved, patient care can easily become fragmented with each professional attending only to his specialized sphere of influence. For example, it is not uncommon for complex and anxiety-generating psychosocial problems such as suicide attempts to precipitate redundant referrals to a number of psychosocial disciplines at the same time (Naylor & Mattson, 1973). The child as a person can get lost in this crowd. For the patient with complex medical problems, the situation is compounded by the need to be attended by a number of medical subspecialists.

The obvious problem in such a multidisciplinary setting is to maintain adequate effective communication among all parties concerned. This is not an easy task in a fast-paced environment where the physician, who ultimately has the authority and responsibility for the patient's care, is likely to be unavailable at times of crucial decision making. Plans for patient care are, at times, made tentatively with the risk of being vetoed by the doctor later. This process leads to confusion, anger, and frustration for patient and staff alike. The tensions that arise among staff members as a result of trying to work in such a complex place under the restrictions of the medical hierarchy of authority frequently contribute to the problems of high staff turnover and professional "burnout" (Bates, 1970).

Professional burnout and high staff turnover among nonphysician health care professionals have significant impact on the quality of patient care an institution is able to offer. In a large hospital where patients have only brief encounters with the physicians in charge of their care, patients come to rely on other personnel, especially nursing, for a sense of continuity of care. Unfortunately, frequent changes of staff create added stress, particularly for the chronically ill. The psychologist in a pediatric setting is frequently called upon to help alleviate stress within the system by facilitating effective communication among staff members and providing emotional support to those coping with the emotionally draining experiences of death and loss (Easson, 1970; Drotar, 1975; Drotar, 1976a). At times, referrals framed by physicians as individual patient problems are actually precipitated by work-related stresses on staff as in the following example:

> Jill, a 19-year-old patient with cystic fibrosis, was referred because of anxiety which was described by the pediatric house staff as pathological. Closer examination of this young woman's problem indicated that she was reacting realistically to an imminently terminal condition which was stressing the entire staff. Members of a number of professional disciplines had tried to provide support for her and her family but without any coherent intervention plan. Rather than providing psychological help for her existential situation, the consultant arranged a meeting to bring relevant caretakers together to discuss the impact of their stresses, and to formulate a plan of action which involved them in providing increased support in line with the stresses engendered by her life-threatening condition.

Physicians' Misperceptions of the Psychologists' Role

The action-oriented medical model is a prime determinant of the physician's perceptions and fantasies about the psychologist's role. The psychologist may be expected to function within the physician's time frame and be available at a moment's notice to provide quick evaluation and treatment of complex problems.

The pediatrician's experience with medical consultations inevitably colors his or her expectations of the psychologist. For example, the consultation request to other medical services is often quite specific with both procedures and required information determined by the referring physician. In a milieu in which ad hoc action is a preferred mode, such consultations are often arranged expeditiously. There may be little concern for, or only an abbreviated attempt at, preparing children and families for the requested consultation. In medical facilities, such consultations are routine and children and their families have some expectation that they will be subjected to medical procedures by other than their primary physician. In this action-oriented, rapid delivery approach, specialists move in on patients quickly and disappear without further patient contact. Despite the fact that this medical consultative model frequently does not mesh well with sound psychological service delivery, physicians' expectations for the psychological consultation may remain based on such a view and may pose difficulties for psychologists unaccustomed to the medical culture.

In medical consultations, patient cooperation and compliance often involve a passive acceptance of procedures and regimens. In contrast, psychological evaluation requires more egalitarian patient-professional transactions. Children and their parents cannot be coerced to relate to psychologists or to participate meaningfully in evaluative procedures. Patients do not reveal their inner lives, their fantasies, anxieties, and feelings upon demand. Thus, in order for effective psychological consultation to take place, children and families should ideally be willing to participate. A specific rationale for the referral and preparation for face-to-face contact with the psychologist is essential.

Often in the pediatric setting, children and families have not yet identified, or at best have tenuously construed, their difficulties as emotionally based. Indeed, in the context of traumatic physical insult or chronic illness, the family's focus is avowedly on somatic issues. For this reason, directing the patient's and family's attention to what the physician discerns as areas which require further psychological evaluation is not easily accomplished. In outpatient medical facilities, several visits may be required with physicians to help the family to contact the consultant psychologist. On hospital wards, where the psychologist has greater access to identified patients and famiies, the need for their preparation by the referring physician is even more imperative. For inpatients, the unannounced appearance of a psychologist can be experienced by patients as invasive and indicative of a further loss of autonomy. Unfortunately, such experiences are all too common for patients and are disruptive, upsetting, and likely to increase resentment and augment resistance. Hollon (1973) has observed the irony that the request for psychological consultation, if not properly framed for the patient, may serve to heighten anxiety and distress, despite the fact it was undertaken to relieve stress.

Pediatricians often expect that psychological evaluation will inevitably generate quantifiable information. The assumption that testing is appropriate in all psychological consultations, or that it is intrinsically therapeutic, is a common misunderstanding. At times, the referral for a narrowly construed psychometric evaluation may represent physicians' attempts to distance themselves from difficult and compelling emotional concerns by focusing on more "manageable" data gathering:

> Donna, a 10-year-old girl, was in a transient remission from a type of leukemia with a very poor prognosis. She had suffered serious CNS side effects from the many chemotherapies to which she had been subjected. Prior to a vitamin-therapy, the hematologist requested "intelligence testing" in order to determine if some of the CNS sequelae were reversible for this child who had at one time well-above average school performace. Testing served to vivify to her and her mother that she was indeed deteriorating. The psychologist quickly realized that the frustration and sadness posed by this confrontation would disrupt the good adaptation mother and daughter had made, and testing was discontinued.

In this illustration, the child and parent had not asked for evaluation or psychological support. It seemed likely that the well-intentioned physician was attempting to offer some concrete and tangible help to a courageous family facing a grave illness. However, the kind of assistance offered was disruptive and tangential to their more immediate and powerful concerns about their child's physical peril.

Another commonly encountered misunderstanding is the expectation that the psychologist can expertly intervene in any problem situation deemed "emotional" by the referring physician. The evolution of such demands is not difficult to fathom. There are relatively few mental health professionals who serve in the highly stressful medical milieu. Overburdened physicians understandably hope that psychological services can always address the diversity of their patients' needs for emotional support and information about their disease. Yet such expectations are often impossible to meet and fuel interprofessional disappointment and disenchantment:

> A pediatric psychologist newly consulting to an ambulatory (outpatient) service on a part-time basis was requested to implement behavioral programs for encopretics and obese children, provide crisis-intervention to sexually abused and physically abused children, treat longer term patients for a variety of neurotic and characterological difficulties, learn hypnotherapeutic techniques to use with pain patients, as well as to teach interviewing techniques and act as a group-process consultant to the ambulatory team. His effectiveness and competence were questioned initially when he set limits on the demands to which he would respond.

ACCOMMODATIONS TO HOSPITAL STRUCTURE

The structure of pediatric settings demands that psychologists alter their traditional styles of mental health intervention. Over the course of time, we have found a number of innovative approaches especially useful in responding to the unique demands of our setting. The strategies outlined below have been shaped by the requirements of the milieu and also by the necessity of achieving our ideal image of the successful "pediatric psychologist" in gradual stages. The development of our service has encompassed the stages of initial entry and solidification of professional credibility and is now entering the phase of true collaborative physical and psychosocial care for pediatric patients.

Entering the Setting

The successful entry into a medical system depends on the psychologist's clear awareness of, and respect for, the culture of the environment. In the action-oriented medical milieu, the consultant's visibility and availability must be established (Bolian, 1971; Naylor & Mattson, 1973). The consultant's physical presence at "natural" intersections such as nurses' stations, conference rooms, or hallway coffee pots communicates to the staff his or her availability. Attendance at medical staff meetings can help the consultant gradually become part of the ward or division activities. In addition, informal conversations can help pediatric staff get to know the psychologist's style, values, and interests (Geist, 1977). Such consistent availability communicates an attitude and style of interested openness, a desire to be of help, and a respect for pediatric colleagues. In entering a setting, we have found it important to be highly flexible and to demonstrate interest in a variety of problems in order to facilitate relationships with pediatric staff. As one gathers experience and becomes more familiar with the new terrain, more specific roles can be shaped and refined through a process of education and negotiation with colleagues.

In addition to establishing his availability, the psychologist must actively work to build relationships with his pediatrician colleagues. The clarification of the psychological consultation with the referring physician can be a relationship-building endeavor. The physician's initial consultation request often takes either a formal, distant form, or communicates in an unstructured, chaotic style. Hesitancy, uncertainty, and lack of personal familiarity with the psychologist may lead some practitioners to have a secretary call the consultant or to send a formal written request. These distant and formal requests can often be taken as an invitation to initiate further contacts and to begin a more informal, personalized relationship. These formal referrals can be quite efficient and appropriate for some purposes: developmental screening, specialized tests for mental retardation placements, periodic reevaluation, and other tasks where the role of the consultant is to provide "expert" and specialized case-oriented information. However, it is advantageous to follow up such distant requests with a personal meeting, which includes further clarification and data gathering concerning the referral. Pediatricians' implicit assumptions of the psychologist-as-tester can be clarified and corrected as the initial relationship with the pediatrician is refined over time. Acting solely as a consultant via written reports can be limiting and self-perpetuating unless strenuous efforts are made to develop personal contacts and establish clear channels of interprofessional communication.

A physician's first request for psychological consultation can often be seen as a "trial by fire" that the psychologist must pass. It is not uncommon for initial referrals to be the physician's most difficult, complex, or most "hateful" patients (Groves, 1978). The doctor may preface his request with "Have I got one for you." Such remarks can reflect a combination of the physician's dismay, helplessness, and anticipatory glee at finding someone to relieve him of the burdensome patient. Given the initial goal of fostering relationships with the pediatric staff, it is often wise to acquiesce to some of their less realistic demands for active intervention and problemsolving. Interested questions, data gathering, supportive empathizing with the physician's predicament, and specifying what psychological consultation can realistically provide are techniques that can gradually help shape mutually adaptive professional roles and foster good working relationships.

The consultant's ability to demonstrate skills in assessment and intervention is crucial to substantiate credibility with pediatric staff. In the initial phases of work, consultants need not worry about overextending themselves and "burning out." Of the first patients referred to the newly available consultant, many will have been inadequately prepared and will not appear for their appointments. In addition, many apparent "emergencies" remit with the pediatrician's attentive concern and "giving" the families knowledge that help is available.

Evolving Consultation Methods to Fit the Setting

Styles of consultation evolve over time and should fit the problems of the patient, the style of the medical consultee, and the setting requirements (Caplan, 1970). Interprofessional problems and dissatisfactions occur most frequently when the fit between the variables of patient, physician, consultant, setting, and phase of the consulting relationship is left to chance rather than to explicit negotiation.

The curbside or hallway consultation is a valuable strategy. Standing in a busy intersection to give advice or clarify a case may appear superficial or vague but has very real value in building relationships and providing effective clinical service. In addition, engaging in off-the-cuff discussions is lively, challenging, and requires a firm knowledge of development, clinical and practical experience, and creativity. Following these informal contacts, through successive approximations, the consultant can begin to sit down with medical colleagues, move into an office, and channel the relationship toward a more collegial one with greater mutual understanding and respect. The curbside consultation is especially appropriate when the physician remains the primary caregiver and can implement his own strategies as shown in the following case vignette:

> The consultant was approached in the hall regarding a difficult school avoidant adolescent. The physician, feeling uncertain about how to proceed, asked for a psychological assessment. He had a good ongoing relationship with the boy and his mother. Clarification, support, and direct advice were given by the consultant to help the doctor interpret the symptom, advise the family, and remedy a problem that could have become more intractable during a full psychological assessment. The doctor was advised about how to enlist the school's support and deal with the mother's ambivalence. The family responded well to the physician's authoritative advice, and the boy continued to be seen by the doctor for brief follow-up visits after his return to school.

Concurrent psychologist-pediatrician collaboration is a strategy which can be particularly helpful in cases such as anorexia nervosa, obesity, learning disabilities, hyperactivity, or complex medical-developmental problems, where judicious diagnosis and treatment require a team of professionals. Developing specific behavior modification plans with the physician, including assessment techniques for baseline and treatment conditions, and working with parents in feedback, can help provide a context for mutual learning between psychologists and pediatricians. The following case example illustrates the effectiveness of this "tandem" approach in the treatment of an underweight adolescent girl:

> The psychologist and a primary care pediatrician worked together to develop a treatment program for a 12-year-old girl who was severely underweight. The physician took the role of firm, demanding authority requiring a given diet and strict caloric intake, while the psychologist dealt with feelings and reactions to the demands. This act of splitting functions nto the "bad" doctor and "good" doctor helped to neutralize the family's role in this girl's illness and set the stage for subsequent weight gains.

Parent guidance, group and family interviews with psychologist and pediatricians acting as co-interviewers and co-therapists also lend themselves to this kind of collaborative approach. This type of therapeutic acivity requires an excellent working alliance, a relatively high level of communicative skills on the part of the pediatrician, and should not be undertaken with medical colleagues prematurely.

CLINICAL INTERVENTIONS TAILORED TO THE PEDIATRIC SETTING

Crisis Intervention

Crisis intervention techniques are useful in both busy ambulatory practice settings and inpatient wards. Given the combination of an emotionally charged, stressful atmosphere and continuous work demands, such techniques as clarifying and specifying a problem, facilitating natural system supports, and planning a specified course of action are helpful to both patients and staff.

> A 19-year-old woman presented in the ambulatory practice with her infant son who was "crying all day and night," keeping everyone in the family awake. The mother became assaultive over an alleged insulting remark by the receptionist. This mother was defensive and hostile, demanding to have the infant hospitalized. In collaboration with the nurse and pediatrician, the psychologist's clarifications, and supportive, crisis work with the mother set the stage for more adaptive care. When the mother was able to rest and receive reassurance that her baby would not be taken away fom her, this at-risk family achieved an equilibrium which was maintaincd in continuing outpatient care.

To provide effective crisis intervention, it is essential to determine if the sense of urgency, speed, and action are dictated by patient needs or are erroneously identified as such by a harried pediatric staff as in the following:

> The consultant was called in on an "urgent" situation of a "psychotic" 15-year-old girl who was mute and catatonic. She would not respond to the physician, her mother or brother, and was physically dragged to the examination room. A brief interview with the mother revealed that her daughter had been behaving this way for over 2 years, was in a program for the severely retarded, and had received no regular medical care for over a year. A subsequent visit to the psychologist led to coordination of infomation, a psychiatric inpatient admission for diagnostic evaluation, and referral to appropriate community services.

It is important to note that the accommodation of crisis intervention has its share of disadvantages. For example, responding to pediatric requests in a crisis-oriented way can lead to frequent calls to extinguish "brushfires," or it can foster requests to deal with difficult patients in magical, unrealistic ways at the expense of addressing their more important needs or concerns. The following is an example of a highly stressed child who required empathy rather than "help" for his noncompliance.

Bobby was a 9-year-old leukemia patient who had a recent relapse and began to "act differently" during his chemotherapy visits. His previous stoic silence gave way to violent screaming episodes, refusals to take his medicine, and defiant opposition to painful bone marrow samples being drawn. The staff wished he would be more compliant and easier to manage. The consultant worked with Bobby and the staff to help them cope with his understandably fearful reactions.

In part, the appeal of brief therapy to physicians and psychologists who work in medical settings stems from its promise to provide economical, explicit, and specific treatment analogous to the prescriptive treatment of the physician. The active and authoritative therapist role implicit in brief therapy is congruent with patients' expectations of yielding to medical authority.

Contracting, focusing problems, and setting the number of sessions are useful interventions to aid in clarifying ambiguous referrals and enhancing patient motivation. Indications for implementing brief therapy include positive family expectations and motivation to support psychological treatment. Many medical patients and their parents have no wish to pursue the emotional dimensions of their problems or their child's problems. For this reason, an initial evaluation and contract for treatment are necessary to insure compliance. This strategy is effective for focal problems in children whose basic adjustment is only moderately compromised. For example, symptoms such as an isolated episode of fire setting or stealing, intermittent bed-wetting, fears, headaches, and stomach aches in an otherwise well-adjusted child can be helpfully resolved in short-term psychotherapy. Where multiple or diffuse symptoms and severe situational stresses are predominant, alternative methods or referral for longer term treatment may be indicated.

There are numerous pitfalls in implementing brief therapy in the medical setting. The therapist can easily succumb to the urgency of a patient's symptom or to a physician's need by being overly problem focused. The total developmental picture may be obscured and the overall influence of an intervention unknown. Parental and family pathology can be overlooked. In addition, there is a strong potential for superficial treatment and mere seduction of a patient into a brief relationship which may in the long run be detrimental. Finally, fragmented and disorganized treatment can result from incomplete data or poorly timed interventions. For these reasons, building continuity and long-term follow-up is critical.

Intermittent Contacts

Intermittent contacts on either a PRN or "as needed" basis, or on a monthly or biweekly schedule of visits is a further clinical modification which can be successfully implemented by the psychologist in the pediatric seting. Many families may live far from a treatment facility or may have insufficient financial resources to engage in frequent therapeutic visits. Treatment continuity can be achieved through phone calls, diaries by parents, or behavioral assessment recording procedures:

Jimmy, an 11-year-old boy with persistent enuresis, was seen for one hour every other week following an initial three-session evaluation. Bladder training techniques were taught and Jimmy kept a cumulative record of dry nights. On alternate weeks Jimmy received a phone call from his therapist to check on his progress. Jimmy had a marked decrease in episodes in the first month of treatment and several dry weeks after six weeks of treatment. Follow-up after two months indicated only one or two episodes per month much to Jimmy's pride and his parents' satisfaction in his newly acquired skill.

Feedback and Follow-Up in Psychological Consultation

The products of consultation include verbal information for doctors and patients, establishment of ongoing relationships, written reports, and letters or referrals to other professionals. Where the medical staff may have blocks of over 100 patients who are seen over varying time spans, the consultant's role in fostering continuity, personalized service, and prompt, relevant help to the patient is especially significant. For this reason, feedback to the referring physician is often most helpful when repeated in several modes. For example, an immediate chart note followed by a brief verbal summary makes use of the medical system's primary information channels. In addition, the formal psychological report that includes a summary of actions already taken serves as a benchmark to plan later care and follow-up.

In light of the inherent discontinuities in the setting, feedback to the child and family needs to be repeated and formalized. The "checkup" visit after an evaluation or treatment is a useful format for follow-up, continuity, and summarizing progress. Letters to parents provide yet another useful adjunct to feedback in that they can provide summaries of important issues, information, or recommendation.

PROGRAMMATIC CONSIDERATIONS IN PEDIATRIC SETTINGS

Impact of Expanding Medical Services and Technology

As the consultation process moves beyond the initial entry phase, pediatric acceptance of psychological services inevitably leads to strenuous service demands. In our setting, rapid expansion of medical subspecialties associated with new treatment programs in ambulatory care, childhood cancer, renal failure, and gastrointestinal disease brought new pediatric faculty and patient populations with complex psychosocial needs. As our Division has evolved, requests from subspecialties have expanded along with those from ambulatory and inpatient units, and have resulted in, at times, counterproductive dispersal of our efforts to a variety of medical services and patient populations.

Problems are not only raised by the sheer numbers of patients but by inconsistent or superficial planning for psychological supports for children and families who are highly stressed by medical technologies (Calland, 1972; Duff & Campbell, 1973;

Shurtleff, Hayden, Laeser, & Kronmal, 1974). In the fast paced and emotionally charged acute-care hospital, severely ill children can be erroneously labeled as "problem" patients in need of special treatment by a mental health professional. Helping nursing staff and physicians to recognize their reactions to childrens' distress, to understand how these reactions affect their perceptions of the child's coping, and to develop more effective ways of providing support to children can often be a more sensitive intervention than direct psychological treatment (Drotar, 1976b, 1977b). Expanding medical technologies can also present difficult ethical dilemmas to psychologists who are asked to provide service that is not meaningfully integrated into programs which address the inherent stresses of medical treatments.

Early in our work with children with end stage renal failure, we received numerous requests from the hospital transplantation committee to evaluate children's adjustment to determine who would be a "good" psychological risk for renal transplant. We found this role neither possible nor desirable from an ethical standpoint. A more suitable role for psychology involved participation in a comprehensive-care program which included anticipatory planning for all patients, not just those who were in the midst of psychological crises (Drotar & Ganofsky, 1976, Drotar, Ganofsky, Makker, & DeMaio, in press).

At other times, adherence to our own professional and ethical standards have precluded participation in treatment programs or collaborations with physicians that do not appear to be in the best interests of child and family:

> A psychologist was requested to consult to the "bone marrow transplant committee" after a leukemic child became psychotic during transplantation. He agreed to help evaluate and prepare potential candidates for what was a harrowing hospital ordeal. It was his intention over time to help physicians better prepare patients for the harsh and grim realities of transplanting procedures. Instead of gaining greater access to physicians and impacting on their abilities to prepare patients, he increasingly met patients who had been given no information, medical or otherwise. He felt it was ethically mandated that physicians present to their patients the medical/technical data, as well as respond to their patients' initial concerns and fears. Over time, the psychologist felt that his role served to help physician's evade this responsibility. In addition, having had no preparation, patients who were already quite anxious from illness-related worries were puzzled and alarmed to initially meet a psychologist. The psychologist withdrew from the consultative relationship with the bone marrow transplant group after efforts to redress this situation failed.

Impact of the Medical Model

Significant problems are posed by adherence to models of pediatric care that emphasize disease rather than health, minimize the social context of problems (Engel, 1977), and label problems that are more properly regarded as social and behavioral as "diseases" which must come under the province of medicine.

Undesirable consequences of a disease-oriented model of care include an underemphasis on preventive approaches, localization of problems within the child rather than the family milieu, and inappropriate, confining expectations for the psychologist's role. For example, psychologists in pediatric settings may be expected to diagnose and provide treatment in line with a model of organic disease that does not recognize the importance of the relationship with a caregiver and ignores the necessity of carefully considering the broader context in which a condition occurs.

For a number of years, children hospitalized for environmentally based failure-to-thrive, a complex condition which poses grave hazards to the child's future development (Hannaway, 1970), were often referred to psychology for evaluation of their intellectual and emotional development. These children were often referred too late in their hospital admission to allow a comprehensive evaluation of the child and the family situation. Since the hospital admission emphasized the diagnosis of organic disease, rather than assessment of family influences which had given rise to the problem, planning for treatment or follow-up in the community was often neglected (Drotar, Malone, Negray, & Dennstedt in press). As a consequence, psychological consultation could not contribute to in-depth understanding of the infant's problem or to planning successful treatment.

In many pediatric settings, it is not uncommon for a variety of psychosocial problems such as hyperactivity, learning disabilities, or child abuse to be handled via approaches which should be reserved for organic disease, despite cogent evidence that disease-focused approaches may contribute little to an understanding of etiology, long-term outcome, or treatment (Newberger & Bourne, 1978; Conrad, 1975). Psychologists must combat the maladaptive application of disease-oriented models by taking the lead in planning treatment programs which more effectively meet the psychological needs of children and their families.

Problems of Maintaining Professional Autonomy

It is imperative that psychologists have the freedom to redefine their roles and functions in ongoing dialogues with their pediatric colleagues in order to change patterns of medical care which ignore psychological needs of patients. In our experience, some physicians remain more invested in defining roles of psychologists and other professions than in developing a true partnership which may result in changes in their own functioning with staff or families. One of the major impediments to effective collaboration is the tendency for the pediatric hierarchy to view psychology as an ancillary service akin to laboratory facilities or physical therapy. The need for psychologists to be involved as professional equals in planning for the psychosocial aspects of pediatric programs is often ignored. Ambiguous administrative arrangements which do not provide clear guidelines for evolving psychologist-pediatrician collaboration complicate conjoint planning efforts. As is true of most psychologists in medical settings, our major administrative appointments are in the Department of psychiatry with secondary administrative appointments in the Department of Pediatrics (Nathan, Lubin, Matarazzo, & Persely, 1979). This alignment has posed a number of disadvantages. Since the lines of administrative responsibility for psychologists working in pediatrics were not clear, our group's interests were sometimes bypassed in regard to critical work supports such as secretarial services and office space. Departmental responsibilities for the funding of new positions in connection with program development were also ill-defined. It has been difficult for the two departments (Psychiatry and Pediatrics) to agree on clear arrangements to jointly finance new positions and to allocate monies generated by psychologists from patient fees.

In order to maintain a reasonable work environment, it is desirable for psychologists to reshape the direction of their clinical responsibilities as time pressures and their professional interests change. Pediatricians need to recognize that the services offered by psychologists in hospital settings are not the only mental health services that are available to them.

We have found it useful to clarify our own limitations in time, interest, and ability with our physician colleagues and to develop guidelines to aid decision making concerning referrals. The physician's willingness to become involved in conjoint medical and psychosocial follow-up is a demonstration of commitment which should be respected. Chronically ill children or children with neurological problems requiring periodic, conjoint medical and psychological follow-up warrant priority. We have chosen to focus our clinical energies on patient groups of interest and to direct our consultative efforts toward physicians who are congenial collaborators who respect our role and who share decision making concerning children and families.

We believe that the opportunity to independently pursue and develop areas of professional interest is a singularly important means of reducing "burnout," which is increasingly recognized as a critical issue in high-stress pediatric settings (Koocher, 1980). We have addressed this problem by individually reserving a portion of our work time for the pursuit of special interest projects. These have included the conducting of independent research studies and the writing of clinical papers on such topics as chronic and acute life-threatening illness, cognitively based disorders, problems of blind children, and aspects of normal child development (Benjamin, 1978; Litt, 1979, in press).

Planning new programs of intervention which are primarily under the aegis of psychologists provides other opportunities for establishing professional autonomy. Our frustrations in trying to provide consultation to the families of infants with environmentally based failure-to-thrive within traditional patterns of hospital-based care represent a case in point. Clinical experiences suggested that a viable alternative for the treatment of failure-to-thrive would involve a marked change in current patterns of hospital-based care to include outreach interventions to help families continue to nurture their children once they returned home (Drotar, Malone, & Negray, 1979). Out of concern for this population, and in order to establish a research focus concerning the psychopathology of infancy, a proposal was funded to study the effectiveness of family-oriented outreach intervention on the growth and development of failure-to-thrive infants. Funds from this grant not only provided staffing to carry out this project but also provided partial support for another psychologist.

The development or expansion of medical programs which require psychological consultation may bring both opportunities and new professional dilemmas. For example, our Pediatric Ambulatory Division's interest in expanding the psychological services and teaching prompted the funding of a new psychology position. On the one hand, this development enabled us to expand our activities in the ambulatory setting; on the other, it created conflict over administrative jurisdiction. In part, the difficulty resulted from the pediatricians' belief that the provision of funds entitled them to unlimited control over the activities of the psychologist. Our experience strongly suggests that to achieve maximum autonomy within a large medical setting, psychologists will have to be increasingly active in developing and maintaining control over their own sources of funding through patient fees and research grants. As the need for psychological services expands, salaries for new positions are not automatically funded by pediatric departments or hospitals. Rather, patient fees, collaborative research, or training grants must provide such funding. Active negotiation for the responsibilities and direction of these positions is critical to maintain professional integrity of psychology in a medical setting. For this reason, the development of structures which increase administrative visibility and autonomy of psychology is critical. In our setting, the Division of Pediatric Psychology is now on a similar administrative footing with pediatric subspecialities such as neurology or cardiology. The division representative participates in departmental executive committee planning meetings. Other members of the Division of Pediatric Psychology are highly visible at departmental meetings. Psychologists in pediatric and medical settings must continue to seek alternatives for maintaining their professional autonomy. Independent medical school departments of Medical Psychology or Behavioral Science may ultimately provide more professionally congenial administrative structures (Nathan et al., 1979).

In order to effectively cope with the stresses posed by patient-care demands and complex administrative dilemmas, pediatric psychologists must maintain choice in the ways in which they are deployed by determining the programs to which they will direct their energies as well as the content of their activities. We believe that these assertions of professional identity are critical to the survival of pediatric psychology as an independent discipline.

REFERENCES

Ack, M. The psychological environment of a children's hospital. *Pediatric Psychology,* 1974, **2,** 3–5.

Bates, B. Doctor and nurse: Changing roles and relations. *New England Journal of Medicine,* 1970, **283,** 129–134.

Benjamin, P. Y. Psychological problems following recovery from acute life-threatening illness. *American Journal of Orthopsychiatry,* 1978, **48,** 284–290.

Bolian, G. C. Psychiatric consultation within a community of sick children. *Journal of the American Academy of Child Psychiatry,* 1971, **10,** 293–307.

Botinelli, S. B. Establishment of an outpatient psychology screening clinic: Preliminary considerations. *Pediatric Psychology,* 1975, **3,** 10–11.

Calland, O. H. Iatrogenic problems in end-stage renal failure. *New England Journal of Medicine,* 1972, **287,** 334–337.

Caplan, G. *The theory and practice of mental health consultation.* New York: Basic Books, 1970.

Conrad, P. The discovery of hyperkinesis: notes on the medicalization of deviant behavior. *Social Problems,* 1975, **23,** 12–21.

Drotar, D. Death in the pediatric hospital: Psychological consultation with medical and nursing staff. *Journal of Clinical Child Psychology,* 1975, **4,** 33–35.

Drotar, D. Mental health consultation in the pediatric intensive care nursery. *International Journal of Psychiatry in Medicine,* 1976, **7,** 69–81. (a)

Drotar, D. Psychological consultation in the pediatric hospital. *Professional Psychology,* 1976, **9,** 77–83. (b)

Drotar, D. Clinical psychological practice in the pediatric hospital. *Professional Psychology,* 1977, **10,** 72–80. (a)

Drotar, D. Family oriented intervention with the dying adolescent. *Journal of Pediatric Psychology,* 1977, **2,** 68–71. (b)

Drotar, D., & Ganofsky, M. A. Mental health intervention with children and adolescents with end stage renal failure. *International Journal of Psychiatry in Medicine,* 1976, **7,** 181–194.

Drotar, D., Ganofsky, M. A., Makker, S., & DeMaio, D. A family oriented supportive approach to renal transplantation in children. In N. Levy (Ed.), *Psychological factors in hemodialysis and transplantation.* New York: Plenum, in press.

Drotar, D., Malone, C. M., & Negray, J. Psychosocial intervention with the families of children who fail to thrive. *Child Abuse and Neglect: The International Journal,* 1979, **3,** 927–935.

Drotar, D., Malone, C. A., Negray, J., & Dennstedt, M. Psychosocial assessment and care of infants hospitalized for nonorganic failure to thrive. *Journal of Clinical Child Psychology,* in press.

Duff, R. S., & Campbell, A. G. M. Moral and ethical dilemmas in the special care nursery. *New England Journal of Medicine,* 1973, **289,** 890–894.

Easson, W. B. *The dying child.* Springfield, IL: Charles C. Thomas, 1970.

Engel, G. L. The need for a new medical model: A challenge for biomedicine. *Science,* 1977, **196,** 127–136.

Geist, R. Consultation on a pediatric surgical ward: Creating an empathic climate. *American Journal of Orthopsychiatry,* 1977, **47,** 432–444.

Groves, J. E. Taking care of the hateful patient. *New England Journal of Medicine,* 1978, **298,** 883–887.

Hannaway, P. J. Failure to thrive—A study of 100 infants and children. *Clinical Pediatrics,* 1970, **9,** 96–99.

Hollon, T. The interaction model of consultation in the general hospital. Paper presented at the annual meeting of the American Psychological Association, Montreal, Canada, 1973.

Johnson, M. Mental health intervention with medically ill children: A review of the literature 1970–77. *Journal of Pediatric Psychology,* 1979, **4,** 147–164.

Koocher, G. P. Pediatric cancer: Psychosocial problems and the high costs of helping. *Journal of Child Clinical Psychology,* 1980, **8,** 2–5.

Litt, C. J. Trichotillomania in childhood: A case of successful short-term treatment. *Journal of Pediatric Psychology,* 1980, **5,** 37–42.

Litt, C. J. The development of transitional objects, a study of two pediatric populations. *American Journal of Orthopsychiatry,* in press.

Nathan, R. G., Lubin, B., Matarazzo, J. D., & Persely, G. W. Psychologists in schools of medicine—1955, 1964 and 1977. *American Psychologist,* 1979, **34,** 622–627.

Naylor, K. A., & Mattson, A. "For the sake of the Children": Trials and tribulations of child psychiatry-liason service. *Psychiatry in Medicine,* 1973, **4,** 389–402.

Newberger, E. H., & Bourne, R. The medicalization and legalization of child abuse. *American Journal of Orthopsychiatry,* 1978, **48,** 593–607.

Pitcher, G. A. Pleasure/pain and primary physicians. *Journal of Clinical Child Psychology,* 1978, **7,** 29–32.

Rothenberg, M. B. The unholy trinity—Activity, authority and magic. *Clinical Pediatrics,* 1974, **13,** 870–73.

Schroeder, C. S. Psychologists in a private pediatric practice. *Journal of Pediatric Psychology,* 1979, **4,** 5–18.

Shurtleff, D. B., Hayden, B. W., Laeser, J. D., & Kronmal, R. A. Meyelodysplasia: Decision for death or disability. *New England Journal of Medicine,* 1974, **291,** 1005–1011.

Smith, E. E., Rome, L. P., & Freedheim, D. K. The clinical psychologist in the pediatric office. *Journal of Pediatrics,* 1967, **71,** 48–51.

Task Force on Pediatric Education. *The future of pediatric education.* Evanston, IL: Author, 1978.

Tefft, B. M., & Simeonson, R. J. Psychology and the creation of health care settings. *Professional Psychology,* 1979, **32,** 558–570.

Toback, C., Russo, R. M., & Gururaj, V. J. Pediatric psychology as practiced in a large municipal hospital setting. *Pediatric Psychology,* 1975, **3,** 10–11.

Tuma, J. M. Pediatric psychologist . . . Do you mean clinical child psychologist? *Journal of Clinical Child Psychology,* 1975, **4,** 9–12.

U.S. Public Health Service. *Grants for residency training in general internal medicine and/or pediatrics: Guidelines prepared by the Department of Health, Education and Welfare.* Washington, DC: Author, 1978.

Wright, L. The pediatric psychologist: A new role model. *American Psychologist,* 1967, **22,** 323–325.

CHAPTER 7

The Role of the Pediatric Psychologist as Consultant to Pediatricians

Michael C. Roberts

Logan Wright

The relationship of psychology with pediatric practice typically has been stronger than with other medical specialties. The development of a liaison relationship occurred as pediatricians, by the force of their clinical practice, recognized that the problems they are called upon to treat require more than just medical and physical interventions; there are emotional and psychological aspects of the problems. Concomitantly, psychologists began to discover the varied types of psychopathology related to organic illness and the utility of behavioral interventions for some medical and pediatric entities. Thus, applied child psychologists began to extend their skills to health-related problems. Consequently, pediatricians and psychologists collaborate to respond to the variety of psychiatric, psychosomatic, developmental, learning, and other illness-related problems that are encountered in children's medical settings.

While this psychologist-pediatrician relationship is growing stronger, given the two disciplines' diverse training and orientation, the liaison is sometimes tenuous. Differences such as mistrust or resentment of intrusions onto professional "turf," language or jargon differences, procedural differences, and certainly differences in knowledge bases often preclude effective functioning. Despite these differences, the collaborations between psychologists and pediatricians have been rewarding to each as well as beneficial to patients.

In this chapter we focus on how a psychologist/pediatrican-consultant relationship can be established and what roles can be assumed in the delivery of health care psychology for children. We first examine some basic information useful to the pediatric psychologist's understanding of the pediatrician and pediatric psychology. Then we turn to the multifaceted roles characterizing the pediatrics/psychology-consultant relationship.

Psychologists and pediatricians collaborate in a wide variety of settings. Pediatric psychology rapidly developed primarily in children's hospitals and developmental centers (Wright, 1979a). Increasingly, however, the physician is accepting the pediatric psychologist as a peer and calling on him or her much as one might request consultation with a cardiologist or other specialist. This is often without the benefit of a suprastructure of hospital departments, although these institutional settings are still prevalent (e.g., Morrison, 1976). Whereas the preceding chapter by Drotar, Benjamin, Chast, Litt, and Vajner covered the hospital settings of inpatient and outpatient services, an additional emphasis in this chapter is placed on working with the pediatrician in the independent practice of pediatric medicine. The acceptance of the pediatric psychologist as a consultant, no matter the type of setting, has been contingent on the provision of competent services. As long as psychology in pediatric practice is competent and providing worthwhile services, the consultant role can be expected to expand vis-à-vis pediatric physicians. We will discuss how the psychologist can work in collaboration with the pediatrician regardless of the setting (hospital, private practice). Most of the factors important to a professional relationship in one setting are applicable to another. Additionally, most of the practice-oriented consultation procedures we recommend may be instituted in some form in all pediatric facilities.

In preparation for consulting in the pediatric setting, the psychologist needs a background in traditional psychological phenomena and practices, and also in the nontraditional areas of medical psychology. For the latter, we suggest several sources in addition to the present handbook. Volumes edited by Magrab (1978) and written by Wright, Schaefer, and Solomons (1979) are useful for pediatric psychology. Summary chapters on pediatric psychology are also available (Christophersen & Rapoff, 1980; Roberts, Maddux, Wurtele, & Wright, in press; Walker, 1979a). General approaches and issues in medical psychology and behavioral medicine are presented in McNamara (1979), Ferguson and Taylor (1980), and Millon, Green, and Meagher (in press). Additionally, access to pediatric medicine textbooks is needed. We recommend several basic texts (Barnett, 1977; Green & Haggerty, 1977; Nelson, Vaughan, & McKay, 1975). Training issues, patterns, and content are presented by Tuma in Chapter 9.

UNDERSTANDING THE PEDIATRICIAN'S ORIENTATION

The consulting psychologist needs to understand the health care perspective before attempting to provide psychological assistance. It is important to note the numerous differences in training for the professions of psychologist and pediatrician, how patients are approached and managed, what aspects of cases are considered significant, among other orientation differences. In this section, we will outline some basic facts about pediatric practice which will aid in understandng the pediatric orientation and subsequently enhance the consultant relationship. An awareness of where pediatricians practice is important. The American Medical Association lists 23,516 physicians who have designated themselves as pediatricians (American Medical Association, 1976, 1977); of these, 21,092 are classified as in patient care. Correspondingly, the American Academy of Pediatrics comprises 14,429 Fellows with only 23% of these in academic medicine, that is, medical schools or teaching institutions (Burnett & Bell, 1978). Thus the vast majority of pediatricians are engaged in office practice, either solo or in a group. In contrast, much of the literature and professional focus in pediatric psychology derives from teaching hospital settings where most of the pediatric psychologists are to be found. Yet most of the pediatricians and patients are not found there. Hence we also want to emphasize and encourage the consultation to the office practice pediatrician.

Pediatricians, regardless of the setting, serve as front-line health-care professionals for a multitude of problems. Salk (1969) stated that a "pediatrician sees more human beings than any other professional during the most crucial stages of early development . . . he is the first to be brought face to face with more developmental, learning, and emotional problems and has the greatest potential influence on child care practices" (p. 2). It is this "front-line" nature of pediatric practice which often permits a consulting psychologist to make maximally effective interventions. Thus psychological services can be focused where the majority of problems are first presented, that is, in medical settings, and not in a psychiatric or mental health center which is away from the site of initial presentation. Early intervention at the pediatric clinic precludes the process of "shaping" the patient to exhibit standardized responses through a series of referrals (Walker, 1979a). Statistics vary, but a conservative finding has been that approximately 50% of child patients have a significant behavioral/psychological problem (Duff, Rowe, & Anderson, 1973; Wright, 1976). Duff et al. (1973) found that only 12% of the patients presenting in the pediatric clinic had purely physical problems; 36% had problems that were considered to be psychological, and the remaining 52% had problems that were both physical and psychological in nature.

The pediatrician is often ill-prepared to meet these demands for psychological advice because medical training emphasizes physical rather than the behavioral aspects. One survey found 54% of graduating pediatric residents reported inadequate preparation in this latter area (Haggerty, 1979). Currently there are efforts to change medical school curricula to include developmental and behavioral pediatric training (Ambulatory Pediatric Association, 1978; Task Force on Pediatric Education, 1978). Yet many practicing pediatricians have only learned psychological techniques through experience or they have to ignore psychological concomitants. Since the pediatrician is used as a source of child management expertise, this aspect of a lack of adequate knowledge and training is a problem. This difficulty can be tactfully ameliorated through a psychological consultantship.

The Nature of Pediatric Practices

Drotar et al., in the preceding chapter, outlined the nature of pediatric practice in the hospital setting. This basic information will be useful in understanding the pediatrician's orientation in the outpatient and inpatient hospital practice. Typically, a neglected area for pediatric psychologists has been in understanding the nature of office-practice pediatrics. One survey of office-practices revealed that 50% of the pediatrician's time is spent on well-child checkups, with an additional 20% for children with minor medical problems (Bergman, Dassel, & Wedgewood, 1966). Another study found that 56% of well-child office visits included advice giving for child management and scholastic performance (McClelland, Staples, Weisberg, & Berger, 1973). The pattern of presenting problems in pediatric offices over a 5-year period appears to be shifting from disease-oriented office visits to contacts regarding academic performance and learning disabilities (up 60%) and behavioral management problems (up 40%) (Burnett & Bell, 1978). This shift is likely caused by improved medical procedures including prevention-immunization and early detection of childhood disease states as well as increased parental interest (Davis, Stone, Levine, & Stolzenberg, 1979).

These statistics suggest that well-child care and its accompanying questions of childrearing take up a large proportion of the pediatrician's time. Understanding the implications of this, for example, the psychologist may wish to focus efforts to assist the pediatrician in anticipatory psychological child guidance. In fact, Brazelton (1975) suggests that up to 85% of the pediatric practice can consist of anticipatory guidance. Unfortunately, it appears that childhood emotional or behavioral problems are underdiagnosed in pediatric offices. A study by Goldberg, Regier, McInerny, Pless, and Roghmann (1979) found only 5% of children seen in 9 practices to be diagnosed by the pediatrician as having psychological problems; this is contrasted with the findings of Duff et al. (1973), noted earlier, that close to 90% of pediatric patients have psychological aspects to their problems.

Studies of pediatric offices have found an average of 13 minutes of the pediatrician's time is spent with each child patient (Bergman et al., 1966; DeLozier & Gagnon, 1975). The pediatrician may see 20, 30 or even 50 patients a day (Wright, 1979a), with the average being 27 patients (Burnett, Williams, & Olmsted, 1978). This has several implications. First, the brevity of contact likely reflects the well-child nature of the office visit, and the time could be used for child management issues. Second, the busy pediatrician has very little free time and must hurry to keep up with the demands of the practice. Suggesting the physician spend more time with patients would probably be a superficial remedy, one few physicians would be likely to adhere to. However, a survey of pediatric practices indicates that the duration of an office visit does increase to 26 minutes when the pediatrician makes interventions which are psychotherapeutically related (Regier & Goldberg, 1976). Third, consultation to the pediatrician needs to be correspondingly brief and to the point. Fourth, pediatric psychological interventions may also need to be briefly implemented and fairly short term. These last two points are particularly important because it is in this area that the pediatric psychologist may have to relinquish some set notions about case treatment in a traditional clinical child psychological perspective (namely, the need for extensive diagnositc assessment and long-term treatment).

Instead, the pediatric psychologist needs to make use of techniques which are economical and more effective. This necessity often is tantamount to emphasizing behavioral techniques and crisis interventions (Harper, 1975; Roberts, Quevillon, & Wright, 1979; Walker, 1979a, 1979b; Wright, 1969, 1979b). Psychological consultations to the pediatrician should be brief and target oriented. For example, in a neurological service in a hospital, Hartlage and Hartlage (1978) suggest short psychological "curbside consultations" to help solve this problem of time and priorities. Correspondingly, to-the-point psychological reports are more likely to be read and considered by the pediatrician than are long, esoteric reports containing confusing jargon. Walker (1979a) recommends action-based reports consisting of "a brief, crisp communication regarding the patient's problem and what should be done about it" (p. 240). Thus understanding the brevity of patient contact in pediatric practice shapes the psychologist's consultation procedures whether in the hospital or office practice of pediatrics.

Pediatric Training

The most obvious difference between a psychologist and a pediatrician is training. The typical clinical psychology training program includes didactic coursework, clinical practica, a research-based dissertation, and an internship year of clinical practice with numerous post-doctoral experiences available (see chapter 9). Familiarity with medical training is less probable but may help the psychologist understand the pediatrician's orientation.

The pediatrician has typically received a baccalaureate degree in a science such as chemistry or biology. A general medical school training is obtained with lecture coursework in a variety of areas including anatomy, pharmacology, diseases and physical states. In the final years of a 4-year basic program leading to the MD degree, clinical clerkships are usually taken with rotations to different specialties and services (e.g., surgery, pediatrics, obstetrics, psychiatry, otolaryngology). A more intensive medical-practical experience is obtained in an internship in one or more areas in the fourth or fifth year. The MD then chooses a specialty area if desired and begins a residency training program ranging from 2 to 5 years. For pediatrics, the residency usually covers 2 years with increasingly independent responsibility for medical cases. Pediatricians have passed a state licensing examination to practice medicine and many become certified as pediatricians by the American Academy of Pediatrics. The latter certification attests to the quality of training and experience. There are, of course, many practicing physicians who restrict their practices to children but who did not go through this type of specialty training, nor are they "board certified."

Private-practicing pediatricians, unlike many of their colleagues at medical centers, do not have a background in research, and many physicians have trouble conceiving of their clinical role as including research (Carey, 1978). The practicing pediatrician's orientation is almost totally clinical with a strong emphasis on the physical components of a patient. The biochemical and bacteriological aspects of a medical problem receive the most emphasis in training. Most of the training is taken in large medical centers where the focus is on inpatient work with children who have serious disease entities. In practice, however, hospitalizations for acute illness have declined 65% (Burnett & Bell, 1978). Yet the physician's interest in physical properties continues on into practice. As noted earlier, though, relatively little of the practitioner's time is spent dealing with physical entities; considerable time is spent on the well-child and child management issues. Realization of this physical emphasis can aid in communication and in conceptualizing the role of the pediatric psychologist. In particular, this is where a consulting psychologist can help the pediatrician to understand psychological concomitants and developmental phenomena.

Case Conceptualization

Another critical difference between psychology and pediatric medicine is in how patient cases are conceptualized. "Differential diagnosis" refers to the process of considering a number of possible causes for a medical symptom and then systematically "ruling out" competing hypotheses until a conclusion is empirically and logically arrived at (Nelson et al., 1975). Although psychology utilizes the term "differential diagnosis," it is rare that systematic assessment is undertaken with the same underlying conceptualization as in medicine. (Psychologists more likely use testing to "rule in" a diagnosis.) Pediatricians may use one of several organizational frameworks for assisting in case conceptualization (Morgan & Engel, 1969). For example, case write-ups may include sections on a child's birth history, nutrition history, immunization history, growth and developmental history, and physical examination findings. Another medical framework for progress notes has the acronym SOAP. Each letter designates a section: subjective data—gathered from the patient; objective data—from physical examination or laboratory tests; assessment—interpretation of the data and goals; plan—diagnostic impressions, treatment interventions, patient or family education, and follow-up.

The Problem-Oriented Medical Record (POR) is a detailed, comprehensive organization of data that is widely used (Weed, 1969). (For a detailed presentation of this method, see Nelson et al., 1975, pp. 221–234; Walker, Hurst, & Woody, 1973). The POR organization is logically structured and can be used in routine practice, but it does generate considerable paperwork.

At the crux of these various organizational schemes is what Nelson et al. (1975) call an "algorithm," which is defined as a "step-by-step plan for proceeding from a clearly identifiable point in diagnosis or management to another identified point at which an objective is achieved or a which clinical judgment or a new algorithm must be applied" (p. 222). The algorithm for differential diagnosis involves weighing evidence for and against a certain disease state as the cause of the presenting symptoms. This consideration is done for three or four disease entities with the priority given to those that are most likely. This "ruling out" process is exemplified by the following excerpt from a differential diagnosis for an infant eventually diagnosed as failure-to-thrive (from the case reported by Roberts & Horner, 1979).

Symptoms	Plan
Weight loss	Hospital admission: adjust diet, decrease diarrhea, and promote weight gain; calorie counting by dietetics; R/O malabsorption problem
Diarrhea	Stool cultures & U/A to R/O organic pathology
Otitis media	Long bone series and skull series-X-ray from bone age
Failure-to-thrive	Neurological exam to R/O petit mal seizures and infantile myoclonic seizures
Maternal deprivation syndrome	Psychological consult for child developmental assessment and mother's depression
Maternal self-reports of depression	Social work consult for family history and home visit
	Begin antibiotics for otitis

Another example of medical differential diagnosis is in the evaluation of potential psychogenic encopresis. The physician and pediatric psychologist must rule out the possibility of physical abnormality causing the chronic constipation symptoms before instituting behavioral procedures for encopresis (e.g., rule out Hirschsprung's disease and spinal cord injury; see Wright & Walker, 1976; 1977; and Nelson et al., 1975, p. 817). This ruling out is necessary because psychological interventions would have little impact on a totally physiologically based problem (and may even exacerbate the problem). A useful reference for the psychologist will be a practical manual on pediatric diagnosis by Athreya (1980).

We have noted the organization and logic of various approaches the pediatrician may utilize in practice. Pediatric psychologists often find it useful to adapt these techniques in consulting with a pediatrician because they are familiar to the physician and provide a systematic approach to patients' problems.

Jargon and Language

Just as psychologists employ jargon, physicians become engrossed in a language peculiar to their profession. Professional jargon, on both sides of a consultant relationship, impedes professional communication. Some basic knowledge of commonly used phrases, jargon, and abbreviations may be helpful to the psychologist. Some examples listed in Table 1 attest to the difficulty the psychologist may have in understanding the pediatrician. To go beyond this brief listing (there are considerably more abbreviations), the pediatric psychologist will need to consult some basic pediatric textbooks (e.g., Barnett, 1977; Nelson et al., 1975).

Table 1.   Common Medical Phrases, Jargon, Tests, and Abbreviations, and their Interpretations

Otitis media—ear infection	PO—by mouth
MS—multiple sclerosis	PRN—as needed; whenever necessary, medicine
HA—headache	to be given when the patient asks for it
URI—upper respiratory infection	stat—immediately
FUO—fever of unknown origin	bid—twice a day, medicine times
PKU—phenylketonuria	tid—three times a day
UCD—usual childhood diseases	q—each or every
PE or Px—physical examination	qam—every morning
R/O—rule out	qd—everyday
I&O—intake and output (e.g., of fluids)	decub—lying down
U/A—urinalysis	OOB—out of bed
BRP—bathroom privileges	Dx—diagnosis
IV—intravenous	Rx—treatment, prescription
IM—intramuscular, injection	prog—prognosis
RBC—red blood count	T&A—tonsils and adenoids
Hgb—hemoglobin	DPT—immunization, injections namely,
GI—gastrointestinal	diphtheria, pertussis, and tetanus vaccines
GU—genitourinary	DOB—date of birth
BUN—blood urea nitrogen test	TOPU—trivalent oral poliomyelitis vaccine
NPO—nothing by mouth, usually no food	ASA—aspirin
or water in preparation for surgery.	T—temperature
	ENT—ear, nose, throat, also known as ORL or
	OTO (otorhynolaryngology)

Summary

The discussion in this section outlines some of what the pediatric psychologist needs to know in order to understand how the pediatrician practices, what training she or he has had, how patient cases are approached, and what language is peculiar to the medical setting. We have found, however, the best teacher of how the pediatrician thinks and acts is the pediatrician.

MODELS OF CONSULTATION TO THE PEDIATRICIAN

Selective Review of Literature on Consultation

Various conceptualizations of roles and functions for the pediatric psychologist have been forwarded. Stabler and Murray (1974), however, note that there is no consensus among professionals in the field as to what skills and functions should be fulfilled. In a seminal paper presenting a role model for the discipline, Wright (1967) proposed the psychologist should be a consultant to physicians and to parents and should be a scientist-practitioner. Schofield (1969) urged that the medical psychologist should have "a particular sophistication in physical illness, equipped to research and consult with regard to the psychological concomitants of physical disease'' (p. 574). Others have also outlined similar functions of a specialist-consultant—resource, educator, facilitator, counselor, and conferring diagnostician (Drotar, 1976; Nixon, 1975; Smith, Rome, & Freidheim, 1967). Salk (1970), in particular, diminishes the role of a pediatric psychologist as a technician who performs extensive direct testing and therapy and encourages the role of consultation for case management. Given these general descriptions of a composite consultant role, there arises a need to further define the consultative process for pediatric psychology.

Several conceptual models have been provided for describing the consultant relationship (e.g., Burns & Cromer, 1978; Caplan, 1970; Platt & Wicks, 1979; Stabler, 1979). In the following section, we describe three general models and approaches of pediatric psychology consultation to pediatricians, applicable to the different medical settings. The three models are simple yet allow us to describe the complexity of psychologist-pediatrician liaisons. Next we present several ways in which the pediatric psychologist can consult effectively following one model or combinations of these models. Our suggestions are oriented to the pediatric practice wherever found, rather than to traditional psychological practices. We do emphasize an orientation to the pediatric office practice rather than practice located in medical centers because an expansion of the latter services is needed.

Three Models of Consultation

We have labeled the three descriptive models of consultation Independent Functions Model, Indirect Psychological Consultation Model, and Collaborative Team Model. In some regards, these models follow those of Stabler (1979) and Burns and Cromer (1978). However, we elaborate on the three basic relationship patterns and emphasize that any pediatric psychology consultantship may involve any one of the three approaches profitably. We do not encourage one particular arrangement over the other models. We do, however, contend that the psychologist should provide service geared to the needs of the pediatrician and patients where they are located. This may require some modification of consultation to fit the setting. The differing views of pediatric psychology require the individual psychologist to determine what are the functions of the consultantship—following his or her own proclivity and the demands of the particular setting. The psychologist can also adapt to the requirements of the situation by redefining her or his role in order to provide more effective services.

Independent Functions Model

When a consultation relationship follows this first pattern, the psychologist acts as a specialist who independently undertakes diagnosis and/or treatment of a patient referred by the pediatrician. Except for exchanges of information before and after referral of a patient, the pediatrician and psychologist work noncollaboratively. This pattern follows the usual establishment of independent practices of two professions with referrals to each other as needed. This model of the psychologist-pediatrician having independent functions has been noted by Drotar (1978) as a "noncollaborative" approach, by Stabler (1979) as "coordination of multiservices."

The diagnostic role of this approach often relegates the psychologist to what Salk (1974) calls the "technician." That is, the psychologist does testing, which may not be needed, which has little impact on patient care, and which often removes the psychologist from active participation.

Pediatricians, in office and hospital practice, dislike reports and procedures filled, for example, with psychological jargon, and speculation regarding intrapsychic dynamics (e.g., Hartlage & Hartlage, 1978; Rie, 1969; Salk, 1974). The role of the psychologist has greatly expanded such that treatment is usually undertaken by the psychologist, especially in this "independent functions" consultation model. However, when independently making pediatric psychological interventions with referred pediatric patients, there are several problems of which the psychologist should be aware.

A first problem is that the psychologist should be careful not to "swallow" the patients up and totally remove responsibility and decision making from the physician. The pediatrician must be informed of what the psychologist is doing, just as the psychologist needs knowledge of what the pediatrician is doing. Obviously, communication is needed—reports, letters, and telephone calls help meet this requirement. Direct contact in conference meetings would be helpful but often is not possible given the busy pediatric practice. A second area of potential problems for the pediatric psychologist is that of "turf issues." The psychologist often is functioning in problem areas typically considered the domain of the pediatrician. For example, the treatment of encopresis requires both physical and behavioral interventions. However, it is often easy for the pediatric psychologist to take over treatment of both aspects and therefore "swallow up" the patient. As an example of the second problem, the physics of enemas, mineral oil, and suppositories in the treatment of encopresis recommended by Wright (1973, 1975) do not require prescription and may be bought "over-the-counter." However, medical/physical prescribing is a privilege assiduously guarded by medical doctors more so than other procedures. The psychologist needs to recognize the concerns of medicine a priori, but without "kowtowing" or employing less than optimal procedures. Again, communication is critical and a clear explanation of the procedures is necessary (perhaps relying on psychological articles in the medical literature to back the psychologist; e.g., Wright & Walker, 1977).

This "independent functions" consultation is likely the most prevalent form of consultation between pediatrician and psychologist because it follows a more traditional pattern of independent professional practice. Many nontraditional problems, however, can be handled in this model. The pediatrician makes a referral and continues to see a patient for medical treatment. The psychologist concurrently sees the patient or family and does what is needed in the psychological realm. The medical and behavioral management of juvenile diabetes exemplifies this arrangement (Lowe & Lutzker, 1979). Additionally, the pediatrician may see problems concomitant to medical disorders which require special psychological interventions and make a referral (e.g., for social skills training, La Greca & Mesibov, 1979; or for multiple problemsolving, Roberts & Ottinger, 1979). Since the pediatrician may be aware of some problems sooner than other professionals, traditional psychological therapy may also be requested (e.g., divorce counseling for the children or help for emotional problems of childhood).

The pediatric psychologist and pediatrician can function effectively in this independent practice arrangement as long as they maintain appropriate communication and mutual respect for expertise. This role may be restrictive if the psychologist permits it. The pediatrician may consider only some types of cases to be appropriate for referral and, as a consequence, the psychologist's role will be limited. In this situation, there probably is no active input in the definition of functions by the psychologist. The psychologist may need to educate the physician about psychological roles beyond the diagnostic one and about what are appropriate referrals.

Indirect Psychological Consultation Model

The second approach to a consultation arrangement is one in which the pediatrician retains the major responsibility for patient management. The psychologist works with the pediatrician to provide indirect psychological services to the patient. The psychologist has limited or no contact with the actual client and usually considers only data gathered by the pediatrician. This pediatric-psychological relationship is more collaborative than the "Independent Functions Model" outlined in the previous section. This second type usually develops in medical-center settings which also have a teaching function (e.g., the psychologist supervises a pediatric resident) since the relative positions of consultee and consultant require an educative stance rather than a true collaboration. Burns and Cromer (1978) suggest that this consultation model will increase given the new emphasis on primary care practitioners providing mental health services (Wright, 1978a). Thus it is likely that more pediatricians currently practicing will request psychological assistance of an educational or supervisory nature. The pediatrician, in turn, carries through on behavioral interventions. This model of indirect psychological contact with patients is similar to the models labeled "Process-educative" (Stabler, 1979) and a combination of "Didactic/Seminar," "Supervision," and "Client-Centered (Case) Consultation" (Burns & Cromer, 1978).

This psychologist consultant arrangement can take several forms. The pediatrician may request brief contact (e.g., by telephone call) for specific information. The brief contact may also come, if the psychologist is available, in "on-the-spot" consultations for particular problems (Salk, 1974). These brief contacts may involve questions of (1) the appropriateness of a child behavior and possible treatments (e.g., bedwetting at age 6 years), (2) the interpretation of test data (e.g., school achievement test scores), (3) community sources of assistance (e.g., for special education classes or tutoring), and (4) appropriateness of a referral (e.g., what can psychology do for an emotionally disturbed retardate?). The psychologist may answer these questions briefly or suggest a more detailed examination.

A second form of indirect psychological consulting can occur through the presentation of information in seminars, conferences, pediatric section meetings, and continuing educational programs. This form of consultation is not case oriented but more oriented to general psychological approaches.

A third approach of "indirect" patient treatment can occur when a mutual trust has developed of the other professional's abilities. In this approach, the pediatrician carries out a psychological intervention recommended by the psychologist consultant who has no direct patient contact. For example, as detailed later, standardized procedures can be established for certain types of behavioral disorders frequently appearing in the pediatric practice. For instance, intervention with enuresis or encopresis can be feasibly made by pediatricians and their staff (Christophersen & Rainey, 1976; Christophersen & Rapoff, 1980). Standardized procedures can also be established for the pediatric practice to deal with psychogenic pain (namely, headaches and stomach aches for which no organic cause is found). Intervention by the pediatrician for these types of patients' problems may be more acceptable and effective because the parents and the child may be more willing to accept the pediatrician's psychological advice for a problem originally seen as physical.

These three forms may be present within the indirect patient contact model of psychological consulting. Some restrictions may arise on this indirect approach. The psychologist may not actually see the patient and must rely on the data gathered by the pediatrician. Problems of the type and reliability of assessment can impede accurate, useful decision making on the part of the consulting psychologist. The pediatrician needs to learn some assessment skills and to be provided with appropriate evaluation devices. Furthermore, resentment may develop in the pediatrician if this role is perceived as subservient to the psychologist. On the other hand, the psychologist may resent relinquishing some cherished aspects of psychological practice, namely, diagnosis and treatment. A final problem is very likely to arise with this mode of psychological service. The pediatrician may not be interested in personally providing the actual service and may not have the time needed to learn and implement it. Thus, training and consulting to support personnel such as nurses, pediatric nurse practitioners, and even clerical staff may be necessary (Wright, 1978a).

Collaborative Team Model

The third major model of psychological consulting to the pediatrician is one of true collaboration. In this approach, the pediatrician and psychologist work together with shared responsibility and joint decision making. Case management is conducted conjointly with the professionals contributing their own unique perspectives and competence. Often in this approach, roles are not clearly demarcated in the provision of any one particular service. A cooperative team is thus the essence of this type of pediatrician-psychologist consulting. In many ways, this model is similar to the "Process Consultation" (Stabler, 1979) and "Collaboration" (Burns & Cromer, 1978) models.

This model represents an optimal situation where professionals coact as functional equals. The team approach of collaboration is more likely to exist in special units or within institutions, such as teams consulting to sections in hospitals of oncology (Koocher, Sourkes, & Keane, 1979; Lewis, 1978), renal dialysis (Berger,

1978; Brewer, 1978; Magrab, 1975), surgery (Geist, 1977), and neonatal intensive care (Magrab & Davitt, 1975). In such settings, teams of social workers, medical doctors, psychologists, clergy, audiologists and speech pathologists, educational experts, and others can collaborate. Such teams are less likely in the private pediatric practice away from teaching/research centers. This is due to the demands of practice which require more independent functioning. Financial restraints also limit such services. Though it is unfortunate that the typical pediatric office practice rarely has extensive personnel resources (Yankauer, Connelly, & Feldman, 1970), several types of problems can be treated with only the psychologist and limited pediatric staff.

Numerous problems which require a psychological and medical coalition are amenable to the conjoint approach, for example, obesity, anorexia nervosa, drug abuse, physical handicaps, and chronic diseases (Walker, 1979a). In the case of anorexia nervosa, for example, the extensive weight loss and accompanying problems—gastric hypoacidity, carotenemia, hypoproteinemia—are medical concerns. Aspects of medical treatment include monitoring these as well as prescribing an appropriate diet (Linscheid, 1978). The psychologist, in conjunction with the pediatrician, can establish behavioral contingencies for eating and weight gain while working with the patient in psychotherapy for increasing self-perceptions of trust and self-control (Bruche, 1977; Garfinkel, Garner, & Moldofsky, 1977; Garfinkel, Kline, & Stancer, 1973).

Chronic diseases such as juvenile diabetes require continual medical overview for diet, insulin intake, urinalysis, and exercise. The consulting psychologist may assist in enhancing the patient's compliance to the medical regimen (Walker, 1979b) and in the adjustment to the disease itself (Garner & Thompson, 1978; Magrab & Calcagno, 1978). As another example of the collaborative approach, LaGreca and Ottinger (1979) reported a case of a child with cerebral palsy whose psychological intervention was made to increase muscle-stretching exercises, while the medical aspects were checked by the conferring pediatrician. Developmental problems also occur frequently which need different resources in a team approach (Walker, 1979a). The failure-to-thrive case reported by Roberts and Horner (1979) demonstrates the collaboration of psychologists, pediatric nurse practitioners, physicians, social workers, and occupational therapists. The psychologist's input to this alliance was developmental assessment of the child and cognitive-behavioral treatment of the mother's depression. Similarly, resources usually exist in the hospital or community even if not directly part of the pediatric section of a hospital or office practice. The psychologist's role may be to coordinate the various services for particular patients.

Another major area for collaborative team efforts is community prevention programs (Peterson, Hartmann, & Gelfand, 1980). These have been relatively untouched by pediatric psychologists who could serve as consultants to teams consisting of several professionals. Such efforts may include assisting disease immunization programs (Peterson, 1980), encouraging proper nutrition and/or breast feeding, alleviating infant mortality, preparing children for physical examinations or dental checkups (Melamed, Hawes, Heiby, & Glick, 1975; Melamed &

Siegel, 1975), screening school children (Durlak & Mannarino, 1977), and child abuse screening and follow-up (Christophersen, Kuehn, Grinstead, Barnard, Rainey, & Keuhn, 1976; Reid & Taplin, 1977).

Burns and Cromer (1978) note that this collaborative approach allows the pediatrician to share responsibility for mental health interventions. The conjoint consultative relationship encourages reciprocal respect for the unique contributions of each profession.

Pediatric Practice-Oriented Consultation

Regardless of which of the three approaches or combinations outlined is followed, there are numerous exciting ways the pediatric psychologist can function to enhance the pediatrician's practice in hospital or office. Thus the psychologist-consultant need not feel constrained into any one of these models. In this section, we present some suggestions about how the psychologist can assume an active and vital role in consulting to the practicing pediatrician. The section heading emphasizes that pediatric psychologists as consultants should direct their efforts to the particular needs of the pediatrician for actual practice.

When psychologists help solve the pediatricians's problems, they enhance the physician's reputation as well as their own. The former effect is likely to open many opportunities for research and service. The pediatrician usually recognizes the patient's needs and wants to provide more comprehensive services; however, time constraints often do not permit direct participation. In particular for the private practitioner, time is money. The pediatric psychologist is most likely to succeed in gaining acceptance if the programs proposed required little of the pediatricians's time but have significant impact on patient care.

Psychological Screening and Referrals

The psychologist, in establishing a consultantship, often finds it useful to teach the pediatrician some basic techniques for screening mental health problems. Since the pediatrician sees many children at critical periods of development, it is logical that the pediatric practice serve as a first line for identifying children with problems. Screening is a concept already familiar to pediatricians—separation of patients on the basis of key indicators of medical problems (e.g., routine blood tests of newborns for phenylketonuria). Data gathered in screens are considered implicative, not diagnostic; in-depth follow-up examination is usually required. Following an algorithm-screening approach, some pediatricians also use protocols for managing telephone calls for medical complaints such as fevers, upper respiratory infections, head injury, abdominal pain, and other frequently phoned-in complaints (Heagarty, 1979; Levy, Rosekrans, Lamb, Friedman, Kaplan, & Strasser, 1979; Strasser, Levy, Lamb, & Rosekrans, 1979). These procedures help screen the calls, improve the patient management, and standardize data gathering.

The pediatrician has already been trained in some psychological screening procedures. For example, most have experience with the Denver Development Screening Test (DDST) which serves as a first assessment of an infant's developmental status with referral for a comprehensive psychological evaluation using a more diagnostic instrument such as the Bayley Scales of Infant Development (Wright *et al.*, 1979; also see chapter 3).

Additional psychological screening procedures may need to be added to the pediatrician's armamentarium (Hartlage & Hartlage, 1978). For example, Metz, Allen, Barr, and Shinefield (1976) report on the development of a general psychological portion to the Pediatric Multiphasic Examination (Allen & Shinefield, 1974). The various sections of this screening test for children ages 4–16 years have been found to screen children for psychological problems with referral for diagnostic testing and treatment. Other screening techniques under development are aimed at specific disorders for identifying infants "at risk" for child abuse, failure-to-thrive, or developmental disorders (Parmelee, Kopp, & Sigman, 1976; Field, Hallock, Ting, Dempsey, Dabiri, & Schuman, 1978), social and school adjustment problems (Durlak, Stein, & Mannarino, in press). The pediatric psychologist may adapt the models of screening protocols exemplified by the medical ones of Levy *et al.* (1979). Flow-chart designs with branching questions may be utilized for a large number of common behavioral problems (for both telephoned and office referred complaints).

As an adjunct to assisting the pediatrician with such screening, the pediatric psychologist may want to prepare descriptions of available resources for potential referral. For example, a list of problems can be paired with agencies or practitioners whose expertise may be needed in treatment. These might include audiologists and speech pathologists, family counseling and mental health centers, crisis intervention centers, educational experts and contacts in school systems for special education, emotional conflicts, or mental retardation classes, social workers, pastoral counselors, youth homes and camps, day-care centers, state and county welfare agencies, charities, among other community and private resources.

Furthermore, the psychologist can help the pediatrician make timely and appropriate referrals for psychological intervention. The psychologist does not want to be overwhelmed with every child with a possible problem since many children are potentially identifiable as such. Thus the pediatrician and psychologist can jointly establish a decision-making framework for determining which cases the pediatrician will handle, which ones need psychological supervision of the pediatrician, and which cases to refer to the psychologist.

Restructuring Pediatric Office Practices

Helping to change procedures in private office or hospital outpatient clinics is one aspect of psychological consulting not often considered by the psychologist and rarely requested by the physician. However, if approached diplomatically, the ramifications of an objective review of office procedures from a psychological perspective may be greatly beneficial. The children and families may benefit from the consultant's efforts and an increase in consumer satisfaction may result.

The psychologist can examine the procedures used by the pediatrician and the office staff in scheduling appointments, in greeting children and parents, in allowing long waits, in gathering data regarding medical problems, in taking medical tests, in making physical examinations, in giving medications, and in explaining medication regimens to parents. The psychologist can observe the waiting room for ways to enhance the aims of the pediatric practice. Can slide-and-narration programs be shown continually for children and parents on a variety of medical and psychological issues? For example, films could be made available on ear infections, choices of children's shoes, and influenza and cold treatments, as well as toilet training, breast-feeding, parent-child interactions, infant stimulation, and many others. Are there toys available which not only entertain the waiting child but also stimulate and educate? Parents may consider the pediatrician's choice of toys and books as an endorsement. This can be used to benefit the child by influencing the parent's toy buying.

Recommendations for remedying problems observed in the examination of the practice may include teaching the staff to model appropriate child care and management to parents, to take every opportunity to educate parents in normal child development, to educate and stimulate children, or to prepare and reassure children in a frightening environment. Thus we are recommending that the psychologist observe who does what, how they do it, what the result is, and how it can be improved. Other articles related to this type of consultation include Ack (1974), Green, Dudding, Viren, and Leake (1977), and Sarata and Jeppersen (1977).

Protocols and Checklists for Referral and Standardized Treatment

The psychologist can provide protocols, checklists, and questionnaires to the pediatrician to assist in screening and referral, and in implementing standardized treatment procedures. In the first instance, the use of one- or two-page assessment devices can identify potential problems rapidly through staff interviews or parental completion of the forms. These diagnostic and treatment protocols should follow the format of an algorithm as noted earlier. The pediatrician should already have some protocols as standard practice for determining the child's growth in comparison to norms on growth curves (height, weight, head circumference; *National Center for Health Statistics Growth Charts,* 1976; Nelson *et al.,* 1975; Wright, 1978b). Comparison of psychological protocols to these existing medical ones may aid in acceptance of additional procedures for screening and referral procedures. The psychologist may recommend assessment protocols already well-established in psychological settings. For example, the staff can be taught to administer the Vineland Scale of Social Maturity (Doll, 1965) and the Minnesota Child Development Inventory (Ireton & Thwing, 1972). Significant developmental milestones can also be charted following the Gesell Developmental Schedules (Gesell & Amatruda, 1947). Results from these sorts of scales are useful for identifying the developmentally delayed child and for requesting a comprehensive evaluation. Some checklists are also useful for suggesting developmentally when to begin intervention (e.g., toilet training, Azrin & Foxx, 1974).

Other standardized scales or protocols may be more diagnostic or predictive for quantifying the degree of hyperactivity (Conners, 1969, 1972), determining the likelihood of child abuse with any given patient (Kempe & Helfer, 1972; see checklist adapted by Wright, 1978b), assessing childhood behavioral disorders (Achenbach, 1978; Miller, Barrett, Hampe, & Noble, 1971; Quay & Peterson, 1967, 1979), diagnosing anorexia nervosa (Slade, 1973; Sours, 1969), and assessing fears and phobias (Scherer & Nakamura, 1968).

The pediatric psychologist may wish to investigate referral protocols and checklists which are still under development but show promise. For example, Wright (1978b) presents several checklists based on reviews of the literature. Similarly, the consulting psychologist may choose to develop particular checklists for the pediatrician. For example, if the patient population comes from a poor or older neighborhood, lead poisoning from old paint chips may be a significant concern. An examination of the literature will reveal important psychological features of lead poisoning and circumstances leading to it. A lead poisoning protocol for psychological concomitants can supplement the medical tests the pediatrician may prescribe. Protocols for other problems may be needed for assessing child eating disorders, school problems, habits and compulsions, or any number of potential disorders.

The psychologist must be cautious in supplying these screening and preliminary diagnostic instruments to the pediatric staff without psychological consultation and supervision. Ultimate responsibility, of course, rests with the psychologist to insure that these procedures are used properly.

A second major way protocols can be used is in the implementation of standardized treatment procedures. As noted earlier, the pediatrician and auxiliary staff can conduct many psychological interventions with the consultation of the pediatric psychologist following a previously designed course of action. The use of established forms permits the controlled treatment by staff or parents for presenting problems that recur frequently. The procedures can include branching decision-making trees where changes in treatment programs should be made to individualize the intervention, or when problems arise. Christophersen and Rapoff (1980) suggest condensing treatment procedures for behavior problems into protocols of one or two pages. The advantage of standardized procedure protocols is that they are immediately present and can be instituted during the presenting clinic visit. Wright (1980) describes the use of such protocols as means of providing standardized compliance procedures. A standardized compliance procedure seeks to achieve the following: (1) *a rationale and procedure* for both the treatment and the compliance aspects of care; (2) *a standardized vehicle* for specifying and recording transactions between the patient or the parent (in child cases), and the therapist; (3) *a means for checking and correcting* the degree of compliance achieved; and (4) *involvement of the therapist* in a formally structured and regular (compliant) manner.

The specific methods whereby the above objectives are both standardized and achieved are as follows:

1. A structured pretreatment interview that explains the rationale and procedure for both the treatment and the compliance methods.

2. Development of a form on which all relevant data can be provided accurately and with as much ease as possible.
3. The requirement that all relevant data be recorded immediately on the form provided and that this form be mailed to the therapist at a precise time and place each week.
4. The requirement that patients or their parents contact the therapist, in person or by phone, on a weekly basis and at a precise time.

During this time, necessary corrections are made in both the treatment and the compliance aspects of the treatment. Following this approach, Wright (1980) published a form for reporting compliance in encopresis treatment. Parents apply the recommended behavioral treatment and record important data which are mailed weekly to the supervising therapist. This procedure indicates how compulsively parents and patients are complying with the *compliance* aspects of the program, which in turn is a good indicator of how well they are adhering to the actual *treatment* procedure.

When toilet training, for example, the psychologist or pediatrician can provide parents with a copy of *Toilet Training in Less Than a Day* (Azrin & Foxx, 1974), and checklists can be drawn from the book for staff to monitor parental actions and child progress (e.g., Christophersen & Rapoff, 1978; Doleys, 1980a; Walker, 1978). The consulting psychologist may wish to design treatment protocols for such pediatric psychological problems as encopresis (Christophersen & Rainey, 1976; Doleys, 1980b), behavioral control problems (Rainey & Christophersen, 1976), anorexia nervosa, medication regimen compliance, obesity, juvenile diabetes, asthma, and so on.

The protocols may be of benefit in organizing the staff or monitoring patients and parents. Brief intervention protocols or brochures for parents can be prepared for simpler problems as well. For example, adapting procedures recommended by Wright, Woodcock, and Scott (1970), instructions can be made to parents about ignoring infant crying at bedtime after checking the physical well-being of the child. Rainey and Christophersen (1976) published protocols for bedtime problems and for temper tantrums under a general framework of "Guidelines for Clinician" and "Guidelines for Parents." Christophersen (1977) and Allen and Bergman (1976) describe procedures for encouraging children to sit appropriately in car safety restraint seats. The program can be promoted by pediatric staff in training parents in the use of fairly simple, yet consistent, actions by the parents. Christophersen and Rapoff (1980) summarize a study which reports that a written protocol describing this car seat program was effective. A similar program, for example, can be adopted for children who misbehave in supermarkets (Barnard, Christophersen, & Wolf, 1977). Similarly, a written outline of procedures can be provided for decreasing thumb or pacifier sucking by contingently reinforcing nonoccurrence of the behavior (e.g., television cartoons, Baer, 1962; bedtime story reading, Knight & McKenzie, 1974). In this way, brief psychological interventions can be made for simpler problematic events in child development which may come to the attention of the pediatrician. Other problems may include weaning from breast or bottle and getting a child to take solid food, food refusal, infant stimulation, and whining, among other events of psychological relevance.

A programmatic approach to psychogenic pain may also be used. Recurrent abdominal pains and/or headaches are often common presenting problems in the pediatric practice. When the physician can rule out physical causes of the pain, then psychological factors become important. An examination of the antecedents-behavior-consequences of the situation (Roberts & La Greca, in press) may reveal that the child's initial problems are precipitated by anxiety-arousing events and are followed by some form of reinforcement (e.g., attention, staying home from school), which perpetuates the pain complaints. Significantly altering the situational sequence can reduce the child's anxiety and spurious reports of physical pain (Miller & Kratochwill, 1979). A standardized approach to these cases can be programmed.

Other standardized procedures can be adapted from the literature in cliniclal child psychology. Forehand and his colleagues, for example, have a well-researched program of parent training for increasing a child's compliance to parental requests (Arnold & Forehand, 1978; Forehand, 1977; Forehand, Sturgis, McMahon, Aguar, Green, Wells, & Breiner, 1979; Gardner, Forehand, & Roberts, 1976; Peed, Roberts, & Forehand, 1977). McMahon and Forehand (1978) presented an experimentally validated 2½-page brochure for parents which described the use of differential attention and time-out for the inappropriate mealtime behaviors of preschool children. Other researchers have developed similar programs for parent training (Christophersen & Barnard, 1978; Christophersen, Barnard, Ford, & Wolf, 1976; Forgatch & Toobert, 1979). Procedures may also be obtained from the literature for school phobia or refusal (Ayllon, Smith, & Rogers, 1970; Kennedy, 1965), obesity (Epstein, Wing, Steranchak, Dickson, & Michelson, 1980), impulsivity/overactivity (Routh, 1978), and eating disorders (Wright et al., 1979).

The type of standardized psychological interventions suggested here should be employed primarily for fairly simple, circumscribed problems. The psychologist should maintain some control to insure appropriateness of application. As a form of consulting to the pediatric practice, however, standardized procedures have the advantages of cost-efficiency, minimizing pediatrician and psychologist time by using existing staff, being very effective, providing needed services, and allowing a focus on more complicated psychological cases as determined by earlier screening. The kinds of treatment protocols developed will depend on the needs of the clinic practice and the particular needs of individual child patients. Christophersen and Rapoff (1980) note that when the psychologist provides treatment protocols, they need to be readily incorporable into the existing practice with a minimum disruption, and they need to be cost efficient.

Educational Programming

We have noted that the pediatric psychologist as consultant may wish to turn the focus from individual case management to a more general provision of information. Obviously, the psychologist needs to serve as a resource or repository of psychological information for quick consultation and questioning. Through a more general, structured forum, the psychologist can educate others on a larger scale. Olbrisch and Sechrist (1979) suggest the specialist in the health care psychology field might design educational programs and train health professionals to help patients. The presentation of psychological material in short courses or conferences, seminars, grand rounds, inservice training or continuing education programs can have considerable effect in enhancing health professionals' functioning with patients (Burns & Cromer, 1978). These types of programs can be used to explain the standardized treatment procedures and protocols. The psychologist can describe what psychological services are available and what types of presenting problems are particularly solicited. Most important, didactic educational programs can be tailored to particular problems for nurses and pediatricians. The psychologist can take a general title of "How to Handle the _____ Patient" and then fill in the blank with relevant adjectives or phrase for which psychology has something to offer (e.g., fill in the blank with "chronically ill," "preschool," "adolescent," "encopretic," "noncompliant," "presurgery"). Other topics might include child management techniques, normal and abnormal child development, basic psychometric and behavioral assessment, and simplified behavioral techniques. A central concern should be that the consulting psychologist provide material which is relevant and useful to the pediatrician's everyday practice. This forum permits a maximum use of the pediatric psychologist as a teacher-resource type of consultant to the pediatrician. Similarly, the pediatric psychologist can make talks to lay groups on a variety of topics (Seagull & Seagull, 1979).

Reading Lists for Pediatricians, Parents, and Children

The psychologist can assist the pediatrician to competently handle many situations through a bibliographic approach. Many books and articles are available commercially for parents and children, and professionally for the pediatrician. The psychologist can help the pediatrician wade through the overwhelming number of books to recommend the parents read for their own use, and the child can read or be read in order to help in adjustment. Most important, the psychologist can use readings to educate and prepare the pediatrician in several psychological areas. In this section, we discuss how the psychologist can prepare booklists for parents, children, and pediatricians.

Numerous questions arise in pediatric practice which are often referred to as "Dr. Spock" or "one hand on the door" questions (Wright, 1979a). These questions often do not lend themselves to 5–10 minutes of advice. Having protocols on hand as described here would obviously help in this situation. However, there is little likelihood that all possible questions can be prepared for in advance. What can be done is to provide bibliotherapeutic assistance. Parents can be given books to read and told to return for extended consultation if they need additional assistance. Several general parenting books are available (e.g., Becker, 1971; Christophersen, 1977; Patterson & Gullion, 1968; Glasgow & Rosen, 1978). Our experience indicates that many parents dislike reading technical/textbookish manuals. If readings are presented in laypersons' language and tied to experience that is familiar to parents, the material seems to be learned better and retained longer. *Parent Power*, by Wright (1978c), covers 20 basic principles of human behavior and is presented in understandable language. This book or others can be recommended for parents requesting general information on child management.

Sometimes parents request information regarding specific psychological/ behavioral problems. Self-help books which are directed at parents for conducting toilet training (Azrin & Foxx, 1974), for remediating obesity (Stuart & Davis, 1972), for handling the child with spina bifida (Swinyard, 1966), for dealing with handicaps (Adams, 1979; Spock & Lerrigo, 1965), for information on diabetes (Joslin Clinic, 1974; Traisman & Newcomb, 1965), and about coping with death or the dying child (Spinetta, Spinetta, Kung, & Schwartz, 1976) are available. Van Vechten, Satterwhite, and Pless (1977) have prepared an extensive list of available brochures and materials for parents of physically handicapped children which provide information and instruction for such disease categories as allergies, asthma, birth defects, cerebral palsy, cleft lip and palate, heart disease, cystic fibrosis, diabetes, and epilepsy, among others. In many cases, this type of information should not take the place of an involved professional but should be complementary in assisting professional educative and treatment effects.

An additional role the pediatric psychologist and pediatrician can take is in providing readings to children on subjects with which they are concerned. A few books by professionals have been prepared for children on specific topics such as divorce (Salk, 1978), leukemia (Aronson & Heifetz, 1980), and hospitalization (see reviews by Altshuler, 1974; Flandorf, 1967). Other books may be found as well.

A profitable approach to children in adjustment or understanding is to provide storybooks of fictional or biographical accounts which deal realistically with problems. Walker (1979a), for example, recommends books about handicapped people and what they accomplish (e.g., Adams, 1979; Bernanos, 1968; Eareckson, 1976; Killilea, 1952). Aradine (1976) has reviewed children's literature on death and suggests several books geared to the child's developmental stage (e.g., *Charlotte's Web,* White, 1952; *About Dying,* Stein, 1974). *Ms.* magazine (1976) also published an annotated booklist on sensitive subjects including numerous books on death, separation and divorce, and adoption. Two excellent books for children regarding mentally retarded children are *My Brother Steven Is Retarded* (Sobol, 1977), and *Mary Fran and Mo* (Lynch, 1979). The psychologist can search out additional books and provide the books or list them for the pediatrician to give to parents. For example, Human Sciences Press (Children's Books, 1980) lists children's books for reading by children who have a new sibling, whose friend has moved, grandparent has died, parents have divorced, or parent has remarried.

The psychologist can further educate the pediatrician by preparing the pediatrician and staff on particular problems through a reading curriculum. Lewis (1978) provides a list of references for professionals on terminal illness, grief, developmental changes in perceptions, reactions by parents, and professionals' own reactions to terminal illness (Spinetta, 1974; Spinetta, Deasy, Koenig, Lightsey, Schwartz, Hartman, & Kung, 1979; Vore & Wright, 1974).

Other reading lists may be prepared on such issues as the psychological adjustment to chronic disease (e.g., Magrab & Calcagno, 1978), hyperactivity (e.g., Routh, 1978), neurological disorders (e.g., Feuerstein, Ward, & Le Baron, 1979; Miller, 1979), numerous other childhood disorders, and behavior therapy in relation to pediatric problems (Walker, 1979b). Indeed, the pediatrician may benefit from a thorough appraisal of the pediatric psychological field through this volume and Magrab (1978), or a pediatric desk manual (e.g., Wright et al., 1979). The pediatrician usually does not have a great deal of time to spend on this type of activity, therefore the summaries should be selectively recommended.

Facilitating Pediatric Treatment Interventions

Our focus in this section is on how the psychologist can help the pediatrician make medical treatment more effective or avoid adverse psychological concomitants. We outline several psychological contributions to furthering medical/pediatric regimens and procedures.

DECREASE MEDICAL FEARS

Many children express considerable fears of medical procedures and personnel. When the fear becomes exaggerated, irrational, or intense enough, it becomes maladaptive and produces conflict with the child's environment. Even minor forms of medical fears may be detrimental to medical treatment and the child's well-being. The remediation of children's medical anxiety may make the pediatrician's treatment more effective. Several procedures have been investigated in the psychological literature which the consultant may wish to consider. There are many books and filmstrips commercially available in wide use which purport to prepare the child for medical procedures or hospitalization. There are coloring books and popular books with a text and photographs or artist representations of hospital scenes. Unfortunately, many of these are inadequate in preparing the child reader and may actually heighten anxiety by providing misinformation (Altshuler, 1974; Roberts, 1979). Some well-controlled empirical research has demonstrated competent anxiety-reducing preparations including puppet play (Cassell & Paul, 1967), information, emotional support, and coping-strategies anticipation (Visintainer & Wolfer, 1975), and filmed modeling (Melamed, Meyer, Gee, & Soule, 1976; Melamed & Siegel, 1975; Roberts, Wurtele, Boone, Ginther, & Elkins, 1981). The psychologist can adapt these types of procedures to the individual practice. Additionally, information protocols can be prepared for children and parents (Roberts, 1979). Indeed, preparation of parents for their child's hospitalization may assist in diminishing the child's anxiety. The psychologist may also choose to assist in tours of the hospital for patient preparation (Bottell, 1977; Ferguson, 1979; Johnson, 1974). A programmatic campaign in schools may be attempted to reduce general medical fears in children (Roberts et al., 1981). In short, the consulting psychologist can use psychological principles to reduce children's anxieties about medical settings which can facilitate the pediatrician's intervention through a happier child, faster recovery, fewer behavior problems, and better cooperation.

PROMOTE MEDICAL REGIMEN COMPLIANCE

Psychology has much to offer the problem of patient compliance to the medical regimen. Presumably, if medical treatments are to be effective, then the patient must be a conscientious partner with the physician. At first thought, this might appear to be less a problem with children than with adults because children are seemingly under the control and management of their parents, or adult caregivers. No doubt every pediatric clinic and hospital has an unwritten list of patients who are notoriously noncompliant and frustratingly make frequent appearances for medical intervention. Estimates of noncompliance often range up to 90% of patients. However, adequate programs are not available for enhancing pediatric compliance to regimens for such medical problems as diabetic diet and insulin self-administration, epileptic seizure medication and self-control, and other complex diseases and treatments. The noncompliance extends even to the seemingly simple act of taking penicillin for uncomplicated infections (see a comprehensive review by Marston, 1970). The consultant to a pediatrician often finds that a great need exists for enhancing compliance in the independent pediatric practice. A needed assistance to pediatric intervention can come from the psychologist attending to this behavioral problem. Studies have shown that regimen compliance can be enhanced by such things as (1) educating a patient (parent) regarding the rationale and need for the treatment, (2) altering the regimen to fit the patient's daily routine, (3) using shaping techniques to approximate total compliance, and (4) causing the patient to perceive greater concern by the professional (Dunbar & Stunkard, 1977; Falvo, 1979; Sackett & Haynes, 1976).

Step-by-step compliance protocols and checklists have proven useful. Data recording of the events and information related to the medical regimen may prove helpful as well. Self-monitoring, which is, in turn, the focus of professional monitoring, can increase adherence to treatment programs. For example, the child with diabetes can keep a daily record of diet, exercise, insulin injections, and urinalysis. Accurate recording and compliance can then be rewarded by parents or the pediatrician. Other psychological interventions can be made utilizing the four points outlined above. The psychologist can establish standardized, general compliance procedures (e.g., develop compliance forms for use by all diabetic patients), and prepare individualized procedures as needed. In the latter case, special intensive programs may be needed for either parents or the patient in cueing medication taking, recording and rewarding compliance, and so on (Lowe & Lutzker, 1979). The area of compliance is of major importance in medicine. The pediatric psychologist can positively affect the pediatric practice by furthering compliance to prescribed medical regimens.

ASSISTANCE IN DIFFICULT INTERPERSONAL SITUATIONS

The pediatrician often is faced with difficult emotional situations in which he or she must deal with reactions of patients, parents, staff, and self. The psychologist can help smooth out these problematic situations by prior consulting or just being present and applying traditional psychological principles. The most traumatic event for all parties is informing parents of the diagnosis of terminal illness and later, at the death of the child patient.

For the needs of the pediatrician, the psychologist can be a much needed support since health-care providers seldom are trained to cope with dying patients. Additionally, the pediatrician may have unresolved personal feelings about death and see a patient's death as a professional failure (Wright et al., 1979). The psychologist can help the pediatrician work through these feelings in order to facilitate the interventions that need to be done. Psychological consultation to parents may be necessary. Certainly, informing the parents and the child in an informative, understanding, and supporting manner is requisite for cases of fatal disease (Coolidge, 1977; Koocher & Sallan, 1978; Schulman & Kupst, 1980; Wright, 1970, 1974). Allowing the child some informed choice in treatment is also helpful for her or his adjustment (e.g., Koocher, 1974; Nitschke, Wunder, Sexauer, & Humphrey, 1977). After the death of a child, pediatric follow-up and contacts should be made. For example, it is recommended that physicians hold at least three conferences with parents of a dead child—at time of death, 2−3 days afterward, and 3−6 months later (Clyman, Green, Mikkelsen, Rowe, & Ataide, 1979; Kennell & Klaus, 1976). Schreiner, Gresham, and Green (1979) suggest that even a 25-minute telephone call one week after an infant's death can often ameliorate serious reactions in the parents.

A second difficult situation is informing parents of mental retardation in their child (Noland, 1970). The psychologist can perform a service in consulting to the pediatrician in such cases for psychometric advice, and how to provide the news to the parents. We have found procedures outlined by Rheingold (1945) in a classic paper to be most helpful in interpreting mental retardation to parents. Miller (1979) discusses a related issue of counseling parents of children with neurological disorders. If this stage is handled properly, later pediatric interventions for medical treatment and/or psychological and educational interventions will be facilitated.

These two examples depict how the psychologist can assist the pediatrician in handling difficult interpersonal situations. Additional ones might include assisting a child in adjusting to the ill or dying relative, in preparing for parents' divorce, in genetic counseling, and in cases of orthopedic disabilities among other stressful circumstances (see Wright et al., 1979).

Assist in Prevention Efforts

We have noted that one major contribution the psychologist can make is to help prevent medical and psychological difficulties from occurring. Prevention has not been a prime concern in the psychological literature, but work is growing (e.g., Gelfand & Hartmann, 1977; Peterson et al., 1980). Numerous opportunities for psychological prevention are present in the pediatric practice. The term "anticipatory guidance" has been proposed to describe the professional's anticipating common psychological/behavioral problems and helping parents avoid them early (Brazelton, 1975; Christophersen & Barnard, 1978; Nelson et al., 1975). The pediatric psychologist can be present, for example, at "well-baby" clinic visits when parents might be most receptive to learning prevention and management information. Protocols are often useful for such anticipatory guidance.

Tefft and Simeonsson (1979) emphasize that resources should be committed to prevention. They particularly encourage early detection through routine screening. Identification of "at-risk" or "vulnerable" children can be appropriately conducted in pediatric clinics (Newberger & McAnulty, 1976). Interventions can then follow. The psychologist's potential in this process has been documented in earlier sections.

Other psychologically assisted prevention efforts can be taken, for example, with such relatively nonpsychological phenomena as promoting the use of car safety restraints for children (Christophersen, 1977), in bathtub drownings (Pearn, Brown, Wong, & Bart, 1979), in poison control, in decreasing adolescent smoking (McAlister, Perry, & Maccoby, 1979), in increasing disease innoculation, in decreasing teenage pregnancies (Magrab & Danielson-Murphy, 1979), and in improving safety of infant's sleeping conditions (Smialek, Smialek, & Spitz, 1977). In the last instance, a safety checklist for determining crib safety has been provided which can be used as a guide for other protocols. There is much the psychologist can do in assisting the pediatrician in prevention of both psychological and medical problems. Careful observation and reviews of the literature will expose additional areas.

Arrange Psychologist Availability

Implicit in previous sections has been that the psychologist must be available and approachable by the pediatrician and ancillary staff as well as by the patients and parents. The pediatric psychologist needs to structure scheduled times of availability for consultation. Scheduled availability guarantees access to the psychologist. Salk (1974) reports that "on-the-spot" consultation is needed so that patient care is continuous and is sensitive to psychological aspects. Additional advantages are noted as well. Hartlage and Hartlage (1978) similarly cite the need for "curbside consultation" in handling target-oriented questions.

The pediatric psychologist who consults to a pediatric practice should maintain a predictable schedule so that staff can check in with the professional on a regular basis. The psychologist may use hospital rounds on the pediatric ward, staff coffee breaks, or use other structures for this purpose.

Availability to families and patients can also be arranged on a regular schedule. A unique model for providing psychological services in a private pediatric office has been described by Schroeder and her colleagues (Mesibov, Schroeder, & Wesson, 1977; Schroeder, 1979; Schroeder, Goolsby, & Stangler, 1975). A call in/come in service was instituted by psychological consultants to several pediatricians. Two hours a week are scheduled for parents to call in to the pediatricians' office for answers to psychological or behavioral questions. Any problems that cannot be handled by the phone call are referred for a come in appointment with the psychologist. Protocols or algorithms may need to be developed for determining how to handle such telephone calls for psychological advice (see Levy *et al.*, 1979, for an example of those developed for medical problems). Schroeder (1979) cites evidence that this approach fills a definite need for psychological availability in the pediatrician's office. Morgan and Cullen (1980) have described a similar pediatric consultation program where the pediatrician refers parents with psychological questions about behavior or management to a psychologist with scheduled hours at the pediatrician's office. These authors conclude that the service is important and well received by parents and pediatricians and makes effective interventions because of its timeliness.

Additional Practice-Oriented Procedures

We have touched on several ways the pediatric psychologist can consult to a private pediatric practice. We have not exhausted the possibilities of pediatric *practice*-oriented consultation. There are considerably more services the psychologist can provide. For example, the psychologist could evaluate day-care centers in the area for recommendation by the pediatrician or help train babysitters for a referral service. Alternatively, the psychologist can serve an important function in enhancing patient-physician communication (DiMatteo & Taranta, 1979; Kupst, Blatterbauer, Westman, Schulman, & Paul, 1977). The immense need for psychological counseling might be most effectively and economically met through groups (e.g., for abusive parents, Savino & Sanders, 1973; for hemophilia, Caldwell, Leveque, & Lane, 1974; Mattson & Agle, 1972; visual handicaps, Keegan, 1974). What the individual does in consultation is limited only by the creativity and ingenuity of the psychologist in determining the needs, developing procedures, and demonstrating psychology's utility in the pediatric setting. We endorse the position of Tefft and Simeonsson (1979) that psychology should help create health care settings.

PUTTING CONSULTATION INTO PRACTICE

In this chapter, we have been discussing the development of psychological consultation arrangements with pediatricians. The information regarding the pediatric orientation should be useful for understanding the physician's thinking and actions. Three types or models of consulting were then examined with a fourth approach elaborated. We believe the pediatric *practice*-oriented consultation approach can be an exciting development with multiple roles to be created. This approach can result in numerous advantages to the psychologist and pediatrician and, most certainly, to the child patients and their families. In this section, we want to briefly note some considerations when attempting to put a consultation into actual practice.

In developing a relationship, the psychologist is advised to go slowly and cautiously in taking cases or providing psychological assistance. The psychologist should be wary of overpromising results which may not be delivered. One might start with a few cases, and after gaining some success where results can be demonstrated, gradually expand to a fuller caseload. The pediatrician is not likely to hand over "lock and key" to her or his practice and clientele. Feedback should be given to the pediatrician regarding what has been done and why, when and how interventions were successful and unsuccessful. This will promote realistic expectations by the physician and perhaps make referrals more appropriate. Thus we are again proposing that communication with the pediatrician is essential. The psychologist needs to diplomatically observe patients' confidentiality as well as the needs of the referring pediatrician (King, 1980). We also propose that the pediatric psychologist will need to successfully employ social skills in negotiating for and carrying on a consultantship. While pediatricians have been found to be most open to liaison relationships, the pediatrician in this regard is a consumer, and the psychologist is a salesperson.

The psychologist may find that only certain types of cases are being referred. These can be expanded through education of the physician and demonstration of capabilities in the area. One type of case is particularly problematic—the difficult case by which the pediatrician has been frustrated for some time. Psychologists may get these cases "dumped on" them. It is often good to take these cases because the pediatric problem and management may have become psychological—no longer requiring medical overview. Additionally, the psychologist may earn the gratitude of the pediatrician by relieving him or her of a particularly burdensome case. We submit, however, that one would not want a psychological consultantship to consist entirely of troublesome, complex cases; expansion into other roles would be more exciting.

Finally, we want to make a strong plea for the psychologist to utilize his or her research training when consulting to the private pediatrician. The problem of establishing an empirical basis for pediatric psychology remains large. Christophersen and Rapoff (1980) argue that only one psychological procedure (for toilet training) has been validated and is feasible for pediatric office use. This may be selling pediatric psychology a little short, but the basic point is well taken— pediatric psychology must concentrate efforts in evaluation and validation if it is going to "earn a permanent position as a pediatric health care provider" (Christophersen & Rapoff, 1980, p. 326). Without an adequate data base, pediatric psychology cannot expand its roles. Many of our suggestions in earlier sections need to be evaluated in practice. The consulting psychologist can provide much of what is needed.

The research aspect of pediatric psychology is well founded in the hospital setting (see chapter 8). Our experience has shown that clinical applications can be made *and* evaluated in the private pediatric practice as well. Case studies reported by Roberts and Ottinger (1979) and La Greca and Ottinger (1979) demonstrate evaluative contributions in a pediatric psychology practicum in a private practitioner's clinic (Ottinger & Roberts, 1980). Larger research projects as well may be undertaken in private practices (e.g., Carey, 1978).

A continuing project to prepare children for hospitalization, and to decrease medical fears in general may be instituted (e.g., Roberts *et al.*, 1981). Additionally, research has been attempting to enhance regimen compliance in juvenile diabetes (Roberts & Wurtele, 1980; Wright & Roberts, 1978). While a service is being provided in these instances, data for evaluation are also being gathered.

We affirm the statement of Wright (1967) that the pediatric psychologist should be a scientist-clinician. So much research is needed in this area, particularly if pediatric psychology is to move beyond the intuitive stage to the empirical. Through research, a better understanding of medical-psychology relationships can be fostered, development of more effective intervention and prevention programs can occur, and more adequate services can be provided to children and their families. Only substantive research can help practitioners achieve the goal of health care—to assist the child to go into adulthood at the optimal stage of development. Numerous areas for further research are outlined in the chapter in this volume by Routh (chapter 8) and in Roberts *et al.* (in press).

One exciting aspect of the pediatric psychology discipline is that there is much to be done in the clinical as well as in the research realms. The pediatric psychologist must innovate, create, adapt, apply, and research to make this profession a live, vibrant, and growing phenomenon. This chapter advocates a fertile setting for this to occur is through consultant relationships with pediatricians.

REFERENCES

Achenbach, T. M. The child behavior profile: I. Boys aged 6-11. *Journal of Consulting and Clinical Psychology,* 1978, **46,** 478−488.

Ack, M. The psychological environment of a children's hospital. *Pediatric Psychology,* 1974, **2,** 3−5.

Adams, B. *Like it is: Facts and feelings about handicaps from kids who know*. New York: Walker, 1979.

Allen, D. B., & Bergman, A. B. Social learning approaches to health education: Utilization of infant auto restraint devices. *Pediatrics,* 1976, **58,** 323−328.

Allen, C. M., & Shinefield, H. R. Automated multiphasic screening. *Pediatrics,* 1974, **54,** 621−626.

Altshuler, A. *Books that help children deal with a hospital experience*. Washington, DC: U.S. Government Printing Office, DHEW Publication No. (HSA) 74−5402, 1974.

Ambulatory Pediatric Association. *Standards for education in ambulatory pediatrics*. January 1978.

American Medical Association. *Profile of medical practice*. Chicago: A.M.A. Center for Health Services Research and Development, 1977.

American Medical Association. *Distribution of physicians in the United States*. Chicago: A.M.A., 1965−1976.

Aradine, C. R. Books for children about death. *Pediatrics,* 1976, **57,** 372−378.

Athreya, B. H. *Clinical methods in pediatric diagnosis*. New York: Van Nostrand, 1980.

Arnold, S. C., & Forehand, R. A comparison of cognitive training and response cost procedures in modifying cognitive styles of impulsive children. *Cognitive Therapy and Research,* 1978, **2,** 183−187.

Aronson, J., & Heifetz, J. *Jordie's present*. Jefferson City: American Cancer Society, Missouri Division, 1980.

Ayllon, A. T., Smith, D., & Rogers, M. Behavioral management of school phobia. *Journal of Behavior Therapy and Experimental Psychiatry,* 1970, **1,** 125–138.

Azrin, N. H., & Foxx, R. M. *Toilet training in less than a day.* New York: Simon & Schuster, 1974.

Baer, D. M. Laboratory control of thumbsucking by withdrawal and re-presentation of reinforcement. In L. P. Ullman & L. Krasner (Eds.), *Case studies in behavior therapy.* New York: Holt, Rinehart & Winston, 1962.

Barnett, H. L. *Pediatrics,* 16th ed. New York: Appleton-Century-Crofts, 1977.

Becker, W. C. *Parents are teachers: A child management program.* Champaign, IL: Research Press, 1971.

Berger, M. The role of the clinical child psychologist in an endstage renal disease program. *Journal of Clinical Child Psychology,* 1978, **7,** 17–18.

Bergman, A. B., Dassel, S. W., & Wedgwood, R. J. Time-motion study of practicing pediatricians. *Pediatrics,* 1966, **38,** 254–263.

Bernanos, M. *The other side of the mountain,* translated by Elaine P. Halperin. Boston: Houghton Mifflin, 1968.

Barnard, J. D., Christophersen, E. R., & Wolf, M. M. Teaching children appropriate shopping behavior through parent training in the supermarket setting. *Journal of Applied Behavior Analysis,* 1977, **10,** 49–59.

Bottell, H. Taking the fear out of hospitals. *Good Housekeeping,* June 1977, pp. 232–234.

Brazelton, T. B. Anticipatory guidance. In S. B. Friedman (Ed.), *The pediatric clinics of North America.* Philadelphia: Saunders, 1975.

Brewer, D. The role of the psychologist in a dialysis and transplantation unit. *Journal of Clinical Child Psychology,* 1978, **7,** 71–72.

Bruche, H. Anorexia nervosa and its treatment. *Journal of Pediatric Psychology,* 1977, **2,** 110–112.

Burnett, R. D., & Bell, L. S. Projecting pediatric practice patterns: Report of the survey of the Pediatric Manpower Committee. *Pediatrics,* 1978, **62** (4, part 2, supplement) 625–680.

Burnett, R. D., William, M. K., & Olmsted, R. W. Pediatrics manpower requirements. *Pediatrics,* 1978, **61,** 438–445.

Burns, B. J., & Cromer, W. W. The evolving role of the psychologist in primary health care practitioners training for mental health services. *Journal of Clinical Child Psychology,* 1978, **7,** 8–12.

Caldwell, H. S., Leveque, K. L., & Lane, D. M. Group psychotherapy in the management of hemophilia. *Psychological Reports,* 1974, **35,** 339–342.

Caplan, G. *The theory and practice of mental health consultation.* New York: Basic Books, 1970.

Carey, W. B. On doing research in office practice. *Pediatrics,* 1978, **62,** 424–425.

Cassell, S., & Paul, M. H. The role of puppet therapy on the emotional responses of children hospitalized for cardiac catherization. *Journal of Pediatrics,* 1967, **71,** 233–239.

Children's Books. *Psychology book catalog.* New York: Human Sciences Press, 1980.

Christophersen, E. R. *Little people: Guidelines for common sense child rearing.* Lawrence, KS: H & H Enterprises, 1977.

Christophersen, E. R., & Barnard, J. D. Management of behavior problems: A perspective for pediatricians. *Clinical Pediatrics,* 1978, **17,** 122–124.

Christophersen, E. R., Barnard, J. D., Ford, D., & Wolf, M. M. The family training program: Improving parent-child interactions In E. J. Mash, L. C. Handy, & L. A. Hameslynck (Eds.), *Behavior modification approaches to parenting:* New York: Brunner/Mazell, 1976.

Christophersen, E. R., Kuehn, B. S., Grinstead, J. D., Barnard, J. D., Rainey, S. K., & Kuehn, F. E. A family training program for abuse and neglect families. *Journal of Pediatric Psychology,* 1976 (Spring), 90–94.

Christophersen, E. R., & Rainey, S. K. Management of encopresis through a pediatric outpatient clinic. *Journal of Pediatric Psychology,* 1976, **1,** 38–41.

Christophersen, E. R., & Rapoff, M. A. Enuresis treatment. *Issues in Comprehensive Pediatric Nursing,* 1978, **2,** 35–52.

Christophersen, E. R., & Rapoff, M. A. Pediatric psychology: An appraisal. In B. Lahey & A. Kazdin (Eds.), *Advances in clinical child psychology,* Vol. 3. New York: Plenum Press, 1980.

Clyman, R. I., Green, C., Mikkelsen, C., Rowe, J., & Ataide, L. Do parents use physician follow-up after the death of their newborn? *Pediatrics,* 1979, **64,** 665–667.

Conners, C. K. A teacher rating scale for use in drug studies with children. *American Journal of Psychiatry,* 1969, **126,** 884–888.

Conners, C. K. In H. C. Quay & J. S. Werry (Eds.), *Psychopathological disorders of childhood.* New York: Wiley, 1972.

Coolidge, C. B. The dying of Robin: A mother's reflections, *Journal of Pediatric Psychology,* 1977, **2,** 79–81.

Davis, J. K., Stone, R. K., Levine, G., & Stolzenberg, J. Child psychology and pediatric medicine. A training program for primary care physicians. Manuscript submitted for publication, 1979.

DeLozier, J. E., & Gagnon, R. O. The national ambulatory medical care survey: 1973 Summary United States, May 1973–April 1974. Vital and Health Statistics, Series 13, Data from the National Health Survey, No. 21. U.S. Department of Health, Education, and Welfare, Publication No. (HRA) 76–1772, 1975.

DiMatteo, M. R., & Taranta, A. Nonverbal communication and physician-patient rapport: An empirical study. *Professional Psychology,* 1979, **10,** 540–547.

Doleys, D. Enuresis. In J. M. Ferguson & C. B. Taylor (Eds.), *The comprehensive handbook of behavioral medicine,* Vol. 1. Jamaica, NY: SP Medical & Scientific Books, 1980. (a)

Doleys, D. Encopresis. In J. M. Ferguson, & C. B. Taylor (Eds.), *The comprehensive handbook of behavioral medicine,* Vol. 2. Jamaica, NY: SP Medical & Scientific Books, 1980. (b)

Doll, E. *Vineland Social Maturity Scale.* Circle Pines, MN: American Guidance Service, 1965.

Drotar, D. Psychological consultation in a pediatric hospital *Professional Psychology,* 1976, **7,** 77–83.

Drotar, D. Training psychologists to consult with pediatricians: Problems and prospects. *Journal of Clinical Child Psychology,* 1978, **7,** 57–60.

Duff, R. S., Rowe, D. S., & Anderson, F. P. Patient care and student learning in a pediatric clinic. *Pediatrics,* 1973, **50,** 839−846.

Dunbar, J., & Stunkard, A. J. Adherence to diet and drug regimen. In R. Levey, B. Rifkind, B. Dennis, & N. Ernst (Eds.), *Nutrition, lipids, and coronary heart disease.* New York: Raven Press, 1977.

Durlak, J. A., & Mannarino, A. P. The Social Skills Development Program: Description of a school-based preventive mental health program for high-risk children. *Journal of Clinical Child Psychology,* 1977, **6,** 48−52.

Durlak, J. A., Stein, M. A., & Mannarino, A. P. Behavioral validity of a brief teacher rating scale (the AML) in identifying high risk acting-out school children. *American Journal of Community Psychology,* in press.

Eareckson, J. *Joni.* Grand Rapids, MI: Zondervan, 1976.

Epstein, L. H., Wing, R. R., Steranchak, L., Dickson, B., & Michelson, J. Comparison of family-based behavior modification and nutrition education for childhood obesity. *Journal of Pediatric Psychology,* 1980, **5,** 25−36.

Falvo, D. Physician behavior and its relationship to patient compliance. Unpublished manuscript. Southern Illinois University School of Medicine, 1979.

Ferguson, B. F. Preparing young children for hospitalization: A comparison of two methods. *Pediatrics,* 1979, **64,** 656−664.

Ferguson, J. M., & Taylor, C. B. (Eds.) *The comprehensive handbook of behavioral medicine.* Jamaica, NY: SP Medical & Scientific Books, 1980.

Feurstein, M., Ward, M. M., & LeBaron, S. W. M. Neuropsychological and neurophysiological assessment of children with learning and behavior problems: A critical appraisal. In B. B. Lahey & A. E. Kazdin (Eds.), *Advances in clinical child psychology,* Vol. 2. New York: Plenum Press, 1979.

Field, T., Hallock, N., Ting, G., Dempsey, J., Dabiri, C., & Shuman, H. H. A first-year follow-up of high-risk infants: Formulating a cumulative risk index. *Child Development,* 1978, **49,** 119−131.

Flandorf, V. F. (compiler) *Books to help children adjust to a hospital situation.* Chicago: American Library Association, 1967.

Forehand, R. Child noncompliance to parental commands: Behavioral analysis and treatment. In M. Hersen, R. M. Eisler, & P. M. Miller (Eds.), *Progress in behavior modification,* Vol. 5. New York: Academic Press, 1977.

Forehand, R., Sturgis, E. T., McMahon, R. J., Aguar, D., Green, K., Wells, K. C., & Breiner, J. Parent behavioral training to modify child noncompliance: Treatment generalization across time and from home to school. *Behavior Modification,* 1979, **3,** 3−25.

Forgatch, M. S., & Toobert, D. J. A cost-effective parent training program for use with normal preschool children. *Journal of Pediatric Psychology,* 1979, **4,** 129−145.

Gardner, H. L., Forehand, R., & Roberts, M. Time-out with children: Effects of an explanation and brief parent training on child and parent behaviors. *Journal of Abnormal Child Psychology,* 1976, **4,** 272−288.

Garfinkel, P. E., Garner, D. M., & Moldofsky, H. The role of behavior modification in the treatment of anorexia nervosa. *Journal of Pediatric Psychology,* 1977, **2,** 113−121.

Garfinkel, P. E., Kline, S. A., & Stancer, H. C. Treatment of anorexia nervosa using operant conditioning techniques. *Journal of Nervous and Mental Disease,* 1973, **157,** 428–433.

Garner, A. M., & Thompson, C. W. Juvenile diabetes. In P. R. Magrab (Ed.), *Psychological management of pediatric problems,* Vol. 1. Baltimore: University Park Press, 1978.

Geist, R. A. Consultation on a pediatric surgical ward: Creating an empathic climate. *American Journal of Orthopsychiatry,* 1977, **47,** 432–444.

Gelfand, D. M., & Hartmann, D. P. The prevention of childhood behavior disorders. In B. B. Lahey & A. E. Kazdin (Eds.), *Advances in clinical child psychology,* Vol. 1. New York: Plenum Press, 1977.

Gesell, A., & Amatruda, C. S. *Developmental diagnosis.* New York: Paul B. Hoeber, 1947.

Glasgow, R. E., & Rosen, G. M. Behavioral bibliotherapy: A review of self-help behavior therapy manuals. *Psychological Bulletin,* 1978, **85,** 1–23.

Goldberg, I. D., Regier, D. A., McInerny, T. K., Pless, I. B., & Roghmann, K. J. The role of the pediatrician in the delivery of mental health services to children. *Pediatrics,* 1979, **63,** 898–909.

Green, H. G., Dudding, B. A., Viren, M. A., & Leake, H. C. The pediatric clinic: Diagnosing inefficiencies and measuring the effects of remedial action. *Clinical Pediatrics,* 1977, **16,** 541–547.

Green, M. & Haggerty, R. J. *Ambulatory Pediatrics.* Philadelphia: Saunders, 1977.

Haggerty, R. J. The task force report. *Pediatrics,* 1979, **63,** 935–937.

Harper, R. G. Behavior modification in pediatric practice. *Clinical Pediatrics,* 1975, **14,** 962–967.

Hartlage, L. C., & Hartlage, P. L. Clinical consultation to pediatric neurology and developmental pediatrics. *Journal of Clinical Child Psychology,* 1978, **7,** 19–20.

Heagarty, M. C. The telephone syndrome. *Pediatrics,* 1979, **64,** 696–697.

Ireton, H., & Thwing, E. *The Minnesota Child Development Inventory.* Minneapolis: Interspective Scoring Systems, 1972.

Joslin Clinic. *Th diabetic handbook.* Philadelphia: Lea & Febiger, 1974.

Johnson, B. H. Before hospitalization: A preparation program for the child and his family. *Children Today,* 1974, **3,** 18–21.

Keegan, D. L. Adaptation to visual handicap: Short-term group approach. *Psychosomatics,* 1974, **15,** 76–78.

Kempe, H. C., & Helfer, R. E. *Helping the battered child and his family.* Philadelphia: Lippincott, 1972.

Kennedy, W. School phobia: Rapid treatment of fifty cases. *Journal of Abnormal Psychology,* 1965, **70,** 285–289.

Kennell, J. H., & Klaus, M. H. *Maternal infant bonding.* St. Louis: Mosby, 1976.

Killilea, M. *Karen.* New York: Prentice-Hall, 1952.

King, H. E. Discussant's comments. In M. C. Roberts (chair), *Psychological intervention in the pediatric setting.* Symposium presented at annual meeting of the Southeastern Psychological Association, Washington, DC, March 1980.

Knight, M. F., & McKenzie, H. S. Elimination of bedtime thumb-sucking in home settings through contingent reading. *Journal of Applied Behavior Analysis,* 1974, **7,** 33–38.

Koocher, G. P., & Sallan, S. E. Pediatric oncology. In P. R. Magrab (Ed.), *Psychological management of pediatric problems*, Vol. 1. Baltimore: University Park Press, 1978.

Koocher, G. P. Talking with children about death. *American Journal of Orthopsychiatry*, 1974, **44**, 404–411.

Koocher, G. P., Sourkes, B. M., & Keane, W. M. Pediatric oncology consultations: A generalizable model for medical settings. *Professional Psychology*, 1979, **10**, 467–474.

Kupst, M. J., Blatterbauer, S., Westman, J., Shulman J. C., & Paul, M. H. Helping parents cope with the diagnosis of congenital heart defect: An experimental study. *Pediatrics*, 1977, **59**, 266–272.

La Greca, A. M., & Mesibov, G. B. Social skills intervention with learning disabled children: Selecting skills and implementing training. *Journal of Clinical Child Psychology*, 1979, **8**, 234–241.

La Greca, A. M., & Ottinger, D. R. Self-monitoring and relaxation training in the treatment of medically ordered exercises in a 12-year-old female. *Journal of Pediatric Psychology*. 1979, **4**, 49–54.

Levy, J. C., Rosekrans, J., Lamb, G. A., Friedman, M., Kaplan, D., & Strasser, P. Development and field testing of protocols for the management of pediatric telephone calls: Protocols for pediatric telephone calls. *Pediatrics*, 1979, **64**, 558–563.

Lewis, S. Considerations in setting up psychological consultation to a pediatric hematology-oncology team. *Journal of Clinical Child Psychology*, 1978, **7**, 21–22.

Linscheid, T. R. Disturbances of eating and feeding. In P. R. Magrab (Ed.), *Psychological management of pediatric problems*, Vol. 1. Baltimore: University Park Press, 1978.

Lowe, K., & Lutzker, J. R. Increasing compliance to a medical regimen with a juvenile diabetic. *Behavior Therapy*, 1979, **10**, 57–4.

Lynch, M. *Mary Fran and Mo*. New York: St. Martin's Press, 1979.

McClelland, C. Q., Staples, W. P., Weisberg, I., & Berge, M. E. The practitioners' role in behavioral pediatrics. *Journal of Pediatrics*, 1973, **82**, 325–331.

McMahon, R. J., & Forehand, R. Nonprescription behavior therapy: Effectiveness of a brochure in teaching mothers to correct their children's inappropriate mealtime behaviors. *Behavior Therapy*, 1978, **9**, 814–820.

McAlister, A. L., Perry, L., & Maccoby, N. Adolescent smoking: Onset and prevention. *Pediatrics*, 1979, **63**, 650–658.

McNamara, J. R. (Ed.) *Behavioral approaches to medicine: Application and analysis*. New York: Plenum Press, 1979.

Magrab, P. R. Psychological management and renal dialysis. *Journal of Clinical Child Psychology*, 1975, **4**, 38–40.

Magrab, P. R. (Ed.) *Psychological management of pediatric problems*, 2 vols. Baltimore: University Park Press, 1978.

Magrab, P. R., & Calcagno, P. L. Psychological impact of chronic pediatric conditions. In P. R. Magrab (Ed.), *Psychological management of pediatric problems*, Vol. 1. Baltimore: University Park Press, 1978.

Magrab, P. R., & Danielson-Murphy, J. Adolescent pregnancy: A review. *Journal of Clinical Child Psychology*, 1979, **8**, 121–125.

Magrab, P. R., & Davitt, M. K. The pediatric psychologist and the developmental follow-up of intensive care nursery infants. *Journal of Clinical Child Psychology*, 1975, **4**, 16–18.

Marston, M. V. Compliance with medical regimens: A review of the literature. *Nursing Research*, 1970, **19**, 312–323.

Mattsson, A., & Agle, D. P. Group therapy with parents of hemophiliacs. *Journal of the American Academy of Child Psychiatry*, 1972, **11**, 558–571.

Melamed, B., Hawes, R., Heiby, E., & Glick, J. Use of filmed modeling to reduce uncooperative behavior of children during dental treatment. *Journal of Dental Research*, 1975, **54**, 797–801.

Melamed, B. G., & Siegel, L. J. Reduction of anxiety in children facing surgery by modeling. *Journal of Consulting and Clinical Psychology*, 1975, **43**, 511–521.

Melamed, B. G., Meyer, R., Gee, C., & Soule, L. The influence of time and type of preparation on children's adjustment to hospitalization. *Journal of Pediatric Psychology*, 1976, **1**, 31–37.

Mesibov, G. B., Schroeder, C. S., & Wesson L. Parental concerns about their children. *Journal of Pediatric Psychology*, 1977, **2**, 13–17.

Metz, J. R., Allen, C. M., Barr, G., & Shinefield, H. R. A pediatric screening examination for psychosocial problems. *Pediatrics*, 1976, **58**, 595–606.

Miller, A. J., & Kratochwill, T. R. Reduction of frequent stomachache complaints by time out. *Behavior Therapy*, 1979, **10**, 211–218.

Miller, L. C., Barrett, C. L., Hampe, E., & Noble, H. Revised anxiety scales for the Louisville Behavior Checklist. *Psychological Reports*, 1971, **29**, 503–511.

Millon, T., Green, C. J., & Meagher, R. (Eds.), *Handbook of clinical health psychology*. New York: Plenum Press, in press.

Morgan, J. R., & Cullen, P. M. Giving (almost) psychology away: A multi-level preventive program for providing child rearing advice to parents of pre-schoolers. Paper presented at the convention of the Southeastern Psychological Association, Washington, DC, March 1980.

Morgan, W. L., & Engel, G. L. *The clinical approach to the patient*. Philadelphia: Saunders, 1969.

Morrison, T. L. The psychologist in the pediatricians office: One approach to community psychology. *Community Mental Health*, 1976, **12**, 305–312.

Ms. Magazine. A new list of books for free children: Sensitive subjects. *Ms.*, 1976, **3**, 95–98.

National Center for Health Statistics Growth Charts. Monthly Vital Statistics Report, Vol. 25, No. 3. 5 pp. (HRA) 76–1120. Health Resources Administration, Rockville, MD, June 1976.

Nelson, W. E., Vaughan, V. C., & McKay, R. J. *Textbook of pediatrics*. Philadelphia: Saunders, 1975.

Newberger, E. H., & McAnulty, E. H. Family intervention in the pediatric clinic: A necessary approach to the vulnerable child. *Clinical Pediatrics*, 1976, **15**, 1155–1161.

Nitschke, R., Wunder, S., Sexauer, C. L., & Humphrey, G. B. The final-stage conference: The patient's decision on research drugs in pediatric oncology. *Journal of Pediatric Psychology*, 1977, **2**, 58–64.

Nixon, G. Systems approach to pediatric consultation. *Journal of Clinical Child Psychology*, 1975, **4**, 33–35.

Noland, R. (Ed.), *Counseling parents of the mentally retarded*. Springfield, IL: Charles C. Thomas, 1970.

Olbrisch, M. E., & Sechrest, L. Educating health psychologists in traditional training programs. *Professional Psychology,* 1979, **10,** 589–595.

Ottinger, D. R., & Roberts, M. C. A university-based predoctoral practicum in pediatric psychology. *Professional Psychology,* 1980, **11,** 707–713.

Parmelee, A. H., Kopp, C. B., & Sigman, M. Selection of developmental assessment technique for infants at risk. *Merrill-Palmer Quarterly,* 1976, **22,** 177–199.

Patterson, G. R., & Gullion, M. E. *Living with children: New methods for parents and teachers.* Champaign, IL: Research Press, 1968.

Pearn, J. H., Brown, J., Wong, R., & Bart, R. Bathtub drownings: Report of seven cases. *Pediatrics,* 1979, **64,** 68–70.

Peed, S., Roberts, M., & Forehand, R. Evaluation of the effectiveness of a standardized parent training program in altering the interaction of mothers and their noncompliant children. *Behavior Modification,* 1977, **1,** 323–350.

Peterson, L. Increasing immunization levels in high risk preschool children. Paper presented at the meeting of the Midwestern Psychological Association, St. Louis, May 1980.

Peterson, L., Hartmann, D. P., & Gelfand, D. M. Prevention of child behavior disorders: A lifestyle change for child psychologists. In P. O. Davidson & S. M. Davidson (Eds.), *Behavioral medicine: Changing health lifestyles.* New York: Brunner/Mazel, 1980.

Platt, J. J., & Wicks, R. J. (Eds.) *The psychological consultant.* New York: Grune & Stratton, 1979.

Quay, H. C., & Peterson, D. R. *Manual for the Behavior Problem Checklist.* Champaign: Children's Research Center, University of Illinois, 1967.

Quay, H. C., & Peterson, D. R. *Revised Behavior Problem Checklist: Rationale and development.* Unpublished manuscript, University of Miami, 1979.

Rainey, S. K., & Christopherson, E. R. Behavioral pediatrics: The role of the nurse clinician. *Comprehensive Issues in Pediatric Nursing,* 1976, **1**(4), 19–28.

Regier, D. A., & Goldberg, I. D. National health insurance and the mental health services equilibrium. Paper read at the annual meeting of the American Psychiatric Association, Miami, May 13, 1976.

Reid, J. B., & Taplin, P. S. A social interactional approach to the treatment of abusive children. Unpublished manuscript, 1977.

Rheingold, H. L. Interpreting mental retardation to parents. *Journal of Consulting Psychology,* 1945, **9,** 142–148.

Rie, H. D. Pediatrics and changing practices in clinical child psychology. In *Issues concerning the expansion of psychology within pediatric settings.* Symposium presented at the 77th Annual Convention of the American Psychological Association, Washington, DC, September 1969.

Roberts, M. C. Psychological preparation for pediatric hospitalization and surgery. Paper presented in M. C. Roberts (chair), *Pediatric psychology: Theory and intervention for psychological-medical problems with children.* Symposium presented at the meeting of the Midwestern Psychological Association, Chicago, May 1979.

Roberts, M. C., & Horner, M. M. A comprehensive intervention for failure-to-thrive. *Journal of Clinical Child Psychology,* 1979, **8,** 10–14.

Roberts, M. C., & La Greca, A. M. Behavioral assessment. In C. E. Walker (Ed.), *Clinical practice of psychology: A practical guide for mental health professionals.* New York: Pergamon Press, in press.

Roberts, M. C., Maddux, J. E., Wurtele, S. K., & Wright, L. Pediatric psychology: Health care psychology for children. In T. Millon, C. J. Green, & R. Meaghor (Eds.), *Handbook of clinical health psychology*. New York: Plenum Press, in press.

Roberts, M. C., & Ottinger, D. R. A case study: Encopretic adolescent with multiple problems. *Journal of Clinical Child Psychology*, 1979, **8**, 15−17.

Roberts, M. C., Quevillon, R. P., & Wright, L. Pediatric psychology: A developmental report and survey of the literature. *Child & Youth Services*, 1979, **2**, 1−9.

Roberts, M. C., & Wurtele, S. K. On the noncompliant research subject in a study of medical noncompliance. *Social Science & Medicine*, 1980, **14A**, 171.

Roberts, M. C., Wurtele, S. K., Boone, R. R., Ginther, L., & Elkins, P. Reduction of medical fears by use of modeling: Applications in a general population of children. *Journal of Pediatric Psychology*, 1981, **6**, 293−300.

Routh, D. K. Hyperactivity. In P. R. Magrab (Ed.), *Psychological management of pediatric problems*, Vol. 2. Baltimore: University Park Press, 1978.

Sackett, D., & Haynes, R. *Compliance with therapeutic regimens*. Baltimore: Johns Hopkins University Press, 1976.

Salk, L. The purposes and functions of the psychologist in a pediatric setting. Paper presented in *Issues concerning the expansion of psychology within pediatric settings*. Symposium presented at the 77th Annual Convention ofthe American Psychological Association, Washington, DC, September 1969.

Salk, L. Psychologist in a pediatric setting. *Professional Psychology*, 1970, 395−396.

Salk, L. Psychologist and pediatrician: A mental health team in the prevention and early diagnosis of mental disorders. In G. J. Williams & S. Gordon (Eds.), *Clinical child psychology: Current practices and future perspectives*. New York: Behavioral Publications, 1974.

Salk, L. *What every child would like parents to know about divorce*. New York: Harper & Row, 1978.

Sarata, B. P., & Jeppersen, J. C. Job design and staff satisfaction in human service settings. *American Journal of Community Psychology*, 1977, **5**, 229−236.

Savino, A. B., & Sanders, R. W. Working with abusive parents: Group therapy and home visits. *American Journal of Nursing*, 1973, **73**, 482−84.

Scherer, M. W., & Nakamura, C. Y. A fear survey schedule for children (FSS-FC). *Behavior Research and Therapy*, 1968, **6**, 173−183.

Schofield, W. The role of psychology in the delivery of health services. *American Psychologist*, 1969, **24**, 565−584.

Schreiner, R. L., Gresham, E. L., & Green, M. Physicians responsibility to parents after death of an infant. *American Journal of Diseases of Childhood*, 1979, **133**, 723−726.

Schroeder, C. S. Psychologists in a private pediatric practice. *Journal of Pediatric Psychology*, 1979, **4**, 5−18.

Schroeder, C., Goolsby, E., & Stangler, S. Preventive services in a private pediatric practice. *Journal of Clinical Child Psychology*, 1975, **4**, 32−33.

Schulman, J. L., & Kupst, M. J. (Eds.) *The child with cancer: Clinical approaches to psychosocial care. Research in Psychosocial aspects*. Springfield, IL: Charles C. Thomas, 1980.

Seagull, E. A. W., & Seagull, A. A. The talk to a lay group as a method of primary prevention. *Journal of Clinical Child psychology*, 1979, **8**, 130−132.

Slade, P. D. A short anorexia behavior scale. *British Journal of Psychiatry,* 1973, **122,** 83–85.

Smialek, J. E., Smialek, P. Z., & Spitz, W. U. Accidental bed deaths in infants due to unsafe sleeping situations. *Clinical Pediatrics,* 1977, **16,** 1031–1036.

Smith, E. E., Rome, L. P., & Freidheim, D. K. The clinical psychologist in the pediatric office. *Journal of Pediatrics,* 1967, **71,** 48–51.

Sobol, H. L. *My brother Steven is retarded.* New York: Macmillan, 1977.

Sours, J. A. The anorexia nervosa syndrome: Phenomenologic and psychodynamic components. *Psychiatric Quarterly,* 1969, **43,** 240–256.

Spinetta, J. J. Adjustment in children with cancer. *Journal of Pediatric Psychology,* 1977, **2,** 49–51.

Spinetta, J. J. The dying child's awareness of death: A review. *Psychological Bulletin,* 1974, **81,** 256–260.

Spinetta, J. J., Deasy, P. M., Koenig, H. M., Lightsey, A. L., Schwartz, D. B., Hartman, G. A., & Kung, F. H. *Talking with children with a life-threatening illness: A handbook for health care professionals.* San Diego: Childhood Adaptation Project, 1979.

Spinetta, J. J., Spinetta, P. D., Kung, F., & Schwartz, D. B. *Emotional aspects of childhood cancer and leukemia: A handbook for parents.* San Diego: Leukemia Society of America, 1976.

Spock, R., & Lerrigo, M. O. *Caring for your disabled child.* New York: Macmillan, 1965.

Stabler, B. Emerging models of psychologist-pediatrician liaison. *Journal of Pediatric Psychology,* 1979, **4,** 307–313.

Stabler, B., & Murra, J. P. Pediatrician perceptions of pediatric psychology. *Clinical Psychologist,* 1974, **27,** 13–15.

Stein, S. B. *About dying.* New York: Walker, 1974.

Strasser, P. H., Levy, J. C., Lamb, G. A., & Rosekrans, J. Controlled clinical trial of pediatric telephone protocols. *Pediatrics,* 1979, **64,** 553–557.

Stuart, R., & Davis, B. *Slim chance in a fat world: Behavioral control of obesity.* Champaign, IL: Research Press, 1972.

Swinyard, C. A. *The child with Spina Bifida.* New York: Association for the Aid of Crippled Children, 1966.

Task Force on Pediatric Education, American Academy of Pediatrics. *The future of pediatric education.* Denver: Hirschfield, 1978.

Tefft, B. M., & Simeonsson, R. J. Psychology and the creation of health care settings. *Professional Psychology,* 1979, **10,** 558–570.

Traisman, H. S., & Newcomb, A. L. *Management of juvenile diabetes.* St. Louis: Mosby, 1965.

Van Vechten, D. V., Satterwhite, B., & Pless, I. B. Health education literature for parents of physically handicapped children. *American Journal of Diseases of Childhood,* 1977, **131,** 311–315.

Visintainer, M. A., & Wolfer, J. A. Psychological preparation for surgical pediatric patients: The effect on children's and parent's stress responses and adjustment. *Pediatrics,* 1975, **56,** 187–202.

Vore, D., & Wright, L. Psychological management of the family and the dying child. In R. E. Herdy & J. G. Gull (Eds.), *Therapeutic needs of the family: Problems, descriptions, and therapeutic approaches.* Springfield, IL: Charles C. Thomas, 1974.

Walker, C. E. Enuresis and encopresis. In P. Magrab (Ed.), *Psychological management of pediatric problems*. Baltimore: University Park Press, 1978.

Walker, C. E. Behavioral intervention in a pediatric setting. In J. R. MacNamara (Ed.), *Behavioral approaches to medicine: Application and analysis*. New York: Plenum Press, 1979. (a)

Walker, C. E. Behavioral intervention in a pediatric setting. In J. R. MacNamara (Ed.), *Behavioral approaches to medicine: Application and analysis*. New York: Plenum Press, 1979. (a)

Walker, H. K., Hurst, J. W., & Woody, M. F. (Eds.) *Applying the problem-oriented system*. New York: MEDCOM Press, 1973.

Weed, L. L. *Medical records, medical education, and patient care*. Cleveland: Press of Case Western Reserve University, 1969.

White, E. B. *Charlotte's Web*. New York: Harper & Row, 1952.

Wright, L. The pediatric psychologist: A role model. *American Psychologist*, 1967, **22**, 23-325.

Wright, L. Pediatric psychology: Prospect and retrospect. *Pediatric Psychology*, 1969, **1**(1), 1-3.

Wright, L. Counseling with parents of chronically ill children. *Postgraduate Medicine*,41970, **47**, 173-177.

Wright, L. Handling the encopretic child. *Professional Psychology*, 1973, **4**, 137-144.

Wright, L. An emotional support program for parents of dying children. *Journal of Clinical Child Psychology*, 1974, **3**, 37-38.

Wright, L. Outcome of a standardized program for treating psychogenic encopresis. *Professional Psychology*, 1975, **6**, 453-456.

Wright, L. Indirect treatment of children through principles oriented parent consultation. *Journal of Consulting and Clinical Psychology*, 1976, **44**, 148.

Wright, L. Primary health care physicians to assume expanded role. *Feelings: And Their Medical Significance*, 1978, **20**, 1-4. (a)

Wright, L. Assessing the psychosomatic status of children. *Journal of Clinical Child Psychology*, 1978, **7**, 94-112. (b)

Wright, L. *Parent power: A guide to responsible childrearing*. New York: Psychological Dimensions, 1978. (c)

Wright, L. A comprehensive program for mental health and behavioral medicine in a large children's hospital. *Professional Psychology*, 1979, **10**, 458-466. (a)

Wright, L. Health care psychology: Prospects for well-being of children. *American Psychologist*, 1979, **34**, 1001-1006. (b)

Wright, L. The standardization of compliance procedures, or the mass production of ugly ducklings. *American Psychologist*, 1980, **35**, 119-122.

Wright, L., & Roberts, M. C. Application of a standardized compliance program to control juvenile diabetes. Funded Grant Proposal to Research Council of University of Oklahoma Health Sciences Center, February 1978.

Wright, L., Schaefer, A. B., & Solomons, G. *Encyclopedia of pediatric psychology*. Baltimore: University Park Press, 1979.

Wright, L., & Walker, C. E. Behavioral treatment of encopresis. *Journal of Pediatric Psychology*, 1976, **1**(1), 35-37.

Wright, L., & Walker, C. E. Treating the encopretic child. *Clinical Pediatrics,* 1977, **16,** 1042−1045.

Wright, L., Woodcock, J., & Scott, R. Treatment of sleep disturbance in a young child by conditioning. *Southern Medical Journal,* 1970, **63,** 174−176.

Yankauer, A., Connelly, J. P., & Feldman, J. J. Pediatric practice in the United States: With special attention to utilization of allied health worker services. *Pediatrics,* 1970, **45,** 321−554.

CHAPTER 8

Pediatric Psychology as an Area of Scientific Research

Donald K. Routh

Pediatric psychology was originally defined (Wright, 1967) on the basis of professional background and work setting rather than as a coherent scientific specialty. Thus while pediatric psychologists may have been trained in any of several different areas of psychology, they almost all work with children in developmental clinics, hospitals, or in pediatric or medical group practice settings.

EMERGENCE OF PEDIATRIC PSYCHOLOGY AS AN AREA OF SCIENTIFIC RESEARCH

The research interests of pediatric psychologists followed naturally enough from those of their parent disciplines, medicine and psychology, which are both research-based professions. Although in earlier days training in medicine was acquired on an apprenticeship basis and through proprietary schools which gave little attention to science, ever since the 1910 Flexner Report (Moll, 1968) medical education has been strongly linked to basic biomedical research. In contrast to fields such as medicine, law, social work, and engineering, psychology was an academic discipline first, and only later a profession. Both the scientist-practitioner model (Shakow, 1947) and the more recent practitioner model (Korman, 1974) of training in clinical psychology are committed to grounding all professionals in the basic scientific aspects of psychology.

Many of the original members of the Society of Pediatric Psychology were faculty members in departments of pediatrics in medical schools. Already in 1970–1971, almost three out of four such departments had psychologists on their faculties (Routh, 1972). Like other faculty members, these psychologists are expected to carry out and publish research in order to be considered for promotion and tenure, and many help support their research activities by grants from private foundations and the federal government. Thus scientific research is part of the job definition of many pediatric psychologists. Of course others work in developmental clinics, hospitals, or medical group practice settings which are not university affiliated. Rendering quality service to children requires these professionals, also, to keep up to date on research findings which have any direct bearing on practice in the field. This need is being recognized increasingly in the continuing education requirements of state licensure laws in psychology. Thus although only some pediatric psychologists must produce research, all should be research consumers.

Pediatric psychologists differ from developmental psychologists (some of whom also work in medical settings) in their research as well as their clinical training. Both groups are child oriented, grounded in research methodology, and trained in general psychology. Pediatric psychologists, however, have also had practicum, internship, and/or postdoctoral clinical training, and are concerned with the effects of illness on the child and with developmental disorders, while developmental psychologists are more concerned with the phenomena of normal development.

Some of the research activities of the pediatric psychologist may at first seem unfamiliar to pediatricians, who when they think of research may envision only a biomedical scientist at the "bench." Pediatric psychology research, true to its behavioral science heritage, is carried out not only in the laboratory but in the pediatrician's office, at the bedside in a children's hospital, and in the child's home, school, or neighborhood. Pediatricians will gradually learn that in the hands of pediatric psychologists, clinical research of this kind is not incompatible with scientific rigor.

Little more than a decade after the 1968 founding of the Society of Pediatric Psychology, a professional journal, and several books have appeared in the field. The *Journal of Pediatric Psychology* began publication in 1976. In 1978 the two volumes on Psychological Management of Pediatric Problems edited by Magrab appeared, and in 1979 the *Encyclopedia of Pediatric Psychology* by Wright, Schaefer, and Solomons was published. The corresponding medical subspecialty of behavioral pediatrics was not far behind in announcing its existence. In 1980 appeared both the first issues of the *Journal of Developmental and Behavioral Pediatrics* and the first volume of the research annual, *Advances in Behavioral Pediatrics*.

The content of these professional journals and books is, to a considerable extent, scientific research. In a first editorial attempt to define the boundaries of pediatric psychology as an area of scientific research, Routh and Mesibov (1979) described it as including developmental disabilities such as mental retardation and autism; the clinical psychology of the infant; problems of the preschool child, including noncompliance, toilet training, and the development of self-help skills; disorders of parenting such as neglect, child abuse, and failure-to-thrive; psychological aspects of physical illness in children; death and the child; preparation for hospitalization and the care of children in hospitals; and child neuropsychology. Obviously, this list of research topics was only a preliminary one, and many others can be expected to emerge as the field defines itself further. The remainder of the present chapter is an attempt to survey some of the principles and major findings of research in these areas, and thus to provide an overview of pediatric psychology as an area of scientific research.

RESEARCH ON ASSESSMENT

The psychological assessment of children has always been one of the professional activities of pediatric psychologists. From a research standpoint, three aspects of assessment which are of particular interest are screening, developmental assessment, and the assessment and monitoring of children's behavior problems.

Screening

Psychologists are probably more likely to do research on screening than to be involved in the actual screening process, which is often the job of nurses or community volunteers. Lessler (1972) provides the following definition:

> Screening is the acquiring of preliminary information about characteristics which may be significant to the health, education, or well-being of the individual and which are relevant to his life tasks. The means of data collection must be appropriate and reasonable with regard to the economics of time, money and resources for dealing with large numbers of persons. (p. 193)

The basic goal of any such screening program is to identify serious or potentially serious conditions in the child before the usual time of diagnosis, in order to intervene at the earliest possible moment, and thereby improve the ultimate outcome for the child. It seems obvious that since pediatricians and other health professionals see literally every child in infancy and during the preschool period, they are in a unique position to carry out screening programs. Well-known examples of biomedical screening procedures include the use of blood tests on newborn infants to identify phenylketonuria (PKU) and the use of serial measures of head circumference to identify developing hydrocephalus. In each case, early identification is crucial to minimizing the impact of the condition on the child (i.e., through a low phenylalanine diet or surgical installation of a shunt).

Screening procedures with a larger psychological component include screening tests of general development such as the Denver Developmental Screening Test and procedures for the preliminary identification of hearing loss, delayed speech and language development, and visual impairment. The basic procedure for validating a screening device involves applying it to a representative population of children under realistic conditions (i.e., in a pediatrician's busy office or a neighborhood health clinic rather than in a laboratory or a highly instrumented tertiary health care center), and then subjecting all of the children (not just those who are positive on the screening measure) to a standard diagnostic procedure.

Table 1 is a worksheet for calculating screening test validity reproduced from Stangler, Huber, and Routh (1980). The information necessary to use this worksheet consists of the following items:

1. Correct referrals, or the number of children who appeared to be abnormal on both the screening test and the diagnostic or criterion test.
2. Overreferrals, or the number of children who appeared abnormal on the screening test but were then diagnosed as normal.

Table 1. Worksheet for Calculating Screening Test Validity

Screening Test	Criterion Test			
	Abnormal	*Normal*		
	a	b	a	b
Referrals (positive)	Correct referrals	Over-referrals		
	c	d	c	d
Nonreferrals (negative)	Under-referrals	Correct nonreferrals		

Rate of referral

$$= \frac{a + b}{a + b + c + d} \times 100$$

Screening test validity

$$= \frac{a + d}{a + b + c + d} \times 100$$

Sensitivity

$$= \frac{a}{a + c} \times 100$$

Rate of overreferral (total sample)

$$= \frac{b}{a + b + c + d} \times 100$$

Rate of overreferral (total number of referrals)

$$= \frac{b}{a + b} \times 100$$

Predictive validity of positive tests

$$= \frac{a}{a + b} \times 100$$

Specificity

$$= \frac{d}{b + d} \times 100$$

Rate of underreferral (total sample)

$$= \frac{c}{a + b + c + d} \times 100$$

Rate of underreferral (total number of underreferrals)

$$= \frac{c}{c + d} \times 100$$

Predictive validity of negative test

$$= \frac{d}{c + d} \times 100$$

3. Underreferrals, or the number of children who appeared normal on the screening test but were diagnosed abnormal by the criterion test.

4. Correct nonreferrals, or the number of children who appeared to be normal on both the screening and the diagnostic tests.

As Table 1 shows, the overall screening test validity is simply the percentage of cases which are correctly classified, considering the different kinds of erroneous classification as having equal weight. In practice, of course, it is much more serious to make errors of underreferral than errors of overreferral. That is, it is more of a fault for the screening procedure to fail to identify children with potentially serious conditions than it is for it to identify, erroneously, too many as having such conditions. That is why it is important to calculate, also, the sensitivity and specificity of a screening measure, as indicated on the worksheet. The sensitivity of a screening test refers to its ability to identify truly abnormal cases as such, that is, to avoid underreferrals. The specificity of a screening test, on the other hand, refers to its ability to identify truly normal cases as such, that is, to avoid overreferrals. In most clinical situations, sensitivity is more important than specificity, though both must be taken into account in considering the cost effectiveness of a screening procedure.

Much of the published research on screening procedures unfortunately neglects to provide the types of information described above, and thus fails to be helpful. It is common in such research to present validity information in terms of correlation coefficients, but for evaluation of screening validity, presentation of the type of fourfold table seen in Table 1 is necessary. In screening programs, after all, a dichotomous decision must be made either to refer a child for a diagnostic workup or not to refer the child; thus validity measures based on a continuum do not represent the way test information must be used in practice. It is even less satisfactory to report only the existence of a statistically significant relationship between a screening measure and a diagnostic criterion. Screeners need to know also the numbers of screening errors which are likely to be made by the test, and what kinds.

An example of this kind of research is provided by the study of Huber, Stangler, and Routh (1978) of the BOEL Test as a screening device for otitis media in infants. The BOEL selective attention screening test, developed at the Karolinska Institute in Sweden, was administered by experienced nurse examiners to patients in two pediatric practices. The patients included were 243 infants with a mean age of 9 months, most of whom had a normal medical history. In the standard administration of the BOEL, the infant sits in the mother's lap facing the examiner. The examiner first makes eye contact with the infant and presents an attractive red stick to gain the infant's visual attention. Then on four occasions novel 30- to 35- decibel sounds are made with tiny bell-like objects hidden in the examiner's hands. The sounds are presented alternatively to the infant's left and right, in order to observe whether the infant visually orients to them (the term BOEL stands for the Swedish words "the glance orients to sound"). Of the 12 items on the BOEL, only the four relating to auditory orienting behavior proved to be discriminative. There was a significant association between the BOEL scores and the presence of otitis media. As a screening device for otitis media, these BOEL items had a validity of 87% correct predictions, with 11% false positives, and only 2% false negatives. The sensitivity of the BOEL was 83% (15 of 18 abnormal cases were correctly identified), while the specificity of the test was 88% (199 of 225 normal cases were correctly identified). Of course, using an otoscope is perhaps as simple a way of identifying otitis media as the BOEL test. The study does suggest that the BOEL has promise as an auditory screening device, warranting further research comparing the BOEL and full-scale audiological evaluations of infants' hearing. Indeed Stensland-Junker, the inventor of the BOEL test, has been involved in such research on a continuing basis in Sweden.

Developmental Assessment

Pediatric psychologists are frequently asked to appraise the developmental status of an infant, and a number of standardized procedures have been devised for doing so. The best known of these are probably the Bayley Scales of Infant Development (Bayley, 1969) and the Brazelton Neonatal Behavioral Assessment Scale (Brazelton, 1973). Ever since the first downward extension of the Binet scale by Kuhlman in 1912, the hope has been that such tests would predict the infant's long-term intellectual development, but that hope still does not appear to be very close to realization, except perhaps in the case of infants with moderate to profound mental retardation (e.g., Vander Veer & Schweid, 1974).

The reasons for the lack of long-term predictive validity may lie not so much in the tests themselves as in the lack of stability in infants' behavior over long periods of time. Both the Brazelton and Bayley procedures have generally good interobserver reliability, and with the Bayley the test-retest reliability tends to be relatively high over short time periods. The same test items which are unstable over time for young infants may show high stability over time when administered to older, handicapped children functioning at infant mental ages (e.g., DuBose, 1976). The infant tests seem to be measuring real, albeit unstable psychological processes, and not just random noise. For example, the Brazelton Scale appears to be a sensitive measure of the effects of some obstetrical pain-relieving drugs on the infant (Aleksandrowicz & Aleksandrowicz, 1974) and of the effects of the infant's prenatal addiction to narcotics (Strauss, Starr, Ostrea, Chavez, & Stryker, 1976). Findings with the Bayley Scales have shown an amazing degree of synchrony in longitudinal studies of monozygotic twin infants (Wilson, 1978).

Perhaps at this point we should acknowledge that the behavior of infants is rather unstable over time. Therefore, rather than measure the infant's behavior directly, perhaps it is a better strategy to measure something which is stable and which affects the infant's future behavior and development—the environment. This is the approach followed by the developers of the Home Observation for Measurement of the Environment (HOME). Elardo, Bradley, and Caldwell (1975) showed, for example, that measures of infants' home environment were more highly related to measures of infant development over a period of 30 months than the correlations typically reported between infant tests or level of parental education and childhood IQ. Bradley and Caldwell (1979), studying the families of children ages 3 to 6 years, found concurrent and predictive correlations between the HOME scales and IQ as high as .58. A similar approach to the assessment of children's environments in the domain of personality is represented by the Home Environment Questionnaire (HEQ) under development by Jacob O. Sines.

Assessment of Children's Behavior Problems

Many children are seen in pediatric settings because their parents or teachers are having difficulty managing their behavior. The most common way of evaluating such problems seems to be a brief interview with a parent, usually the mother, supplemented by any impressions gleaned during the medical examination of the child.

Direct observation of the child's behavior in the unfamiliar setting of the clinic or hospital does not seem to be a totally satisfactory way of gauging what problems the child might be having at home or at school. Even a well-standardized interview with the child which generates measures with good interrater reliability may produce information that has no relationship to estimates of behavior disorder derived from mothers and teachers (Berg & Fielding, 1979). Clinicians seem to be aware of this problem in that they place much more credence in information from parents than that derived from observation of the child in an unfamiliar context. McCoy (1976) provided psychology graduate students with films of several children's behavior and written behavioral descriptions of the children by their parents. Judgments of the children's need for treatment and level of adjustment depended almost entirely on the content of the parental reports, not on the films of the children's behavior.

What about the validity of the parent interview as a means of assessing children's behavior problems? Well-standardized procedures have been developed by Graham and Rutter (1968) for using the parent interview in the assessment of the child. These could be supplemented by parent checklists or rating forms which have been developed in recent years, for example, the Personality Inventory for Children (Wirt, Lachar, Klinedinst, & Seat, 1977) or the Child Behavior Profile (Achenbach, 1978; Achenbach & Edelbrock, 1979). Unfortunately, there are also difficulties in relying on the parent as the sole source of information about children's behavior problems. The parent's statements about the child may be biased by the parent's own emotional problems. Also, the parent may not have an adequate comparative framework within which to evaluate the child's problems. Griest, Wells, and Forehand (1979) found that, among mothers of clinic-referred children, maternal depression (measured by the Beck Depression Inventory) was the best predictor of maternal perception of the children's problems. Child behavior as assessed by direct home observations was unrelated to maternal perception of the children's problems. Rapoport and Benoit (1975) obtained information from a variety of sources on a group of children being evaluated for hyperactivity, including teacher questionnaires, ratings by clinical examiners, and parent questionnaires. They also made home visits, obtaining counts of children's spontaneous activity shifts in play and the number of negative interactions, as well as global observer ratings of hyperactivity at home. In addition, they had mothers complete a standardized four-day diary of the child's behaviors and activities. The information from the teachers, clinical examiners, and the home observers was in good agreement. However, the parent questionnaires were completely unrelated to other sources of information about the children. But the mothers' diaries were related to the home observations and to clinic and school ratings. The culprit in this study therefore seemed to be the form of the parent questionnaire. Perhaps parents do not have an adequate frame of reference to deal with the requested judgments such as "just a little," "pretty much," or "very much" concerning the child's behavior. With the diary they did not have to make such comparative judgments but could simply record descriptive information. Therefore, the use of simple parent diaries to record child behaviors at home which are of concern has much to recommend it.

For school-age children referred because of behavior problems, ratings by one or more teachers of the child's behavior should be regarded as an indispensable part of the evaluation of the child. Teacher ratings of this kind are well standardized, have acceptable interrater and test-retest reliability, and seem to be the most valid of the measures that can be obtained at relatively low cost. Quay (1979) provides a detailed and comprehensive review of the psychological dimensions usually found in studies of such rating scales. The two most common of these dimensions, Conduct Disorder and Anxiety-Withdrawal, seem to be literally ubiquitous in rating scale studies, regardless of the particular scales used. The scale that seems to be the most firmly established in clinical use is the Conners Teacher Rating Scale (Conners, 1969). This scale is standardized, has been validated, particularly as a measure of hyperactivity (attention deficit disorder), and is sensitive to the effects of both pharmacological and behavioral treatment (Routh, 1978; Routh & Mesibov, 1980). Although teacher rating scales should be a crucial part of the evaluation and monitoring of the behavior problems of children seen in pediatric settings, their use is far from universal. Sprague and Gadow (1977), for example, deplore the fact that although most elementary school teachers have had children in their classes who receive stimulant drugs, it is still a rare event for them to be requested by a physician to help evaluate the behavior of such a child. Given that classroom behavior is a key bit of diagnostic information, and one of the main indices of drug effectiveness, this is disturbing information. Johnson, Kenney, and Davis (1977) argue that if such a drug is to be used with a child, the school should, as a matter of policy, agree to observe, record, and report behavior changes to the physician. The pediatric psychologist, as a person knowledgeable concerning the research literature on the use of teacher rating scales, could be a key liaison person in helping to put such a practice into widespread use.

RESEARCH ON TREATMENT

Developing and evaluating treatment procedures for children has always been a high priority area in pediatric psychology. The following topics will be discussed under this heading: primary prevention; early intervention; treatment approaches to common problems of the preschool child; the use of behavioral treatment procedures with children; parent counseling; and family therapy.

Primary Prevention

One important type of primary prevention research in which pediatric psychologists might become involved is related to genetic counseling. It has been estimated that 90% of the solid information concerning human genetics is the product of the most recent 30 years. In the times before Mendel, only three hereditary diseases were known—hemophilia, Huntington's chorea, and congenital deafness. We now have a strong biochemical foundation for clinical applications in genetics: the knowledge that chromosomes consist of DNA, which via RNA provide the template for the production of the enzymes which in turn regulate the metabolism of all cells in the body. Hundreds of genetic diseases have now been identified, and the mapping of human chromosomes is proceeding at a rapid pace. It is clear that in the next few years hundreds of new genetic diseases will be found which affect children, many of which will turn out to be preventable through appropriate genetic counseling. Already, about 10% of admissions to pediatric services are considered to be due to genetic disease, and another 25% are related to the child's genotype (Neel, 1976). How can parents or potential parents be informed most effectively in cases where there are significant genetic risks to their offspring? How can they be helped to take appropriate action based on such knowledge? The implications of such research for the prevention of genetic disease are evident.

A current example of research-based, psychosocial primary intervention is provided by the trend toward encouraging the parents of low-birth-weight newborn infants to spend as much time as possible in direct contact with their babies, participating in their care. Parents are being encouraged to become, in effect, part of the staff of neonatal intensive care units where they previously had been excluded. This policy resulted from the work of such researchers as Klaus and Kennell (1976) suggesting that contact of mother and infant during the first postpartum days is important to the formation of the mother's affectional bond to the infant and that the mothers who do not visit their hospitalized newborns are at greater risk than others for child abuse, neglect, and having infants with failure-to-thrive syndrome.

Early Intervention

One of the most successful examples of a biomedical early intervention is the use of the low phenylalanine diet in infancy and early childhood to prevent the adverse effects of phenylketonuria on brain growth and development, and hence to prevent the severe form of mental retardation that would otherwise result. This is regarded as a form of early intervention rather than prevention in that even after exposure to the special diet, the child at a genetic and biochemical level still has PKU, which can be transmitted to subsequent offspring or can affect a fetus in utero should a female with PKU become pregnant.

An interesting example of a psychosocial type of early intervention is provided by the Townsend and Flanagan (1976) study. These investigators worked with 61 severely and profoundly retarded children under age 6, whose parents had applied to have them placed in a state institution. Children in both the experimental group (N = 31) and control group (N = 30) received the usual preadmission counseling over a 12-week waiting period (office interview, tour of the institution, family history, collection of information for the staff conference, etc.). The experimental group received, in addition, home treatment consisting of instruction in child training, discussion of relevant community resources, and counseling about mental retardation, the needs of the child, and homemaking. The treatment required three or four meetings with the parents, each two to three hours long, spread over an eight-week period. The treatment resulted in significant changes in the amount of objectionable behaviors of the child. Of the experimental group, 53% reported a decrease in such behaviors, as compared to only 20% of the control group. The degree of marital conflict, however, went up to 57% in the experimental group, compared to 30% in the control group. Evidently, when the child's behavior improved and it seemed possible that the child could continue to stay at home, disagreements between the spouses ensued. Of those parents who initially said that they definitely planned to institutionalize the child, none changed their minds, despite some instances of the child's behavioral improvement. Similarly, those who initially said that they simply wanted temporary respite care also did not change their minds. It was only in the group of parents who had some hope of taking the child back home, but were uncertain, that the treatment program reduced the prevalence of long-term institutionalization of the child. Although this intervention program was not intended to have effects as dramatic as the low phenylalanine diet for PKU children mentioned above, it did appear to prevent some children from being placed in a type of living arrangement which is both very expensive financially and less adequate than good home care. These are worthy objectives for early intervention research.

Treatment Approaches for Common Problems of the Preschool Child

Mesibov, Schroeder, and Wesson (1977) reported on children's problems for which parents requested help from a call-in and come-in service offered to them through a group pediatric practice. The peak age of children complained about was 2 to 3, and the most frequent concern was about negative behaviors such as noncompliance. Other frequent concerns were about toilet training and procedures for training self-help skills.

When a parent brings a child to the clinic because of the child's noncompliant behavior, it is possible to deal with the problem by the use of straightforward behavioral techniques. For example, Forehand and King (1974) demonstrated that parents could be taught to provide positive reinforcement when their preschoolers complied with commands, and to use a time-out procedure when the children did not comply. This resulted in significantly greater compliance by the child in a clinic playroom, which also seemed to generalize to the child's behavior at home.

However, there appears to be something of a paradox here. On one hand, behavioral procedures such as those just described seem to be very effective in helping parents control unruly children. On the other hand, studies reviwed by Hoffman (1975) indicate that the use of such power-assertive techniques by parents may be associated with subsequent conduct disorder in the child. Hoffman favors the use of what he calls inductive techniques by parents, that is, pointing out the consequences of a child's behavior for others and encouraging the child to develop empathy with others' feelings.

Contemporary research is beginning to suggest that the techniques actually used by parents in controlling their children's behavior effectively are more complex than had been assumed. Peele and Routh (978), for example, devised a situation in which mothers were asked to control the behavior of their 3-year-old children, expecting to find that the mothers used such well-known psychological principles as positive reinforcement (praise), punishment (disapproval and criticism), or modeling of appropriate behavior. Very little use of these techniques was seen. Instead, mothers used such strategies as distracting the child by engaging in dramatic play, verbal reasoning with the child, and bargaining.

In a recent sophisticated analysis of control techniques used by mothers with their preschool children, Schaffer and Crook (1980) concluded that maternal controls were most likely to succeed in gaining compliance if they were properly timed in relation to the child's ongoing activities and if they formed part of a sequential strategy, first getting the child's attention, then encouraging the child to make contact with the desired materials, and finally encouraging the desired action. It seems likely that clinical procedures for dealing with children's noncompliance will be even more effective and lasting if they are based on a fuller knowledge of the actual techniques used by parents who are successful in raising well-behaved children. The same principle would seem to apply to research dealing with tantrums, toilet training, and helping preschool children to develop self-help skills.

Use of Behavioral Treatment Procedures with Children

It is of course far beyond the scope of a single chapter even to sketch current research issues concerning behavioral treatment of children. This literature continues to increase, with new journals and books constantly appearing on the subject. The behavioral literature presently overshadows research on all other types of psychological treatment. For example, when Routh and Mesibov (1980) were assigned the task of reviewing psychological and environmental interventions for helping children with so-called minimal brain dysfunction (MBD), they found themselves discussing behavior modification approaches and very little else. This happened by default, simply because most of the published research literature focused on behavioral approaches.

In their review chapter, Routh and Mesibov concluded that, indeed, behavior modification works with children, especially when one is concerned with circumscribed behaviors in particular situations. Behavioral techniques can be used to induce children to sit still, reduce their disruptive behaviors in class, pay attention, and improve their academic performance. Parents can be taught behavior modification procedures to use in dealing with children's behavior problems at home.

In fact, behavioral techniques have been elaborated which have such power that it causes one to pause and reconsider some issues of human values, beyond the purely technical domain of what techniques are effective. These techniques vary not only in their efficacy in changing behavior but also in their degree of coerciveness. For example, while it might be pleasant for everyone around for a child to sit still and be less disruptive, what is the maximum amount of pressure that should be exerted in producing such a result? There may come a point when the value of the changed behavior does not equal the objections that might be raised to the degree of coercion research, though researchers must be very aware of them. In thinking about such issues, Routh and Mesibov (1980) suggested that one might wish to place reinforcements and punishments in a hierarchy of the following kind:

1. Intrinsic rewards and punishments (those that are inherent in an activity).
2. Rewards and punishments that are a natural consequence of the action.
3. Extrinsic rewards and punishments that are culturally normative for persons in a given situation.
4. Extrinsic rewards that are culturally normative for persons in some situations but unusual for the individual in those particular situations.
5. Unusual or needlessly coercive rewards and punishments.

Other things being equal, the incentives at the top of this list are to be preferred to those nearer the bottom, and rewards are in general preferable to punishments. Thus, in teaching children to read, it would seem desirable when possible to rely on the intrinsic value of being able to decipher an interesting story from a book. Not having money to spend on a shopping errand teaches a child to be more careful with loose change. Food may be an appropriate reinforcer for a toddler learning the correct use of a fork, but not for controlling the behavior of a junior high school student. And in ethical terms, there may be few circumstances when certain types of corporal punishment are justified, even if they might be effective in changing behavior.

Parent Counseling

The idea of dealing with children's problems through counseling or instructing the parents is not new and seems to be endorsed by therapists of every theoretical persuasion. This was Freud's (1909/1959) method of attempting to treat the fear of horses of his most famous child patient, Little Hans. Carl Rogers encouraged his daughter, Natalie Fuchs (1957) to undertake play therapy sessions with her own child at home. The corresponding classic from the behavioral literature is the study by Hawkins, Peterson, Schweid, and Bijou (1966) using the parent as therapist to ameliorate a problem in parent-child relations.

It seems to add greater efficiency to deal with parents in groups rather than individually. In one of the best known studies of the effectiveness of parent group counseling, Tavormina (1975) worked with 51 mothers of mentally retarded children with behavior problems. They were assigned to one of three types of group. Those in the reflective counseling groups read Ginott's (1965) book *Between Parent and Child* and engaged in two months of group discussions on reflecting feelings, setting appropriate limits, providing alternative activities for their children, andso on. Those in the behavioral counseling groups read Becker's (1971) book *Parents Are Teachers: A Child Management Program* and engaged in group discussions and role playing of the use of praise, the use of positive rather than negative contingencies, the need to specify the behaviors to be changed, and related topics. The other groups served as a waiting list control condition. In general, the behavioral counseling groups had significantly better results than the reflective groups, which did significantly better than the controls on a variety of measures that included parent attitudes, children's behavior checklists, and direct observations of the children's behavior.

Still greater cost effectiveness seems at least potentially possible through the use of books, manuals, and other such means of training parents to facilitate development and manage their children's behavior problems. These could be used either as a supplement to or a substitute for contact between parents and professionals, depending on the complexity of the problems dealt with. Reviewing popular primers for parents, Clarke-Stewart (1978) presented evidence that more and more of these books are being published in the U.S. each year (42 new ones were published in 1975 alone), and that today almost all parents read at least one such book. Thus, if such books are really effective, they might constitute the treatment equivalent of the universal screening programs mentioned under the heading of research on assessment.

What is largely missing at this point is rigorous research on the efficacy of such written materials (or of audio or video tapes) in changing parents' behavior and preventing or ameliorating children's behavior problems. In a pioneering study of this kind, Heifetz (1977) found that training manuals alone were surprisingly effective in helping parents teach their retarded children self-help skills; in fact, the manuals-alone condition was not only better than the control group but was as effective as more expensive formats involving training groups, home visits, and telephone consultations. More such research needs to be done.

Family Therapy

When the clinical problem seems to lie in the relationship system rather than in the child or any other family member as an individual, some kind of family therapy would seem to be the preferred treatment approach. This type of situation is familiar to every pediatric psychologist either in pure form or as a complication in the family's response to medical problems. For example, at the outset, one parent may be overinvolved with the child and his or her problems (which could be anything from difficulty with spelling to diabetes); the other parent is rather detached from the situation, and often the child is not relating well to peers. Family therapy aims to produce an outcome in which the child's problem is not only in hand but the parents are relating better to each other and the child is more involved with peers. Another area where family therapy seems to be a rational approach is in the problems of adolescents. Here there is a need for fostering reciprocal communication and negotiation between parents and the teenager. One should not simply work to help the parents control their offspring in authoritarian fashion.

Family problems appear to be epidemic at this time. One index of them is the high rate of marital distress, divorce, and the difficulties of adjustment in second marriages where one or both partners brings children along. The growing medical specialty of family practice tries to deal with such problems in addition to providing primary health care. Surely pediatricians and pediatric psychologists also need to be alert to new developments in family therapy.

From a research point of view, the field of family therapy is chaotic. In fact, little credible research is being done in the area.

In this field there is no standard body of knowledge with agreed-upon goals and defined limits; there is a diversity of approaches; there is no one right way to do family therapy or marital therapy; there is no comprehensive theory; and there is no one way to train. (Framo, 1979, p. 869)

One would hope that behavior therapy researchers, with their rigorous methodological standards, would be attracted to this field. However, as Werry (1979) points out, behavioral researchers have so far been slow to adopt the idea of the family as a system, preferring to concentrate on the behavior of the individual or a dyad such as the married couple or parent-child interaction.

A few promising signs are beginning to appear of behavioral researchers working with families or family therapists publishing research results. For example, Robin, Kent, O'Leary, Foster, and Prinz (1977) trained parents and adolescents in problemsolving and communication skills, and found that this significantly increased their problemsolving behaviors in structured discussions compared to a waiting list control group. No clear evidence of generalization to their behavior at home was presented, however. Minuchin, Rosman, Baker, and Liebman (1978), using family therapy, reported an impressive 88% recovery rate in adolescent females with anorexia nervosa. They obtained psychosocial as well as medical data at follow-up. This study has been properly criticized because it lacked a control group and because it confounded the effects of family therapy with those of the behavioral treatment which was also part of the package. Nevertheless, their results are considerably better than the usual outcome of treatment studies with anorexia nervosa.

Pediatric psychologists should get involved in family therapy research. Their unique background may be able to produce, at last, the combination of rigor and clinical relevance now absent from the literature on family therapy.

RESEARCH ON PSYCHOLOGICAL ASPECTS OF HEALTH AND ILLNESS IN CHILDREN

As a researcher, the pediatric psychologist needs the perspective to stand back a bit from the everyday demands of assessment and treatment. Research on psychological aspects of health and illness in children goes beyond psychosomatic medicine to encompass psychological aspects of all kinds of physical disease and the broader areas of health-promoting behaviors. A few representative research topics within this area are discussed below.

Long-Term Outcome of High-Risk Infants

Longitudinal study of children from conception through maturity is a most important research tool for the pediatric psychologist. The events of interest range from the early spontaneous abortion of the fetus through survival of the individual into adulthood. The continuum of possibilities in between includes fetal or neonatal death; gross malformation evident at birth; severe neurobehavioral handicap such as autism, mental retardation, cerebral palsy, or seizure disorder; milder behavioral difficulties in childhood such as learning disabilities or emotional problems; versus academic and social competence predictive of a satisfying and useful adult life.

It is possible to view this entire spectrum from a strictly biological standpoint. Lilienfeld and Parkhurst (1951) used the term "continuum of reproductive wastage" to refer to the spectrum extending from perinatal death and abortion through cerebral palsy and epilepsy but also including learning disability (considered to be a subtle form of cerebral dysfunction). Pasamanick and Knobloch (1960) advocated a somewhat broader though still exclusively biological concept of a "continuum of reproductive casualty" which included in addition minor motor, perceptual, intellectual, and behavioral difficulties. In a review of their own and others' retrospective studies, Pasamanick and Knobloch (1966) found evidence for a significant association between complications of pregnancy and prematurity and such outcomes as cerebral palsy, mental deficiency, behavior disorders, and reading disabilities.

Sameroff and Chandler (1975) broadened these concepts considerably in their review of "reproductive risk and the continuum of caretaking casualty." They pointed out that in longitudinal, prospective studies the strictly biological predictors such as anoxia or other perinatal complications had proven to be of limited value. Social status and ethnic group membership seem to be important mediator variables. As Sameroff and Chandler note, the typical 3- to 5-point mean IQ difference found at school age between children with histories of reproductive complications and those without such histories is much smaller than the 15 points typically found between blacks and whites and the 50 points between adults at the top and bottom of the socioeconomic scale. The Kauai study of Werner and her colleagues (Werner, Bierman, & French, 1971; Werner & Smith, 1977) provided an especially clear example of the importance of caretaking variables as predictors of long-term outcomes. In the Kauai study, complications of pregnancy and delivery were somewhat predictive of later difficulty in children whose families were of low socioeconomic status and provided little educational stimulation or emotional support. In middle-class families which were educationally stimulating and emotionally supportive, however, biological complications during infancy had little predictive value. In fact, 10 times as many children in the Kauai study had problems attributable to the effects of a poor psychosocial environment than had problems attributable to the effects of perinatal stress.

A recent study by Zeskind and Ramey (1978) has produced experimental confirmation of what would be predicted from Sameroff and Chandler's hypothesis of a transactional relationship between biological and psychological factors in development. Zeskind and Ramey worked with infants from families of a low socioeconomic level. Some of the infants had been fetally malnourished as measured by a low ponderal index (the ratio of birth weight to the cube of birth length), and others had normal fetal nutrition as measured in this way. All infants were randomly assigned either to an instructional day-care program designed to prevent mental retardation or to a nonintervention control group. At three months of age, infants with low ponderal index were significantly below those with normal ponderal index in terms of their Bayley Mental Development Index scores. Mothers of low ponderal index children in the control group had less involvement with their infants than other mothers. At both 18 and 24 months, the ponderal index had continued predictive value only for children in the control group. In the instructional day-care group, low ponderal index children scored as well on the Bayley and Stanford Binet tests as children with a normal ponderal index. Thus, as in the Kauai study, a stimulating psychosocial environment seemed to be able to compensate for initial biological disadvantage.

Severe Problems of Parenting: Child Abuse, Neglect, and Nonorganic Failure-to-Thrive

The problem of child abuse continues to be one with high public visibility. The most widely accepted definition of an abused child seems to be that of Parke and Collmer (1975):

> Any child who received nonaccidental physical injury (or injuries) as a result of acts (or omissions) on the part of his parents or guardians that violate community standards concerning the treatment of children. (p. 513)

The National Center of Child Abuse and Neglect was established by federal legislation in 1974. In 1977 an international journal, *Child Abuse and Neglect,* which publishes research in this area, began appearing in print.

Nonorganic failure-to-thrive in infants, which after all may involve simply inadequate feeding of the infant as one aspect, is a phenomenon at least conceptually related to child abuse and neglect.

A large number of demonstration treatment projects have been put in motion, but an evaluation of 11 such programs by the National Child Abuse Program

Evaluation (described by Cohn, 1980) produced discouraging results. In general, these demonstration projects lacked control groups. Only 42% of the approximately 1700 adult clients studied were less likely to reabuse or neglect their children by the end of treatment. Indeed, 30% of the parents studied were said to have severely reabused or neglected their children even while they were receiving active treatment services.

It is clear that we have much to learn before we will be able to create treatment or prevention strategies that will stand up under rigorous evaluation. Thus child abuse and neglect may be one of those problems for which an indirect research approach will be more productive in the long run than a direct frontal assault, so to speak. Parke and Collmer (1975) described three different approaches commonly taken in child abuse research: personality (what is wrong with the parents or with the child-victim), sociological (situational or stress factors), and social-situational (the interaction of personality and situation). Some very good research continues to be done but more under the separate personality and sociological headings than the interactive one. For example, Burgess and Conger (1978) collected observational data in the homes of abusive, neglectful, and normal families. Interestingly, the neglectful parents appeared to be more deviant in their behavior than the abusive ones, relative to the control group. Both abusive and neglectful parents demonstrated lower rates of interaction, and the neglectful parents were more likely to emphasize the negative in their relationships with their children. Rather than studying the parents, George and Main (1979) studied abused children age 1-3 years in a day-care setting and compared their social behavior with that of other nonabused toddlers. The abused children were more aggressive in their interactions with both peers and caregivers, and also more avoidant in response to friendly overtures by others. Turning to studies with a more sociological approach, Garbarino and Crouter (1978) used child abuse report rates under a state mandatory reporting law to study 20 neighborhood areas and 93 census tracts in a Nebraska county. They found a strong relationship between reported child abuse and socioeconomic indices such as income levels, type of housing, neighborhood transiency, and so on, and argued that the effects were real ones and not simply due to any socioeconomic bias in reporting. Gaines, Sandgrund, Green, and Power (1978) found that family life stresses such as unemployment, illness, arrest, and eviction were the most important variable in separating abusing, neglecting, and normal mothers in a multiple discriminant analysis. As in the Burgess and Conger study, the neglect group was more deviant than the abuse group, compared to controls.

Another worthwhile development in child abuse research is that of studies which attempt to predict child maltreatment in advance. Obviously, "high risk" factors will have to be identified and confirmed in prospective studies before preventative research will be a practical possibility. Altemeier, Vietze, Sherrod, Sandler, Falsey, and O'Connor (1979), for example, followed up a subsample of an initial group of 1400 expectant mothers an average of one year after the birth of their infants to identify those with problems of child abuse, neglect, or nonorganic failure-to-thrive. A group of 273 mothers expected to be at high risk for such parenting disorders was indeed found to have a higher incidence of such disorders than a group of 225 randomly selected from the remainder of the sample. The best predictor on their high-risk index was found to be the mother's history of being abused during her own childhood. This factor predicted both abuse/neglect and nonorganic failure-to-thrive. In a similar prospective follow-up study of a high-risk group of mothers and infants, Egeland and Brunnquell (1979) attempted to validate a Child Care Rating Scale based on a home visit. They estimated a base rate of child abuse of 1 to 2% in their population of primiparous women receiving prenatal care at a Public Health Clinic, but were surprised to learn that by going into the homes and taking a more careful look, they found rates closer to 10%.

Accidents

Accidents are different from child abuse and neglect in that the caregiver cannot be held legally responsible for a child's accidental injury. However, the distinction is in many cases relative rather than absolute. Gregg and Elmer (1969) in a study comparing child abuse and accidental injuries to infants remarked that most of the accidents could have been prevented by commonsense safety measures. Although the injuries of the abused group were more severe, Elmer (1978) found the abused/neglected and accidental injury groups practically indistinguishable in outcome eight years later in a follow-up study. Children in both groups were frequently behind in language and intellectual development and had behavior problems.

According to the National Center for Health Statistics (1978) accidents continue to be the leading cause of death in children past infancy. For this reason alone research on the causes of such injuries and on appropriate countermeasures deserves high priority. It might be thought that the main accident hazards are due to physical environmental dangers, and therefore an engineer is a better choice for such research than a psychologist. Certainly, the engineer has a role. Oglesbay (1969) reported that there was a female-to-male death ratio of 31:1 among burn victims under 12 years of age, simply because of the greater flammability of girls' clothing compared to that of boys. But cultural changes including the women's liberation movement would seem to have lessened the problem by making it more acceptable for girls to wear clothing other than dresses.

In other cases, what appears to be a problem of environmental engineering turns out to be more one involving relationships in the family. Sobel (1970) conducted a house-to-house study involving the unannounced appearance of interviewers and their assistants who completed an index of household poison hazards. It was found that the household hazard index had no relationship to the occurrence of poisoning among the children in the families. Instead, the incidence of accidental poisoning was found to be highly related to psychopathology in the mother and the father, to the presence of marital difficulty, and to a history of stressful life events such as a death in the family, loss of a job, or others requiring major family readjustment.

The child's personality also has a role to play in the likelihood of accidents. In a study of 684 children who were representative of high-, intermediate-, and low-accident liability levels among a larger population, Manheimer and Mellinger (1967) found that males, highly active children, those who were socially extroverted, and children described as "daring" were more likely than others to have accidents. In explaining these findings, the authors noted that extroversion can be regarded as an index of amount of contact with other people, and activity and daring as indices of amount of contact with certain aspects of the nonhuman environment. In both cases, increased contact would increase the exposure of the child to various risk conditions. An analogy might be made between the child who frequently engages in roughhousing with peers or in walking along high railings and the adult traveling salesman who interacts with hundreds of customers and logs thousands of miles per year on the highway. Both are at higher risk for accidents if only because of greater exposure to the conditions in which accidents are likely to occur.

Retrospective research such as the above study, informative as it has been, has serious limitations. People's attributions of certain traits to children may, for example, be influenced by the very fact that the child had certain types of accidents. If a child got hurt, the child must have been an active, daring extrovert, or so it might seem after the fact. It is therefore gratifying that, to an increasing extent, prospective studies are now beginning to appear. Matheny, Brown, and Wilson (1971), as part of their research on twins, found that 1-year-olds identified as having high activity level, short attention span, or as being temperamental had significantly more accidents on follow-up than their co-twins. Among 43 twin pairs discordant on activity and accident frequency, the more active twin was found to account for 71 out of 89 accidents reported at follow-up. In a more recent prospective study, Matheny (1980) found a negative relationship between twins' scores on Elkind's visual-perceptual exploration test at age 6 years and the number of accidents recorded between 6 and 9 years of age. Matheny interpreted his results to mean that such accident-liable children not only were likely to expose themselves to risk more often but also were likely to assess the situation and its potential for harm differently and be less likely to learn from their accidents than their less-liable co-twins.

Psychological Aspects of Infectious Disease in Children

There are several important relationships between the behavior of children and their families and the phenomenon of infectious disease, ranging all the way from the pathways through which such diseases are transmitted to and by the child through the behavioral reactions of children to infectious illness, parents' decisions to use home remedies with the child or consult a physician, to factors affecting compliance with doctors' prescriptions of medication, not to mention the role of central nervous system infections in producing behavioral disability. One ordinary child behavior which affects disease rates is going to school. Children are more susceptible to infectious disease than are adults, and those in day-care or school settings are the most likely of any family member to acquire common infectious diseases from each other and to transmit them to others, according to the data of the classical longitudinal family study by Dingle, Badger, and Jordan (1964). Preschool children in families with school children are therefore more likely to have respiratory disease than preschoolers with no school children in their families.

Having an acute, febrile infectious illness in itself has predictable effects on the behavior of the child. According to the study of Mattson and Weisberg (1970) practically all young children show some temporary loss of age-appropriate behavior during an illness, for example, refusal to assist in dressing and undressing, and may show an increase in thumb sucking and the use of various comforters at nighttime. There seem to be important differences in the reactions of younger versus older children, with the 2-year-old typically showing a clinging, whiney dependence in reaction to the illness, which the child over the age of 3 was more likely to retreat into a self-centered, rather undemanding state. Interviewing older children in the hospital for a short-term illness, Campbell (1978) found that a "Spartan" orientation characterized by a refusal to show emotion and rejection of the sick role was especially characteristic of older children, boys, and children of parents with higher social status.

Mothers seem to vary considerably in their attitudes and behaviors related to their children's illness (the child-health-related attitudes and behaviors of fathers have bcen very little studied). According to the data of Becker, Nathanson, Drachman, and Kirscht (1977) some mothers have an active orientation toward health care, believing in the value of preventive health measures and having positive feelings about the sources of health care. Women in this group were found to be high users of preventive services (such as well-child visits to the clinic) and generated few visits for the child's illness or accidents. Presumably the children of these mothers would have received all appropriate immunizations, and thus would be less likely to be affected by a major contagious disease should they encounter it. Another group of mothers had a much more passive, fatalistic attitude toward health and disease. They were less likely to bring their children in for preventive visits but significantly more likely to bring their child in because of illness or accident. It would be interesting to know the patterns of these two groups of mothers with respect to the use of over-the-counter medications for their children and their levels of compliance with medically prescribed treatment regimens.

The problem of noncompliance with prescribed courses of treatment seems to be an ever-present one. In a classic study, Bergman and Werner (1963), using interviews, counts of pills, and biochemical assays of urine specimens, found that even though 95% of parents were familiar with the proper directions for giving a course of penicillin to their children—three times a day for a full 10 days—very few parents actually complied with the instructions. By even the most liberal criteria of compliance, 71% had stopped administering the antibiotic by the sixth day, and 82% by the ninth day. Charney, Bynum, Eldredge, Frank, MacWhinney, McNabb, Scheiner, Sumpter, and Iker (1967) found that in a more socially advantaged group of families, compliance with an oral penicillin regimen was correlated with the mother's (not the physician's) estimate of the severity of the child's condition, with whether or not their usual doctor prescribed the medicine, and with favorable personality traits of the mother as rated by the pediatrician. Gordis, Markowitz, and Lilienfeld (1969), working with a population of black inner-city youngsters, developed a list of six risk factors. When four or more of these factors were present, the probability of noncompliance was .90.

The area of psychological aspects of infectious disease is thus potentially very fertile field of research for behavioral scientists. Fuchs (1972) made a statement that applies here, that the greatest potential for improving health, in the absence of dramatic breakthroughs in medical science itself, is through changes in what people—both children and parents—do or do not do for themselves.

Stressful Aspects of Health Care Procedures

The child's encounters with health care settings, whether as a hospital patient or as an outpatient, often involve various kinds of stress such as separation from familiar persons, painful experiences such as injections, and the need to cooperate with various unfamiliar and sometimes frightening medical procedures.

Such stresses can even have long-term adverse impact on the child. The well-known studies of Douglas (1975) reported a 26-year follow-up of children brought up in England at a time when most hospitals had policies greatly restricting parental visits to their children in the hospital. The children's age at the time of hospitalization was an important factor in this study, in that children under 6 months of age or over 4½ years were little affected by the experience. Those aged 6 months to 4½ years tended to deteriorate in their behavior at home upon discharge, especially if they had been in the hospital a week or longer. Children admitted to hospitals with less restrictive visiting policies were less likely to show such problems. The children whose behavior deteriorated at home continued to have trouble later in life. At age 13−15 years they tended to be rated by their teachers as troublesome and nervous. At age 15 they performed relatively poorly in measured reading ability (though this was explainable partly on the basis of their degree of physical impairment). They had a higher number of contacts with the police and the courts for delinquent behavior at age 17. Finally, those who were not in school at age 15−18 years had a higher number of job changes.

What is so stressful about hospitalization and other experiences undergone by children in health care settings? One component as already indicated as simply the separation from mother and other familiar caregivers. In the past, excluding parents and other visitors was justified partly on the grounds that "young children are more easily upset emotionally and cry longer and more loudly when their mothers are absent" (Shirley & Poyntz, 1941, p. 251). Indeed this seems to be true for brief aversive procedures. Shaw and Routh (1980) found that children receiving routine injections in a pediatric office cried more when the mother was present than when she was absent from the examining room. However, the children in such a situation seem to be, if anything, more emotionally upset when their mothers are absent, but inhibit expression of distress if the time is brief and the pain not overwhelming. In longer and more frightening medical procedures, the effects of the presence of the mother seems to lessen the amount of stress involved. Vernon, Foley, and Schulman (1967), for example, studied the effects of separation from mother on the behavior of two to five year olds during anesthesia induction. Interestingly, the significant effect was not for the first phase of induction, when the mask was placed and held over the child's face, but only the second phase, from one minute after the mask was placed until a surgical level of anesthesia was reached. During this excitement phase of anasthesia, the children whose mother was absent showed more unhappiness, whining, and so on, than those whose mother was present. Similarly, Frankl, Shiere, and Fogels (1962) concluded that children were less negative and more cooperative when the mother was in the dental operatory with the child than when she was absent.

A second stressful aspect of medical procedures for the child is the amount of pain involved. One of the most common medical experiences is for children evidently one of the most painful. Of 119 children asked "Of all the things that have ever happened to you, what hurt you the worst?" 65 replied "a shot" or "a needle" (Eland & Anderson, 1977, p. 463). Researchers and clinicians, being adults themselves, seem to be rather insensitive to the importance of pain for children. Eland and Anderson (1977) reviewed the medical literature from 1970 to 1975 and found that of 1380 articles on pain, only 33, or 2% dealt with pain in children. In a study of 18 adults and 25 children hospitalized with identical diagnoses, these same investigators reported that the adults received a total of 671 doses of analgesic medications, while the children received a total of only 24 doses of analgesics. The children seemed to be either less able or less willing to verbalize their pain in such a way as to obtain the relief available. One factor seemed to be that the children were afraid to describe their pain for fear of receiving an injection as a result.

In terms of helping the child cope with painful experiences, peer or even sibling modeling seems to be one useful approach. However, the model should not give an unrealistic portrayal of the amount of pain involved in the procedures the child is later to experience. Vernon (1974) found that observing another child receive an injection, wince, and say "ouch" did help children cope with their own subsequent injections. However, it was positively unhelpful if the model acted as if the injection did not hurt at all; children who observed this model were the most upset of the three groups when they received their own injections. Ghose, Giddon, Shiere, and Fogels (1969) found that, at least for 4-year-olds, the experience of watching an older sibling in the dental operatory helped the children behave more cooperatively themselves in a later dental experience.

A third source of stress involved in hospitalization and to a lesser extent in the care of a sick child at home is the restriction in the child's ordinary activities of play, peer interaction, and participation in school. At the extreme, deprivation of such normal activities among children in long-term residential care has been associated with deterioration in children's social interests and skills and the emergence of, for example, rocking and other types of maladaptive stereotyped behaviors (Klaber & Butterfield, 1968). It is the purpose of "child life" and educational programs in hospitals—volunteers, play leaders, and teachers—to try to normalize the everyday lives of children who must be confined to a hospital. Although there has so far been little research on these matters, at least some initial studies have been carried out (Hall, 1977).

In part as a result of some of the research discussed here, hospitals and pediatric and dental offices have introduced quite a number of innovations which undoubtedly help children cope with some of the stresses in being a child patient. Many hospitals have liberalized their visiting policies even to the extent of allowing a parent the option of "rooming in" with a young child and the more frequent use of day hospitalization for surgery as opposed to the traditional overnight or long-term stay. According to a recent survey (Peterson & Ridley-Johnson, 1980), 70% of nonchronic care pediatric hospitals in the United States offer prehospital preparation programs to both parent and child. Commercial modeling films are used in many pedodontic waiting rooms. Most large hospitals have full-time child life staffs and teachers who come in to provide educational experiences for children. Much research remains to be done, however, before we will be able to understand how to minimize the stress of hospitalization and other health care procedures.

Life-Threatening and Chronic Illness in Children

It was not too many years ago that a clear distinction had to be drawn between life-threatening and chronic illnesses in children. Leukemia, for example, was almost invariably fatal. A major research issue was whether children age 6–10 years who had terminal cancer were aware of their prognosis despite the fact that everyone tried to keep it from them. A study by Bluebond-Langner (1974) which involved participant observation by an anthropologist on a pediatric hematology/oncology ward suggested that such children were indeed quite preoccupied with the likelihood of their death. This was confirmed by studies using psychological measures such as the themes in stories child cancer patients told in response to sets of pictures or their placement of figures in a three-dimensional model of a hospital room (Spinetta, Rigler, & Karon, 1973, 1974; Waechter, 1968). In these studies there was a clear difference between the reactions of children with cancer and those with non-life-threatening illness. The children with cancer were more anxious and more isolated than other ill children, increasingly so as they neared death. These studies paved the way for a policy of more open communication with these children by both their parents and health-care personnel. Nitschke, Wunder, Sexauer, and Humphrey (1977) even demonstrated that children as young as 6 years of age were able to be meaningfully involved in the decision of whether to try experimental drugs or to end active chemotherapy after all conventional treatments had failed. There was no change in the proportion of families who opted for such experimental drug treatment before and after the children themselves began to be involved in this decision.

Now, because of advances in medical technology, children with cancer have a much better chance of survival. The present clinical and research issues in their psychosocial care concern ways of helping them cope with living rather than dying: dealing with the social impact of the effects of chemotherapy or surgery, relating to family and peers, and other such issues (Spinetta, in press). Thus leukemia has come to be much more like the chronic but non-life-threatening illnesses with which it was once so strongly contrasted. O'Malley, Koocher, Foster, and Slavin (1979) have documented the fact that not just some but most survivors of childhood malignancies have emotional and behavioral problems. Deasy-Spinetta and Spinetta (1980) have provided a teacher's eye view of these children as having difficulty concentrating, lacking energy, and not reaching out to others. Indeed Lansky, Lowman, Vats, and Gyulay (1975) found school phobia to be a common problem in children with cancer. Lansky, Cairns, Hassanein, Wehr, and Lowman (1978) found childhood cancer to be associated with marital disharmony in the parents. Kalnins, Churchill, and Terry (1980) described a whole array of concurrent stresses in the families of leukemic children, including the illness of other family members, occupational problems, financial difficulties, and other events such as moving or changes in vocational plans.

In dealing with both life-threatening and chronic illnesses in children, then, we are concerned not only with survival but with a very broad range of outcomes. Starfield (1974) has succinctly listed them as what one might call the six Ds: death, disease, disability, discomfort, dissatisfaction, and (social) disruption. For each one, a positive alternative may be stated: instead of death, longevity; instead of disease, an absence of symptoms; instead of disability, functional capacity and achievement; instead of discomfort, comfort; instead of dissatisfaction, satisfaction; and instead of disruption, harmonious relationships with family and society. Actually, three of Starfield's outcome categories (disability, dissatisfaction, and disruption) are familiar to any student of psychopathology. Listing all six categories together emphasizes the inseparability of the physical and behavioral aspects of human outcomes. Future research must deal with this entire spectrum of effects and correlates of all types of chronic illness in childhood.

Research in Developmental and Learning Disabilities

Pediatric psychologists, especially those who work in developmental clinics, find it most important to stay current with research in developmental disabilities—mental retardation, cerebral palsy, seizure disorders, autism, learning disabilities, attention deficit disorder, and related problems. Many of the research contributions of pediatric psychologists have been in this area. It is, however, simply not possible in a single chapter such as this to give more than the most cursory overview of the broad field of developmental and learning disabilities. Since research in developmental disabilities is generally better established than many of the research areas which have been discussed above, however, the reader can simply be referred to good sources of current information in this field.

Psychologists interested in mental retardation will no doubt keep up with current issues of such journals as the *American Journal of Mental Deficiency* and will have on their bookshelves such recent volumes as the Ellis (1979) *Handbook of Mental Deficiency*. Those interested in cerebral palsy, seizure disorders, and child neuropsychology in general should become familiar with the journal *Developmental Medicine and Child Neurology*. A key resource for those concerned with infantile autism is the *Journal of Autism and Developmental Disorders*. The field of learning disabilities, attention deficit disorder, and related phenomena is unfortunately much more chaotic (e.g., see the review by Routh, 1978). One good journal that publishes a number of articles in this area is the *Journal of Abnormal Child Psychology*. There is no doubt that children's academic and behavioral problems in school will continue to be of high interest to the pediatric psychology researcher.

FINANCIAL SUPPORT FOR PEDIATRIC PSYCHOLOGY RESEARCH

Most pediatric psychologists who are at all well known as researchers seem to work in university (usually medical school) settings. Routh (1980) collated the reference citations from the extant issues of the *Journal of Pediatric Psychology* and found 166 individuals whose first-authored articles received two or more reference citations and who were listed in the *Directory of the American Psychological Association*. Of this group 91 (55%) were full professors, 27 (16%) associate professors, 16 (10%) assistant professors, and 2 (1%) instructors in universities. Only 30 (18%) were employed in other settings.

Pediatric psychologists who are medical school faculty sometimes have the opportunity to supervise the research of psychology graduate students, for example, MA theses and PhD dissertations. Such research supervision opportunities are unfortunately not as commonly available to psychologists on medical school faculties as to those teaching graduate psychology departments. It therefore seems to be the case that the progress of systematic programs of research in pediatric psychology depend to a large extent on the availability of external funding, either from private foundations (such as the March of Dimes) or the government (i.e., the National Institutes of Health). The National Institute of Child Health and Human Development would seem to be the prime Institute at NIH with an interest in this area of research, but many of the other Institutes are involved as well, and for the last several years an ad hoc review group known as the Behavioral Medicine Study Section has existed within the NIH to review between 250 and 300 grant applications per year with behavioral science as well as medical aspects. Thus, assuming no precipitous changes in the support of health research by Congress, a considerable amount of funds will continue to be available for pediatric psychology and other behavioral medicine research of high scientific merit.

SUMMARY AND CONCLUSION

Pediatric psychology, like its parent disciplines, medicine and psychology, is a research-based professional specialty. Thus pediatric psychologists, especially those who are on medical school or other university faculties, are expected to carry out and publish research as part of their ordinary duties. Other psychologists who work in developmental clinics, hospitals, or medical group practice settings must also keep up to date on research findings relevant to the field in order to render quality service to children and their families. The past decade has already seen the emergence of a number of books, journals, and other outlets for the publication of such research and of federal and other sources of funds to support it. A brief overview has been presented of some of the research issues being dealt with currently by pediatric psychology researchers. It is hoped that the reader has been able to form from this a clear impression of some of the important questions addressed by such research today.

REFERENCES

Achenbach, T. M. The child behavior profile: I. Boys aged 6 through 11. *Journal of Consulting and Clinical Psychology,* 1978, **46,** 478—488.

Achenbach, T. M., & Edelbrock, C. S. The child behavior profile: II. Boys aged 12—16 and girls aged 6—11 and 12—16. *Journal of Consulting and Clinical Psychology,* 1979, **47,** 223—233.

Aleksandrowicz, M. K., & Aleksandrowicz, D. R. Obstetrical pain-relieving drugs as predictors of infant behavioral variability. *Child Development,* 1974, **45,** 935—945.

Altemeier, W. A., Vietze, P. M., Sherrod, K. B., Sandler, H. M., Falsey, S., & O'Connor, S. Prediction of child maltreatment during pregnancy. *Journal of the American Academy of Child Psychiatry,* 1979, **18,** 205—218.

Bayley, N. *Bayley Scales of Infant Development.* New York: Psychological Corporation, 1969.

Becker, W. C. *Parents are teachers: A child management program.* Champaign, IL: Research Press, 1971.

Becker, M. H., Nathanson, C. A., Drachman, R. H., & Kirscht, J. P. Mothers' health beliefs and children's clinic visits: A prospective study. *Journal of Community Health,* 1977, **3,** 125—135.

Berg, I., & Fielding, D. An interview with a child to assess psychiatric disturbance: A note on its reliability and validity. *Journal of Abnormal Child Psychology,* 1979, **7,** 83—89.

Bergman, A. B., & Werner, R. J. Failure of children to receive penicillin by mouth. *New England Journal of Medicine,* 1963, **268,** 2334—1338.

Bluebond-Langner, M. I know, do you? A study of awareness, communication, and coping in terminally ill children. In B. Schoenberg, A. Carr, D. Peretz, A. Kutscher, & I. Goldberg (Eds.), *Anticipatory grief.* New York: Columbia University Press, 1974.

Bradley, R. H., & Caldwell, B. M. Home observation of the environment: A revision of the preschool scale. *American Journal of Mental Deficiency,* 1979, **84,** 235—244.

Brazelton, T. B. *Neonatal Behavioral Assessment Scale.* Philadelphia: Lippincott, 1973.

Burgess, R. L., & Conger, R. D. Family interaction in abusive, neglectful, and normal families. *Child Development,* 1978, **49,** 1163—1173.

Campbell, J. D. The child in the sick role: Contributions of age, sex, parental status, and parental values. *Journal of Health and Social Behavior,* 1978, **19,** 35—50.

Charney, E., Bynum, R., Eldredge, D., Frank, D., MacWhinney, J. B., McNabb, N., Scheiner, A., Sumpter, E. A., & Iker, H. How well do patients take oral penicillin? A collaborative study in private practice. *Pediatrics,* 1967, **40,** 188—195.

Clarke-Stewart, K. A. Popular primers for parents. *American Psychologist,* 1978, **33,** 359—369.

Cohn, A. H. The pediatrician's role in the treatment of child abuse: Implications from a national evaluation study. *Pediatrics*, 1980, **65**, 358—360.

Conners, C. K. A teacher rating scale for use in drug studies with children. *American Journal of Psychiatry*, 1969, **126**, 884—888.

Deasy-Spinetta, P., & Spinetta, J. J. The child with cancer in school: Teacher's appraisal. *American Journal of Pediatric Hematology/Oncology*, 1980, **2**, 89—94.

Dingle, J. H., Badger, G. F., & Jordan, W. S. *Illness in the home*. Cleveland: The Press of Case Western Reserve University, 1964.

Douglas, J. W. B. Early hospital admissions and later disturbances of behaviour and learning. *Developmental Medicine and Child Neurology*, 1975, **17**, 456—480.

DuBose, R. F. Predictive validity of infant intelligence scales with multiply handicapped children. *American Journal of Mental Deficiency*, 1976, **81**, 388—390.

Egeland, B., & Brunnquell, D. An at-risk approach to the study of child abuse. *Journal of the American Academy of Child Psychiatry*, 1979, **18**, 219—235.

Eland, J. M., & Anderson, J. E. The experience of pain in children. In A. K. Jacox (Ed.), *Pain: A source book for nurses and other health professionals*. Boston: Little, Brown, 1977.

Elardo, R., Bradley, R., & Caldwell, B. M. The relation of infants' home environments to mental test performance from six to thirty-six months: A longitudinal analysis. *Child Development*, 1975, **46**, 71—76.

Ellis, N. R. (Ed.) *Handbook of mental deficiency*, 2nd ed. Hillsdale, NJ: Lawrence Erlbaum Associates, 1979.

Elmer, E. Effects of early neglect and abuse on latency age children. *Journal of Pediatric Psychology*, 1978, **3**, 14—19.

Forehand, R., & King, H. E. Preschool children's noncompliance: Effects of short-term behavior therapy. *Journal of Community Psychology*, 1974, **4**, 42—44.

Framo, J. L. A personal viewpoint on training in marital and family therapy. *Professional Psychology*, 1979, **10**, 868—875.

Frankl, S. N., Shiere, F. R., & Fogels, H. R. Should the parent remain with the child in the dental operatory? *Journal of Dentistry for Children*, 1962, **29**, 150—163.

Freud, S. Analysis of a phobia in a five-year-old boy. In E. Jones (Ed.), *Sigmund Freud: Collected papers*, Vol. 3. New York: Basic Books, 1959.

Fuchs, N. R. Play therapy at home. *Merrill-Palmer Quarterly*, 1957, **3**, 89—95.

Fuchs, V. Health care and the U.S. economic system: An essay in abnormal psychology. *Milbank Memorial Fund Quarterly*, 1972, **50**, 211—237.

Gaines, R., Sandgrund, A., Green, A. H., & Power, E. Etiological factors in child maltreatment: A multivariate study of abusing, neglecting, and normal mothers. *Journal of Abnormal Psychology*, 1978, **87**, 531—540.

Garbarino, J., & Crouter, A. Defining the community context for parent-child relations: The correlates of child maltreatment. *Child Development*, 1978, **49**, 604—616.

George, C., & Main, M. Social interactions of young abused children: Approach, avoidance, and aggression. *Child Development*, 1979, **50**, 306—318.

Ghose, L. J., Giddon, D. B., Shiere, F. R., & Fogels, H. R. Evaluation of sibling support. *Journal of Dentistry for Children*, 1969 **36**, 35—49.

Ginott, H. G. *Between parent and child*. New York: Macmillan, 1965.

Gordis, L., Markowitz, M., & Lilienfeld, A. M. Why patients don't follow medical advice: A study of children on long-term antistreptococcal prophylaxis. *Journal of Pediatrics,* 1969, **75**, 957–968.

Graham, P., & Rutter, M. The reliability and validity of the psychiatric assessment of the child: II. Interview with the parent. *British Journal of Psychiatry,* 1968, **114**, 581–592.

Gregg, G. S., & Elmer, E. Infant injuries: Accident or abuse? *Pediatrics,* 1969, **44**, 434–439.

Griest, D., Wells, K. C., & Forehand, R. An examination of predictors of maternal perceptions of maladjustment in clinic-referred children. *Journal of Abnormal Psychology,* 1979, **88**, 277–281.

Hall, D. J. *Social relations and innovation: Changing the state of play in hospitals.* London: Routledge & Kegan Paul, 1977.

Hawkins, R. P., Peterson, R. F., Schweid, E., & Bijou, S. W. Behavior therapy in the home: Amelioration of problem parent-child relations with the parent in a therapeutic role. *Journal of Experimental Child Psychology,* 1966, **4**, 99–107.

Heifetz, L. J. Behavioral training for parents of retarded children: Alternative formats based on instructional manuals. *American Journal of Mental Deficiency,* 1977, **82**, 194–203.

Hoffman, M. L. Moral internalization, parental power, and the nature of parent-child interaction. *Developmental Psychology,* 1975, **11**, 228–239.

Huber, C., Stangler, S., & Routh, D. K. The BOEL test as a screening device for otitis media in infants. *Nursing Research,* 1978, **27**, 178–180.

Johnson, R. A., Kenney, J. B., & Davis, J. . Developing school policy for use of stimulant drugs for hyperactive children. In J. J. Bosco & S. S. Robin (Eds.), *The hyperactive child and stimulant drugs.* Chicago: University of Chicago Press, 1977.

Kalnins, I. V., Churchill, M. P., & Terry, G. E. Concurrent stresses in families with a leukemic child. *Journal of Pediatric Psychology,* 1980, **5**, 81–92.

Klaber, M. M., & Butterfield, E. C. Stereotyped rocking—a measure of institution and ward effectiveness. *American Journal of Mental Deficiency,* 1968, **73**, 13–20.

Klaus, M. H., & Kennell, J. H. *Maternal-infant bonding.* St. Louis: Mosby, 1976.

Korman, M. National Conference on Levels and Patterns of Training in Psychology. *American Psychologist,* 1974, **29**, 441–449.

Lansky, S. B., Cairns, N. U., Hassanein, R., Wehr, J., & Lowman, J. T. Childhood cancer: Parental discord and divorce. *Pediatrics,* 1978, **62**, 184–188.

Lansky, S. B., Lowman, J. T., Vats, T., & Gyulay, J.-E. School phobia in children with malignant neoplasms. *American Journal of Diseases of Children,* 1975, **129**, 42–46.

Lessler, K. Health and education screening of school-age children: Definition and objectives. *American Journal of Public Health,* 1972, **62**, 191–198.

Lilienfeld, A. M., & Parkhurst, E. A study of the association of factors of pregnancy and parturition with the development of cerebral palsy. *American Journal of Hygiene,* 1951, **53**, 262–282.

Magrab, P. (Ed.) *Psychological management of pediatric problems,* Vol. 1. *Early life conditions and chronic disease.* Baltimore: University Park Press, 1978.

Magrab, P. (Ed.) *Psychological management of pediatric problems,* Vol. 2. *Sensorineural conditions and social concerns.* Baltimore: University Park Press, 1978.

Manheimer, D. I., & Mellinger, G. D. Personality characteristics of the child accident repeater. *Child Development,* 1967, **38**, 491–513.

Matheny, A. P. Visual-perceptual exploration and accident liability in children. *Journal of Pediatric Psychology*, 1980, **5**, 343−351.

Matheny, A. P., Brown, A. M., & Wilson, R. S. Behavioral antecedents of accidental injuries in early childhood: A study of twins. *Journal of Pediatrics*, 1971, **79**, 122−124.

Mattson, A., & Weisberg, I. Behavioral reactions to minor illness in preschool children. *Pediatrics*, 1970, **46**, 604−610.

McCoy, S. A. Clinical judgments of normal childhood behavior. *Journal of Consulting and Clinical Psychology*, 1976, **44**, 710−714.

Mesibov, G. B., Schroeder, C. S., & Wesson, L. Parental concerns about their children. *Journal of Pediatric Psychology*, 1977, **2**, 13−17.

Minuchin, S., Rosman, B. L., Baker, L., & Liebman, R. *Psychosomatic families: Anorexia nervosa in context*. Cambridge, MA: Harvard University Press, 1978.

Moll, W. History of American medical education. *British Journal of Medical Education*, 1968, **2**, 173−181.

National Center for Health Statistics, Division of Vital Statistics. *U.S. national health survey*. Washington, DC: U.S. Government Printing Office, 1978.

Neel, J. V. Human genetics. In J. Z. Bowers & E. F. Purcell (Eds.), *Advances in American medicine: Essays at the Bicentennial*, Vol. 1. New York: Josiah Macy Foundation, 1976.

Nitschke, R., Wunder, S., Sexauer, C. L., & Humphren, G. B. The final-stage conference: The patient's decision on research drugs in pediatric oncology. *Journal of Pediatric Psychology*, 1977, **2**, 58−64.

Oglesbay, F. B. The flammable fabrics problem. *Pediatrics*, 1969, **44** (Supplement), 827−832.

O'Malley, J. E., Koocher, G., Foster, D., & Slavin, L. Psychiatric sequelae of surviving childhood cancer. *American Journal of Orthopsychiatry*, 1979, **49**, 608−616.

Parke, R. D., & Collmer, C. W. Child abuse: An interdisciplinary analysis. In E. M. Hetherington (Ed.), *Review of child development research*, Vol. 5. Chicago: University of Chicago Press, 1975.

Pasamanick, B., & Knobloch, H. Brain damage and reproductive casualty. *American Journal of Orthopsychiatry*, 1960, **30**, 298−305.

Pasamanick, B., & Knobloch, H. Retrospective studies on the epidemiology of reproductive casualty: Old and new. *Merrill-Palmer Quarterly*, 1966, **12**, 7−26.

Peele, R. A., & Routh, D. K. Maternal control and self-control in the 3-year-old child. *Bulletin of the Psychonomic Society*, 1978, **11**, 349−352.

Peterson, L., & Ridley-Johnson, R. Pediatric hospital response to survey on prehospital preparation for chidren. *Journal of Pediatric Psychology*, 1980, **5**, 1−7.

Quay, H. C. Classification. In H. C. Quay & J. Werry (Eds.), *Psychopathological disorders of childhood*, 2nd ed. New York: Wiley, 1979.

Rapoport, J. L., & Benoit, M. The relation of direct home observation to the clinic evaluation of hyperactive school age boys. *Journal of Child Psychology and Psychiatry*, 1975, **16**, 141−147.

Robin, A. L., Kent, R., O'Leary, K. D., Foster, S., & Prinz, R. An approach to teaching parents and adolescents problem-solving communication skills: A preliminary report. *Behavior Therapy*, 1977, **8**, 639−643.

Routh, D. K. Psychological training in medical school departments of pediatrics: A second look. *American Psychologist*, 1972, **27**, 587–589.

Routh, D. K. Hyperactivity. In P. R. Magrab (Ed.), *Psychological management of pediatric problems*, Vol. 2. Baltimore: University Park Press, 1978.

Routh, D. K. Research training in pediatric psychology. *Journal of Pediatric Psychology*, 1980, **5**, 287–293.

Routh, D. K., & Mesibov, G. B. The editorial policy of the Journal of Pediatric Psychology. *Journal of Pediatric Psychology*, 1979, **4**, 1–3.

Routh, D. K., & Mesibov, G. B. Psychological and environmental intervention: Toward social competence. In H. E. Rie & E. D. Rie (Eds.), *Handbook of minimal brain dysfunctions*. New York: Wiley, 1980.

Sameroff, A. J., & Chandler, M. J. Reproductive risk and the continuum of caretaking casualty. In F. D. Horowitz (Ed.), *Review of child development research*, Vol. 4. Chicago: University of Chicago Press, 1975.

Schaffer, H. R., & Crook, C. K. Child compliance and maternal control techniques. *Developmental Psychology*, 1980, **16**, 54–61.

Shakow, D. Recommended graduate training program in clinical psychology. *American Psychologist*, 1947, **2**, 539–558.

Shaw, E. G., & Routh, D. K. Children receiving injections cry more when mother is there. *Bulletin of the Psychonomic Society*, 1980, **13**, 255. (Abstract)

Shirley, M., & Poyntz, L. The influence of separation from the mother on the children's emotional responses. *Jounal of Psychology*, 1941, **12**, 251–282.

Sobel, R. The psychiatric implications of accidental poisoning in childhood. *Pediatric Clinics of North America*, 1970, **17**, 653–685.

Spinetta, J. J. Psychosocial issues in childhood cancer: How the professional can help. *Advances in Behavioral Pediatrics*, 1982, **3**, in press.

Spinetta, J. J., Rigler, D., & Karon, M. Anxiety in the dying child. *Pediatrics*, 1973, **52**, 841–845.

Spinetta, J. J., Rigler, D., & Karon, M. Personal space as a measure of a dying child's sense of isolation. *Journal of Consulting and Clinical Psychology*, 1974, **42**, 751–756.

Sprague, R. L., & Gadow, K. D. The role of the teacher in drug treatment. In J. J. Bosco & S. S. Robin (Eds.), *The hyperactive child and stimulant drugs*. Chicago: University of Chicago Press, 1977.

Stangler, S. R., Huber, C. J., & Routh, D. K. *Screening growth and development of preschool children*. New York: McGraw-Hill, 1980.

Starfield, B. Measurement of outcome: A proposed scheme. In G. D. Grave & I. B. Pless (Eds.), *Chronic childhood illness:Assessment of outcome*. Washington, DC: U.S. Government Printing Office, 1974.

Strauss, M. E., Starr, R. H., Ostrea, E. M., Chavez, C. J., & Stryker, J. C. Behavioral concomitants to prenatal addiction to narcotics. *Journal of Pediatrics*, 1976, **89**, 842–846.

Tavormina, J. B. Relative effeciveness of behavioral and reflective group counseling with parents of mentally retarded children. *Journal of Consulting and Clinical Psychology*, 1975, **43**, 22–31.

Townsend, P. W., & Flanagan, J. J. Experimental preadmission program to encourage home care for severely and profoundly retarded children. *American Journal of Mental Deficiency,* 1976, **80,** 562−569.

Vander Veer, B., & Schweid, E. Infant assessment: Stability of mental functioning in young retarded children. *American Journal of Mental Deficiency,* 1974, **79,** 1−4.

Vernon, D. T. A. Modeling and birth order in responses to painful stimuli. *Journal of Personality and Social Psychology,* 1974, **29,** 794−799.

Vernon, D. T. A., Foley, J. M., & Schulman, J. L. Effect of mother-child separation and birth order on young children's responses to two potentially stressful experiences. *Journal of Personality and Social Psychology,* 1967, **5,** 162−174.

Waechter, E. H. *Death anxiety in children with fatal illness.* Doctoral dissertation, Stanford University. Ann Arbor, MI: University Microfilms, 1968.

Werner, E. E., Bierman, J. M., & French, F. E. *The children of Kauai.* Honolulu: University of Hawaii Press, 1971.

Werner, E. E., & Smith, R. S. *Kauai's children come of age.* Honolulu: University Press of Hawaii, 1977.

Werry, J. S. Family therapy: Behavioral approaches. *Journal of the American Academy of Child Psychiatry,* 1979, **18,** 91−102.

Wilson, R. S. Synchronies in mental development: An epigenetic perspective. *Science,* 1978, **202,** 939−948.

Wirt, R. D., Lachar, D., Klinedinst, J. K., & Seat, P. D. *Multidimensional evaluation of child personality: A manual for the Personality Inventory for Children.* Los Angeles: Western Psychological Services, 1977.

Wright, L. Pediatric psychology: A role model. *American Psychologist,* 1967, **22,** 323−325.

Wright, L., Schaefer, A. B., & Solomons, G. *Encyclopedia of pediatric psychology.* Baltimore: University Park Press, 1979.

Zeskind, P. S., & Ramey, C. T. Fetal malnutrition: An experimental study of its consequences on infant development in two caregiving environments. *Child Development,* 1978, **49,** 1155−1162.

CHAPTER 9

Training in Pediatric Psychology

June M. Tuma

Since its formulation in 1968, the Society of Pediatric Psychology has expressed interest in the training of pediatric psychologists. As the roles and skills of the pediatric psychologist developed through years of experience in pediatric settings, these training ideas became more focused. Today, the *Journal of Pediatric Psychology, Professional Psychology,* and other journals are scattered throughout with descriptions of programs. These expositions typically consider the kinds of settings in which psychologists work in conjunction with pediatricians, the kinds of training experiences typically offered, and the kinds of services offered to children and their families. Most of these descriptions are of training at the internship or the postdoctoral levels, with notable absence of doctoral program description. The reason for that is because there are *no* doctoral programs in pediatric psychology.

As the practice of pediatric psychology became more defined and developed, and pediatric psychologists found themselves in new roles, the field of pediatric psychology became more firmly established. The viability of the field of pediatric psychology was first marked by the beginnings, and then rapid growth of journal articles, then by the establishment of the *Journal of Pediatric Psychology* in 1976, and more recently by a rash of books. Wright, Schaefer, and Solomons (1979) compiled the *Encyclopedia of Pediatric Psychology,* an impressive review of the literature on the management of problems typically seen by pediatric psychologists. Other books containing detailed expositions of the management of illness-related problems are now appearing in print (e.g., Magrab, 1978), and an annual volume of advances in pediatric psychology is proposed. The 1970s indeed marked the beginning of an era of more precise formulation of the practice of pediatric psychology.

As the area becomes more established, training in pediatric psychology is an increasing concern of those who practice the specialty. Concurrently, the growing popularity and appeal of pediatric psychology increasingly stimulate questions from students of psychology about routes to follow for preparation for pediatric psychology. In their search for training, they are eagerly seeking current information about established and developing training centers for pediatric psychology training. The need to inform students about possible training opportunities led to a directory of pediatric psychology practicum training facilities in 1976 (Tuma, 1976) This directory was revised in 1980 and is now available (Tuma, 1980b).

CHILDREN AND NATIONAL POLICY: INCREASING INTEREST IN CHILD TRAINING

Training in all areas of child psychology, not only pediatric psychology, has been receiving increasing attention in recent years. A great deal of concern has been expressed about the supply and demand for child services, which naturally led to investigation about availability of training with an effort to predict psychology's ability to bridge the wide gap between supply and demand of manpower to fill these needs.

These concerns come from a number of sources. The 1970 President's Commission on Mental Health reported that children and youth are among the unserved and underserved populations. Recommendations from that Commission included that new services be established and that a strategy for prevention be developed. The report documents a shortage of specialists trained to work with children and adolescents and the lack of access to appropriate services to children. The Commission further recommended increases in training child specialists in all mental health disciplines, including psychology, in established training programs.

In response to the alarming nature of the need for more services to children, the National Institute of Mental Health (NIMH) adopted guidelines for funding additional training programs and/or revised training programs which address the recommendations of that Commission. A new and exclusive emphasis on priority-based training as a basic condition for NIMH support of training in the future was presented in the fiscal year 1980 (Denham, 1979). The NIMH objectives include policies which seek to influence preparation of personnel for specific priority areas of service need, and promote support of specific rather than generic curriculae. These developments in many ways especially address needs of children, and imply a demand that psychologists take the initiative in the preparation of definitions of adequate programs to train psychologists to provide services to children and youth, and, perhaps even more important, to develop standards for training.

In response to these demands and indications of psychology's reluctance to address the issue of child training as a specialty to date (e.g., Wellner, 1978; APA, 1977), a proposal for a training conference designed to discuss issues, share information, and explore approaches to the training of child psychologists has been submitted to NIMH for consideration for funding (Tuma, 1980a). This proposal is currently being pursued.

Present Status of Mental Health Services to Children

The 1977 U.S. census data indicate that children under 18 comprise roughly 30% of the total population. A detailed APA report documents that less than 1% of all psychological service providers are primarily devoted to serving this population

(VandenBos, Nelson, Stapp, Olmedo, Coates, & Batchelor, 1979). A number of high-risk groups can be clearly identified, including children and adolescents of disturbed parents, chronically mentally ill children, those from poor single-parent families, minority group children, those living in rural settings or depressed inner-city neighborhoods where services are limited or nonexistent, physically handicapped children, and victims of child abuse.

In spite of the needs of this population for mental health services, only about 10% of American children and adolescents in need of care or treatment are served by the present mental health system (ADAMHA, 1978). Some of the more important factors accounting for underservice are related to service availability and methods of service delivery. However, basic to the underservice is also a severe shortage of appropriately trained psychologists.

Supply of Child Health Service Psychologists

The first survey of all licensed and/or certified health service providers in psychology (Mills, Wellner, & VandenBos, 1979) estimated that almost 19,000 psychologists were licensed/certified, relevantly trained, and actively providing mental health services. Less than 1% of the health service provider psychologists, however, spent a majority of their time (over 75%) providing services to children. About 5000 doctoral level psychologists provide some service to children as part of their clinical practice (Denham, 1979), and this appears to equal about 1000 full-time equivalents (VandenBos, 1979). Membership in professional organizations focused around services to children provide similar estimates of the number of health care providers. Recent surveys of three organizations within the APA structure (the Section on Clinical Child Psychology, the Society of Pediatric Psychology and the Division on Children and Youth) obtained a return rate of 26% of the 2300 members (Tuma & Cohen, in preparation; Tuma & Pratt, in preparation; Tuma & Salcedo, in preparation). Taking the overlapping memberships into account (40%), membership involve approximately 1300 psychologists. Since 63% of the sample indicate that they are certified health care providers, these surveys also estimate that approximately 800 psychologists provide services to children.

The current supply of fully trained psychologists (those who have completed an organized program in clinical child psychology with a specialized child-oriented internship) has been estimated at less than 500 (VandenBos et al., 1979). This figure is supported by the surveys by Tuma and her students mentioned above. Respondents indicated that 26% of the sample had completed in an organized graduate program in clinical child psychology, 50% had completed a child practicum, 38% had completed a specialized child-oriented internship and 22% had completed a child-oriented postdoctoral fellowship. The comparison of the known need for service of child populations shows the need for an estimated 5000 additional fully trained, doctoral-level clinical child psychologists within the next decade (VandenBos et al., 1979). Furthermore, the survey revealed that the majority of psychologists who do serve children are located in large urban areas and generally serve a very narrow subset of the total population. Thus the manpower shortage is magnified by unequal distribution of psychologists. Intensified efforts are needed to correct this situation by promoting new and/or revised training programs in psychology to alleviate this gross shortage of manpower.

Child Psychology Training Programs: Current Status

In addition to the need for more child health service providers in psychology, there exists a need for the establishment of standards for training psychologists offering services to children. It has been pointed out that psychologists offering services to children require special skills that go beyond adult work (Wohlford, 1979), and that clinical child psychology should be recognized as a specialty in its own right (Wenar, 1979; Wohlford, 1979). This recognition would promote training standards more specific to the skills and knowledge required for its particular demands for service. The NIMH emphasis on priority-focused training is one early step in the direction of providing governmental support of such specialty development. The priority-focused training NIMH will fund in the future requires demonstration of curriculum, practicum, internship, research, and student identification pertinent to the priority area of training (Denham, 1979).

Psychologists who have interests in addressing children's needs have had very few options for obtaining training designed to address their future professional functioning. The small number of doctoral programs in clinical child psychology even today (Fischer, Mannarino, & Magnussen, 1979; Roberts, 1979) point to a possible preponderance of reliance on informal educational pursuits. Because of the variability of intensity and depth such informal pursuits permit, the quality of that preparation is variable, to say the least.

The number of programs offering clinical child training remains small. Ross (1972) noted the existence of very few programs in 1968, Fischer (1978) listed 12, and Roberts (1979) identified 15 programs offering clinical child psychology training in some variety. More recently, however, Fischer et al. (1979) identified 34 formal programs in clinical child psychology and an additional 52 "informal" specialty training sequences, and in 1980, Tuma and George (in press) identified 40 formal programs.

At least four models of training for clinical child psychology have been reported in the recent literature;

1. Specialized training in child and adolescent mental health within the context of general or adult clinical psychology (Roberts, 1979; Wohlford, 1979).

2. Specialty clinical child psychology programs (Roberts, 1979; Wohlford, 1979).

3. Specialty training in clinical child psychology within the framework of developmental, school, or other types of training programs (Roberts, 1979; Routh, 1977).

4. Supplementary postdoctoral training of a continuing education nature in clinical child psychology for adult, developmental, or other kinds of psychologists (Tuma, 1975).

These models have developed independently in response to a demand for clinical child psychology training. Although some similarities appear in the programs when they are compared, at least at the doctoral level (Fischer *et al.,* 1979; Roberts, 1979), there are currently no agreed-upon criteria for the adequate training of clinical child psychologists.

The Fischer *et al.* (1979) survey reveals some confusion about training content and, indeed, definitions of clinical child psychology. The survey team discovered that many of the respondents described programs that were gravely deficient in their offerings, that is, deficient from the standpoint of offering sufficient course work or experiences to prepare students to work competently with children. They concluded that serious confusion exists in the academic community regarding necessary and sufficient elements of clinical child training. The surveyors' impression was that increasing demands for clinical child specialists and decreasing graduate school applications were leading a number of these departments to make unsupportable claims of having clinical child training programs. The new priorities of NIMH that emphasize specialty training rather than generic training appear to cast additional light on these findings. These claims of specialty training appear to be an early, possibly opportunistic, response to funding pressures at the federal level. This reaction is encouraging from the standpoint of indicating that the availability of increased funding for specialty training though federal agencies can stimulate the academic community to consider training psychologists with the necessary skills for clinical child psychological work. On the other hand, the confusion about what constitutes adequate clinical child psychology education at the doctoral level underscores the need to focus on and delineate the desirable product of specialty clinical child training and design the training format, for example, the content, the sequences, the practicum experiences, the internship experiences, and the alternatives to achieving such a product. Without adequate understanding of appropriate training models, the availability of funding will do little to improve the quality of training in the child area.

The rate of production of PhD clinical child psychologists by existing programs is alarmingly low. The survey by the Section on Clinical Child Psychology reports that the formal and informal training programs produce graduates at the rate of 88 and 93, respectively, in an average year (Fischer, *et al.,* 1979). At this rate, the production of PhD clinical child psychologists falls short by about 80% of the 10,000 clinical child psychologists projected to be needed within the next decade (VandenBos *et al.,* 1979).

Pediatric Psychology Training Programs: Current Status

With regard to pediatric psychology, some information exists in the literature concerning the current status of training. The role models and training in clinical child psychology and pediatric psychology have been contrasted (Tuma, 1975) and two surveys of pediatric psychology training offered in medical schools across the United States have been accomplished (Routh, 1970, 1972). Additionally, a survey (Tuma, 1977) identified 28 internship and 9 postdoctoral settings offering training in pediatric psychology. In the 1980 survey (Tuma, 1980), the number of training settings increased to 33 at the internship level and 18 at the postdoctoral level. As already noted, directories are available for student use.

A very serious question which influences decisions about appropriate training in pediatric psychology has been debated. It is, simply stated: "How do pediatric psychologists differ, if at all, from clinical child psychologists?" This question is important from the standpoint of designing an appropriate training model for pediatric psychology. Is the standard model for clinical child psychology doctoral training sufficient to prepare the pediatric psychologist, or should there be an entirely different set of courses? Some psychologists take the position that clinical training is necessary to pediatric psychology (Drotar, 1977; Stabler & Whitt, 1980; Tuma, 1975), while others are critical of this stance (Tefft & Simeonsson, 1979). The boundary issues implied by this question cause confusion even at the level of those who offer training in both areas. For example, the respondents to the above-mentioned survey (Tuma, 1977) who identified their programs as having a pediatric psychology focus were essentially indistinguishale from those claiming a clinical child focus. Approximately half of the 63 respondents indicated each focus, and 4% claimed to have both foci of training with an emphasis of about 50% on each. Yet the fact that they responded to a survey indicating that pediatric psychology training was offered and were aware of the stated purpose of inclusion of information in a directory of pediatric psychology training programs points to some basic questions. Rapid perusal of the information contained in the directory appears to point to the training *setting* as the distinguishing factor.

The second survey (Tuma, 1980b) was more sensitive to this question and asked that respondents clearly identify their programs as pediatric psychology or clinical child training programs. Again, the programs were about equally divided between pediatric psychology (40%) and clinical child psychology (42%) training programs. In this survey, however, respondents were given the opportunity to indicate whether they offered a combined program. The combination was offered by 23% of the respondents. Respondents were also asked to give their definitions of both areas. The responses were categorized into three major characteristics: setting, population, and theoretical orientation. The ranking for pediatric psychology was population, setting, theoretical orientation; for clinical child psychology the ranking was theoretical orientation, population, and setting, in that order. The definition, then, is still not clear and the question must be addressed. If there is no differentiation between the two areas, then there is no need to have separate training formats. However, if there is a difference, and it is assumed that there is, then this difference must be identified. Surely there are points of convergence, but the boundary issues obscure precise definition of training format.

As previously mentioned, there are no specific training programs for pediatric psychologists at the doctoral level. Routh (1977), however, provides data to indicate that basic doctoral training in pediatric psychology is primarily developmental and clinical psychology but, in addition, can be other areas of psychology. The applicability of developmental psychology to pediatric psychology and clinical child psychology has always been emphasized. Presently, however, there are increasing efforts to define an area designated as applied developmental psychology. Wertlieb (1979) advocates a critical base in applied behavioral science and developmental psychology for clinical child and pediatric psychology which he believes would place both areas in important positions in many health care, education, human service, and public policy settings. In fact, Wertlieb (1979) advocates a marriage between clinical and developmental psychology under the umbrella of the applied developmental psychologies. This rapprochement between basic and applied research would be consistent with the thrust of the "new medical model" (Engel, 1977) by involving clinical child psychologists more into basic research, and it would permit the application of clinical skills by the pediatric psychologist.

Within the present scheme of training for pediatric psychologists, Tuma (1975) advocates that pediatric psychology be regarded as a subspecialty of clinical child psychology that logically should evolve from basic training in clinical child psychology at the doctoral level. However, with the increased emphasis on medical psychology and other health psychological applications as a separate specialty, more training in health-related areas of investigation will become available at the doctoral level. There is also the possibility that the thrust of applied developmental psychology can provide an avenue of appropriate doctoral training. These are the areas of uncertainty in the training for a professional role as new as pediatric psychology.

One of the functions of the pediatric psychologist which has never been questioned is that of consultation and collaboration with pediatricians. Many models of consultation have been presented in the literature, and ever-broadening roles are being emphasized (Koocher, Sourkes, & Keane, 1979). The consultation skill training offered at the doctoral and internship levels necessary for such collaboration was the question of two recent surveys. It was found that doctoral programs primarily offer consultation training with school systems (94%), and only 42% of the programs offer consultation training to primary-care physicians (Schwartz & Tuma, 1978). Internship settings, however, offer medical consultation training more frequently (74%), closely followed by school consultation (71%) (Tuma & Schwartz, 1978). Training in collaborative efforts with primary health-care providers appears to be more universally offered at the internship level. Although information about course work involving medical-psychological topics, such as biological aspects of development, child neuropsychology, biopsychology, is not currently available, it would appear that offerings in these areas at the doctoral level are relevant to pediatric psychology training and perhaps may be a useful addition to the training of the clinical child psychologist as well.

Conclusions on Current Status

The foregoing discussion of current training opportunities highlights several important facts. Many doctoral programs of clinical psychology are ill-equipped to offer curricula for the development of skills and knowledge base required by psychologists who offer services to children. Furthermore, there is an absence of specific criteria of minimal and optimal training in clinical child psychology, including pediatric psychology. Granted, there are exceptional programs that offer well-conceived sequences of training experiences, a laudable combination of core and specialty curriculae, and appropriate collaboration with service delivery facilities which expose students to the target populations of interest to their specialty. There are also training pockets which seem to have anticipated the national need for training for specific services such as medical collaboration and for integrated affiliation with service delivery facilities. The number of programs designed to train psychologists who work with children are too few, however, to influence the manpower requirements of children in need of services. Federal funding will have little impact on increasing this manpower without appreciable consciousness-raising about the grave issues involved in training pediatric and clinical child psychologists who are competent to the task of service to children and their families.

THE ESSENTIALS OF PEDIATRIC PSYCHOLOGY TRAINING

The central issue in the training of pediatric psychologists is how to provide the didactic and experiential background for the many professional roles that have arisen. Related to this, and equally important, is the issue of whether there exists a core of knowledge and skills that can serve as a common denominator for all or most of the developing roles. Finally, there is the question of the locus of professional training—in the university or in the practicum setting.

Professional Roles

Pediatric psychology, in its broadest sense, as the child component of medical psychology, has many different roles and thus requires a broad array of skills. It can be noted from the various chapters in this book that the area of influence of the pediatric psychologist extends beyond the bounds of traditional clinical skill-application of assessment, treatment, consultation, and research. The areas of psychological concern range from health care practices and health care delivery systems, to the management of acute and chronic illness, to the psychology of management of acute and chronic illness, to the psychology of medication and pain.

The specific activities of the pediatric psychologist are those categorized by Wertlieb (1979) as the traditional liaison-consultation and mental health services, changing patient attitudes and behavior, changing health care provider attitudes and behavior, and changing health care services. Thus pediatric psychology can be conceptualized as an area of psychology which embraces the skills, techniques, and knowledge base of both clinical psychology and health psychology as they relate to children.

The Common Denominator

The core of knowledge and skills which serve as a common denominator for all developing roles of pediatric psychology encompasses four areas of psychology. These include basic psychology training (core courses), clinical psychology (mental health), health psychology (medical psychology), and child psychology (developmental perspective). Within the context of the roles pediatric psychologists usually assume, all four areas are necessary for adequate performance.

Basic Training in Psychology

Most psychologists agree that the basic courses within all psychology training programs are important to the preparation of health or medical psychologists (Olbrisch & Sechrest, 1979; Swan, Piccione, & Anderson, 1980) and to pediatric psychologists in particular (Roberts, 1979; Routh, 1977; Tuma, 1980a). This core training provides a solid foundation in the major areas of endeavor of the psychologist working in a health setting but also gives the student a strong sense of identity. This is particularly important for the health care psychologist because of the identity confusion that is likely to be engendered by interdisciplinary collaboration necessary in most medical settings. Even those who propose a program which will be more specialized and deemphasize these core areas raise as an issue how a strong identity will be maintained in the student because of this factor (Stone, 1979). This has also been expressed in discussions of specialized training in other areas of psychology, for example, clinical child psychology (Roberts, 1979).

Morc important, however, is the fact that these core areas serve the pediatric psychologist well in the application of skills to the medical arena. The APA Task Force on Health Research (1976) enumerated several ways in which the various areas of psychology could contribute to health care settings. It follows that the student well steeped in these areas could use that information. For example, organizational psychology and social psychology have especially been suggested as being meaningful in program design and evaluation of the health care delivery system. Physiological psychology would indeed have relevance for the research and understanding of the psychosocial factors of physical illness. Research methodology and design has immense importance as the pediatric psychologist designs new applications of old techniques and new techniques for the evaluation and treatment of pediatric patients and new health care practices. As the areas of involvment of the pediatric psychologist increase, as surely they will, the possibilities of the relevance of as yet unexplored areas of interface between psychology and medicine are enormous.

The usual core areas of psychology include physiological, social, developmental, learning, cognition, personality, research methodology, and statistics. All have been emphasized in basic training in psychology and are considered equally important in the training of the pediatric psychology.

Clinical Psychology

It is repeatedly illustrated in all the chapters of this book and most expositions about the role of the pediatric psychologist that clinical skills are important to functioning within medical settings. Roles which involve application of skills of assessment, intervention, consultation, and research in a medical setting which serves children are very important to the practice of pediatric psychology. Putting aside the issue of whether pediatric psychology in its broad sense would emcompass the specific roles presented here (Tefft & Simeonsson, 1979), in the practice of this specialty area, several skills related to clinical psychology are necessary for adequate performance (Drotar, 1977; Stabler & Whitt, 1980; Tuma, 1975; see also chapters 3 and 4). Recognition that clinical skill training is necessary for the psychologist in interface with medicine is not limited to pediatric psychology but extends to discussion of training in behavioral medicine in psychology (medical psychology) (Belar, 1980; Swan, Piccione, & Anderson, 1980; Sladen, 1979). Clinical psychology is assumed to be the area of psychology which has first expanded its horizons into the area of integration of psychology and medicine (Belar, 1980; Swan *et al.,* 1980; Sladen, 1979). In fact, the first description of health care psychology emphasized clinical psychology as a health science (Schofield, 1969). It has also been pointed out that clinical psychology, with its application exclusively to mental health, has restricted its area of influence unnecessarily and has not become adequately involved in other areas of health-oriented psychological activities (APA Task Force on Research, 1976). This Task Force urged psychologists to acknowledge that they are life scientists and, consequently, health scientists.

Health Psychology

Since pediatric psychology is viewed as a component of medical psychology, it is possible that the future pediatric psychologist will increasingly gain most of the basic knowledge and practicum work at the doctoral level within a program developed for medical psychology (sometimes still referred to as behavioral medicine; see chapter 1). There are some reports in the literature of programs offering research and/or application of health psychology, medical psychology, or behavioral medicine (e.g., Stone, 1979). The prospect of more emphasis on this kind of training at the doctoral level will prove very valuable to the quality preparation of pediatric psychologists in the future.

Pediatric psychologists must choose between a major commitment to practice or research in basic areas of pediatric psychology. Those who elect to practice must have a broader-based training experience than those who choose to practice in a traditional mental health setting, because the area of influence of the pediatric psychologist extends beyond the bounds of traditional skill-application of assessment, treatment, consultation, and research. The areas of psychological concern include all areas of health care, health maintenence, and health service delivery.

Pediatric psychology, within this framework, is an area of psychology which embraces the skills, techniques, and knowledge base of both clinical psychology and health psychology. Thus clinical psychology training prepares the student for the design (see Chapters 5, 6, and 7) and execution of assessment and treatment of children based on the lore of clinical methodology (see Chapters 3 and 4), and medical psychology presents the language and culture of the health care institutions, the psychology of the physically ill, the knowledge of psychosocial determinants of onset, course, and outcome of diseases, and the psychosocial consequences of physical illness, medical treatment procedures, hospitalization, disability, and rehabilitation (see Chapters 1 and 2). The strength of this combination of training consists of the integration of the understanding of clinically relevant issues and the psychological components of physical illness with the knowledge of the course and outcome of physical illness and its treatment within the health care delivery system.

There are many types of health psychologists and many types of health research. No single narrowly conceived program is going to suffice for training pediatric psychologists. Research on the psychosocial factors associated with illness such as asthma is very different from research on unmet health needs in a community (see Chapter 8), or on the provision of play space for children while in a hospital (see Chapter 2). The student cannot be trained for any and all roles within the health system that might ever become available. Programs offering health psychology will and do specialize in the manner of conceptualization of health psychology and the courses that are needed. However, the student too must delineate a particular direction for research and practice. Because the field is still so new to psychology, particularly in its training components, there is no agreed upon curriculum; however, a number of courses have been suggested as appropriate. These include introduction to health psychology, physiological aspects of health psychology, health systems, psychology of stress and coping, health transactions, stress and bodily disease, reproductive behavior, health psychology colloquiums. Course work should be augmented by research and practicum placements in medical settings to enable the student to learn about the medical aspects of the problem area, to learn about the culture and language of the medical environment, and to become involved in interdisciplinary collaboration.

Child Psychology

The psychologist working with children and in children's medical settings must have a base of knowledge of principles of development and change (see preceding section). Most psychologists involved in training students to work with children have acknowledged this assumption. For example, in clinical child training, the Section on Clinical Child Psychology (Section I of Division 12 of the APA) publicized its conviction that those who work clinically with children should have special training for their profession which emphasized the developmental perspective (Cass, 1974). The Society of Pediatric Psychology (Section V of Division 12 of the APA) and the Division on Children and Youth (Division 37 of APA) joined forces with Section I around this issue to organize a training conference for training psychologists who work with children (Tuma, 1980a). Wohlford (1979) has stressed that clinical work with children is qualitatively different from work with adults and requires special training. Thus the training that the student pursues in primarily clinical and/or medical psychology must obtain training in child psychology if the intent is to enter pediatric psychology.

The particular arrangement of training depends, of course, on the kind of training program the student enters. For example, with the availability of a clinical child specialty doctoral program, the student could augment training with medical psychology courses and have all three specialty areas integral parts of the training content. Alternatively, if a medical psychology program which emphasizes child content and practica is entered, general clinical psychology courses would suffice with the addition of courses in developmental and clinical child courses such as child psychopathology, child treatment approaches, and child assessment. The third possibility would involve major emphasis on medical psychology from an adult perspective which could then be augmented with a secondary emphasis on clinical child psychology. The fourth possibility would be an adult clinical program in the absence of a child focus in either clinical child or medical psychology in which case child courses and child medical practica placements would suffice. In all of these training possibilities, an integral part of proper training would involve internship placement in a medical school or other pediatrically oriented training setting.

The minimum courses that would prepare the student have generally been listed as follows: child development, child assessment, child intervention, child psychopathology. The minimum practicum experiences would include at least a year in practicum placement in a child setting and a year's placement within a pediatric internship setting.

Locus of Training: University or Practicum Setting

There has been much controversy about specialty training within psychology. In clinical psychology, for example, which is itself considered to be a "specialty" area of psychology, much attention has been placed on whether other areas, such as clinical child psychology, should be considered a specialty in its own right. Some have contended that it is a specialty (Cass, 1974; Tuma, 1975; Wohlford, 1979), and should therefore have programs for training at the doctoral level, and that its practitioners should have licensure and its training programs should be accredited to insure that certain standards are met. This has been part of the contention of the proposal for the national training conference (Tuma, 1980a). This proposal included pediatric psychology as an application area of child psychology. The gist of the proposal is that the child areas have their own core knowledge and that service to children requires special skills and techniques.

The general point that special training is necessary for work with children is recognized. However, the controversy centers around the necessity of specialized training and the sequence of specialty training best suited to achieve a viable product. Should the specialty training be offered throughout graduate training or should it be placed at an advanced level of training during the graduate sequence, or should such training be reserved for application in the practicum and internship placements? Thus the sequence issue involves the locus issue: is the university doctoral program or the practicum and internship facility most appropriate, and is the student best prepared for the specialty training at one point in the training rather than the other? Another argument enters from the postdoctoral training position: should specialty training follow generic training after doctoral work is completed?

The issues involved in this argument include economics of training and educational philosophy. Financing students at both the doctoral and internship levels usually depends on outside sources. In regard to clinical psychology training, the source is usually NIMH. Since most funding agencies allocate funds according to established priorities, training programs usually design their training programs to take advantages of this funding. Thus, within clinical psychology, a recent development of funding priorities of NIMH switched from generic clincal psychology funding to specialty area funding, which includes child and health care psychology in the list of priorities (Denham, 1979). While such a switch in policy would seem to indicate that clinical psychology training would design specialty programs of training in these two areas, what seems to be happening on a larger scale is that most programs are designing a specialty track program, for example, specialty courses taken in conjunction with a generic program of clinical psychology. In a recent survey (Tuma & George, in preparation), 40 ($N = 56$) doctoral programs in psychology indicated that they have clinical child specialty offerings, and 25 have health care psychology offerings. In the same survey, 87 ($N = 140$) internship facilities indicated that they offer clinical child specialty training, and 56 offer health care psychology training. This development is not surprising in view of the fact that revamping a clinical psychology training program would be expensive both in terms of number of faculty and other resources required. It is much more feasible to add a few faculty and resources and build on an established structure of a broader training program. Most programs also have continued loyalty to more traditional training formats. What is clear, however, even in spite of a lack of information about similar statistics about the number of programs in clinical child and health care psychology in the past, is that the number of programmatic offerings in these areas is responsive to the NIMH guidelines and priorities. The availablity of training positions for interested students is, therefore, increasing.

The issue involved in educational philosophy consists of determining the best method of preparing the student well. When the student is given the opportunity to enter a specialty program, either in health psychology or clinical child psychology, early in the doctoral sequence, the basics of psychology and psychological research methods can be taught within the context of the specialty area. The student is also sensitized to the issues related to the specialty area and develops a commitment to work on problems in that area. On the negative side, however, early immersion in a specialty area limits the time students are able to devote to gaining breadth and depth in the discipline of psychology.

Specialty training beginning only at the postdoctoral level has the advantage of starting with a student who has the basic knowledge and skills of psychology and only requires guidance and introduction to the culture of the specialty area. The advanced student at this level also is more likely to grasp quickly the relevance of areas of knowledge to his or her basic skill training. On the negative side is the prolonged period during which the student interested in a specialty area has to wait to get training related to the area of interest. This is frustrating for the student and perhaps even detrimental to a student's continuance.

THE TRAINING SEQUENCE

Pediatric psychologists have been trained in the typical sequence which has been designed to train clinical psychologists. The four- (or five-) year doctoral training program involves three years basic training within the university doctoral psychology department, a year-long internship at an internship facility, and award of the doctoral degree upon completion of the dissertation. Some programs require that the internship follow the completion of the dissertation, such that the degree is conferred upon completion of the internship. Those programs that usually require the internship be completed prior to the dissertation sometimes permit students to follow a course of internship after completion of the dissertation, as well. Training in pediatric psychology, likewise, requires the two major components of training; (1) course work within the university, also including practica placements, and (2) an internship. These components of training and their availability will be summarized as well as postdoctoral training programs which are also a possible route for training in pediatric psychology.

Formal Doctoral Programs in Psychology

There are no doctoral programs in pediatric psychology. However, because traditions of both clinical psychology and health psychology are integral in the development of their skills, two kinds of training exist which may be relevant to the student interested in a career in pediatric psychology. One is a specialty or subspecialty or track program in clinical child psychology and the other is a subspecialty in health psychology.

Clinical Child Psychology

As noted in a previous section, the number of clinical child doctoral training programs has always been small, and they consist of essentially three types of programs: (1) specialized training in child and adolescent mental health within the context of general or adult clinical psychology; (2) specialty clinical child psychology programs, and (3) specialty training in clinical child psychology within the framework of developmental and other types of training programs. The student usually finds all three types available. In training at the doctoral level, regardless of what kind of format the program follows (specialty, subspecialty within general or adult, subspecialty within developmental and other), the clinical skills and knowledge base will be provided the student. This covers clinical training. The second component of interest to the future pediatric psychologist is health psychology training. The clinical child program of study could be augmented in areas within the department, the university, the community, as suggested by Olbrisch and Sechrest (1979) with courses, workshops and practica, and internship and research in health-related areas. Particularly relevant would be collaborative arrangements with pediatricians in private practice or children's units in hospitals, involvements with community groups of parents of children with specific chronic diseases, and so on. Thus the student following this route would be trained in the traditional areas of clinical child psychology with a compendium of medically related courses and practical application at the practicum and internship levels to children in the health delivery system. Dissertation research could be on a relevant area of health maintenance, delivery, prevention, or similar areas.

Health Psychology

As the availability of health psychology subspecialties within clinical psychology increases, health psychology doctoral training will become a readily available option for the student interested in pediatric psychology. The student choosing to follow an emphasis on health psychology, even in programs not child-oriented, can then through course work in developmental, child courses in psychopathology, assessment, psychotherapy, and behavior modification, obtain the combination of clinical and child courses which would prepare for pediatric psychology practice. Practicum experiences could be sought in a pediatrics unit in a hospital or medical school or pediatric private practice setting. In this manner the basic knowledge about substantive areas, the culture and the language of health care would be obtained. Following this sequence of training, an internship in a medical school setting or similar setting in pediatrics or family practice would be appropriate. The number of doctoral training programs in health psychology is on the increase following the new priority-based training guidelines issued by NIMH (Denham, 1979). A recent survey, for example, identified 25 (Tuma & George, in preparation) existing training sequences and indications from respondents that seven more are in some stage of development.

Adult (General) Clinical Programs

Even if specialty programs in pediatric psychology, medical (health) psychology, and clinical child psychology, which seem most directly related to the training needs of the pediatric psychologist, continue to grow, only a limited number of persons can be trained in this manner, and it is more likely that the traditional graduate programs in psychology will continue to train students who eventually work in medical and health areas. Making note of that fact, Olbrisch and Sechrest (1979) have made some valuable suggestions about how existing programs can produce psychologists from various areas of psychology in the preparation of psychologists to work within a subspecialty of health psychology. This, of course, would include pediatric psychology. Olbrisch and Sechrest propose that programs can work within their present format by coordinating available resources and specifying specialized training goals. The resources that can be used by most programs include resources in the department, resources in the university, and resources in and beyond the community.

RESOURCES IN THE DEPARTMENT

In a program that does not have a specialty training program in health psychology, faculty can be utilized in creative fashion to provide important content and experiences. Olbrisch and Sechrest (1979) suggest that psychologists of other specialties may have expertise in relevant areas. For example, the social psychologist can help the student understand issues of attitude change in the design of health education programs, the physiological psychologist has relevant information concerning the ramifications of working with patients with neuromuscular disease or neurological disease, the community psychologist can contribute to the understanding of the linkages between various services in the health care setting; the sensory psychologist who does biofeedback research can help the student with clinical application of these methods, and the clinical psychologist can help identify the key issues of the targeted patient groups as well as offer courses in clinical skills. For pediatric psychology training, the child-related courses should also be pursued by the student. As new vistas are opened up, no doubt other kinds of information emanating from other psychology areas will become important as well. This expansion of all areas of psychology into the health arena is what has been suggested by the APA Task Force on Health Research (1976).

With the clinical psychology teaching-research clinic, often a part of psychology departments, invaluable experiences for the health student can be provided in delivery of services and practice of research skills. If the clinic has strong ties to the community, appropriate populations of patients could be obtained through outreach to families that have a child with chronic physical diseases such as juvenile diabetes, cancer, and so on. If the quality of service is high and the participants are assured of viewing the benefits of participation positively, these pilot projects designed for the students' needs can lead to continued referrals and training opportunities. These continued referrals can then provide the basis for planning a long-range research program and data collection procedures which would then be invaluable for future students.

RESOURCES IN THE UNIVERSITY

Several course offerings within other departments of the university have relevance for preparation for a health career in psychology. Medical sociology, for example, can give a perpective on the organization of the health care delivery system and introduce the student to the largest available body of literature contributing to a social and psychological perspective on health and illness. It would furthermore sensitize the student to the political factors that influence delivery of medical care and health services. Courses within anthropology can give the student a cross-cultural perspective, which can illuminate underlying assumptions and values inherent in the dominant systems within the student's own culture. Courses in physical education, economics, biology, nursing, home economics, urban and regional planning have also been suggested to have relevance (Olbrisch & Sechrest, 1979). If the university has a school of medicine in the vicinity, numerous courses offered in the biomedical sciences have immediate relevance. The health services that are available to the student body have also been considered to be relevant, giving the student access to possibilities for health services and program evaluation.

RESOURCES IN AND BEYOND THE COMMUNITY

Faculty of the department of psychology can also draw upon sources within the community. Private practitioners in various specialties often are available to students interested in health care. Dentists also have been receptive, particularly as student activities may address and modify children's fears of dental procedures, a serious problem in providing dental services. Hospitals, community clinics, public health clinics can provide opportunities to develop students' skills and research projects. In addition, school health and safety programs, programs or agencies organized to assist specific patient groups (e.g., American Cancer Society, Epilepsy Foundation of America) are sometimes willing to sponsor projects and help students gain access to patients. Numerous opportunities exist in the community, and each community possesses a different array of the kinds of settings in which the student can enter once the faculty has initiated the possibility.

It has also been suggested that there are opportunities beyond the community for the student to develop skills (Olbrisch & Sechrest, 1979). The clinical student can choose a medical center for internship which allows rotations in various departments where health and clinical interests overlap. The student can also be encouraged to attend lectures, workshops, short courses, symposia, and so on, which may not be in the immediate community.

With this combination of resources within the department, university, and community, the student should be able to approximate the kinds of experiences and knowledge base which will undoubtedly be offered in specialty programs of health psychology in a more focused manner. The crucial variable in making this a possibility in the adult clinical program is faculty interest and willingness to supervise and encourage the student's continued involvement.

Predoctoral Internship

The internship is a year the clinical doctoral student spends in an agency which delivers services to clients. It is required by the APA Education and Training Board for the doctoral degree during either the third or fourth year of doctoral training, and it provides the clinical student the opportunity to apply the knowledge and skills obtained at the university setting. While practicum training during the first two years of a clinical student's graduate training is considered to be aimed at developing basic skills, the internship is aimed at developing skills beyond those beginning levels so that when doctoral training is complete, the student will be competent for independent function.

Pediatric psychology, because of its close development from clinical child psychology, has followed a similar format for doctoral training, including the internship year. Usually, however, the internship year is based in a setting nonpsychiatric in nature, that is, in a pediatric or family practice department of a medical school or a developmental clinic. The collaboration is with a physician rather than a psychiatrist (and social worker), the patients are referred primarily for physical rather than behavioral problems, and the setting, of course, is a medical unit rather than a psychiatric unit. In addition to the traditional assessment and intervention techniques utilized by the clinical child psychologist, the pediatric psychologist administers a myriad of assessment, intervention, consultation, and educational techniques designed for physically ill children. The student trained in a specialty area of psychology other than clinical typically follows a course of internship training after the doctoral degree is conferred; this is referred to as a postdoctoral internship, to be considered later.

Availability of Predoctoral Internships

Two recent surveys (Tuma, 1976, 1980b) of predoctoral internship programs listed by the Association of Psychology Internship Centers (APIC) yielded some information about formal internship programs in pediatric psychology. The first survey, which yielded a directory (Tuma, 1976) for students' use in selecting internship placements, identified 28 settings which offered predoctoral internships in pediatric psychology. A second survey, resulting in a second directory (Tuma, 1980b), indicates that the number of programs currently offering training at the predoctoral internship level is 33. It must be stressed, however, that with the increased emphasis on funding health programs as well as psychology's increasing awareness of the vast opportunities in health care settings, this is now a period of rapid development and change which will influence the establishment of new programs.

Internships designed for clinical child psychologists may also be an option for the pediatric psychology aspirant. Most internship programs which are located in or near a medical facility provide, or will allow rotations and/or experiences in medical settings where children are seen. The availability of clinical child internships is increasing. Recently, 87 internships which offered clinical child training were identified (Tuma & George, in preparation).

Medical psychology or health psychology internships constitute a third option for the pediatric psychology student. Fifty-six health psychology internships were recently identified (Tuma & George, in preparation). Although these typically will not focus on physically ill children, some of them might. In addition, those programs that do not provide child experiences may permit such experiences at the student's request.

Postdoctoral Internship

The postdoctoral internship is at the same level of training as the predoctoral internship just considered. The term "postdoctoral" designates the sequence of training rather than the level of training obtained. It differs from the postdoctoral fellowship by virtue of the fact that postdoctoral fellowship training is training offered at an advanced level, that is, postinternship. Students who apply for postdoctoral internships are those who choose to complete their dissertation and other requirements for the doctoral degree prior to internship placement (universities vary as to whether the degree is actually conferred prior to completion of internship). If the internship is regarded by the psychology department to be a requirement of the doctoral degree, then the award of the degree may be withheld until the internship is completed. However, as far as the internship facility is concerned, the student may be considered postdoctoral. For example, stipends are sometimes the same for the postdoctoral and predoctoral interns but are higher for the postdoctoral fellow. Other facilities tend to award a higher stipend to both the postdoctoral intern and fellow than to the predoctoral intern. The actual practice depends more on the relative value placed on the level of knowledge and experience, and therefore skills, or the level of the formal educational advancement.

Availability of Postdoctoral Internships

The first survey (Tuma, 1976) mentioned above identified four postdoctoral internships available in pediatric psychology, whereas the second (Tuma, 1980b) listed seven. The availability for this level of training does not seem very encouraging in spite of the increase in the number of programs in the four years. However, the confusion of terms between the postdoctoral internship and fellowship even at the training director level may contribute to this low number. For example, it may be that when a training director of a program offering a postdoctoral fellowship receives an application from a person who would qualify only for a postdoctoral internship according to the definition noted above, the fellowship position might be offered. This arrangement would not affect the student if the program is flexible enough to provide training opportunities appropriate to the level of skills of the student. The low number of programs may also relate to the fact that with the present format of training sequence, that is, internship prior to award of the doctoral degree, this may be the slot least in demand. The person trained in another area, such as developmental psychology, would normally apply for this position, however. It should be noted that the postdoctoral intern has the same options for training in clinical child or health psychology internships as the predoctoral intern mentioned in the preceding section. Tuma (1980b) listed 9 postdoctoral internships in clinical child psychology.

Postdoctoral Fellowship

As mentioned above, the postdoctoral fellowship is awarded to students who have (1) completed all requirements for the doctoral degree and (2) completed a year-long internship at an acceptable facility. As already mentioned, this level of training is often confused with the postdoctoral internship. The postdoctoral fellowship is a program of study and practice in an area, usually a specialty area, like clinical child psychology or pediatric psychology, and in the context of clinical training, usually involves two years of training rather than the one-year commitment usually associated with internship training. It is sometimes possible, however, to obtain a one-year postdoctoral fellowship, although this varies among programs.

Fellowships in pediatric psychology are usually found in departments of pediatrics or developmental disability centers, although they could be in other settings like departments of family practice, or even others. Training is at a higher level of functioning for the fellow than for either the predoctoral or postdoctoral intern. The skills and knowledge the fellow obtained during the internship year are built upon, and specialization in a more focused area is sometimes permitted by the training program. Programs vary in their requirement for research involvement at this level of training, but because of the longer time commitment, research becomes more viable than within a one-year program. As in most practicum and internship programs, the crux of the training is intensive supervision of all the trainee's activities. Oftentimes, various supervisors supervise specific activities, for example, assessment, parent education and counseling, consultation, or pain management. Supervisors are typically assigned to work with the trainee in accord with their special interests and the nature of the activity. Thus the trainee who is involved in a variety of activities may work with a number of different supervisors, sometimes obtaining many different points of view. This has proven to be confusing for the trainee at times, but in the long-term, this diversity is the strength of the training period. Premature decisions regarding the preferred viewpoint or procedure are as limiting and constricting as premature decisions on specilization. Development of breadth and depth of knowledge and skill training at a high level is the goal of most postdoctoral training programs. This philosophy of training stands the trainee in good stead because it is the constraint of the job which the psychologist finally accepts that often delimits his/her role and function. The student who pursues too narrow a course will find many job opportunities closed. The goal of the student should be to maximize her or his ability to perform many functions, and therefore to be prepared for a number of different kinds of jobs in a variety of job settings.

Availability of Postdoctoral Fellowships

Postdoctoral fellowships in pediatric psychology have also increased, from 9 programs to 18 from the first survey (Tuma, 1976) to the second (Tuma, 1980b). This increase, along with the increase in programs for predoctoral and postdoctoral interns, indicates an increase in opportunities for training in pediatric psychology. The second survey also lists 8 postdoctoral fellowships in clinical child psychology. The number of recent postdoctoral fellowships in the health psychology area is unknown, since the previously mentioned survey (Tuma & George, in preparation) did not attempt to identify postdoctoral training in this area. However, with the overall increase of total development in the area of health psychology, it is conceivable that new program offerings at the postdoctoral level will be forthcoming. Some have already been reported in the literature. As is the usual case, some of these programs will either specialize in work with children's health problems and/or have experiences with this age group within an adult emphasis. Thus the student who elects to obtain specialized training in pediatric psychology after the award of the PhD, either because of lack of training possibilities before this level of training or because an interest in the area developed late, has opportunities open for obtaining such training at the postdoctoral fellowship level.

Characteristics of Pediatric Predoctoral Internships

The current survey of pediatric training programs (Tuma, 1980b; Tuma & Grabert, in preparation) provide information about the characteristics of pediatric psychology internship facilities and training characteristics. The pediatric department is the setting of most pediatric psychology training programs (32%). Pediatric outpatient clinics for developmental and learning disorders (18%), pediatric outpatient clinics (14%), comprehensive child health centers (9%), the hospital medical unit (11%) and psychiatric departments (9%) are also often listed as the major setting for training pediatric psychologists. Some involvement in all these kinds of settings are typical in the programs in addition to the major setting listed.

The most frequently seen kind of disorder of the patients are learning disabilities (32%), conduct disorders (26%), mental retardation (11%), developmental delays (11%), medically related disorders (11%), neuroses (5%), and adjustment reactions (5%). The most frequently seen child in pediatric settings (learning-disabled children) contrasts with conduct disorders most frequently seen in clinical child psychology programs. Most program respondents of both varieties list by overwhelming margin the psychotic/autistic child as the least frequently seen child. The range of children seen by these facilities include, in addition to those listed, genetic defects, physically handicapped, abused children, and children with speech prob-handicapped, abused children, and children with speech problems.

The student typically spends 3.7 hours in intake/screening evaluations, 6.9 hours administering psychological tests, 7.6 hours in intervention, 5.3 hours intervention with parents, 4.2 hours in seminars, 2.8 hours in clinical conferences, and 5.4 hours in supervision. Priorities for pediatric training are assessment, treatment, consultation, and research, in that order. This is another area that was different for clinical child programs, which reversed the priority of the first two activities.

The techniques stressed by these pediatric settings were intelligence techniques (71%), projective techniques (71%), objective personality techniques (47%), developmental tests (41%), interview techniques (24%), school achievement tests (18%), and neuropsychological techniques (6%). Intervention techniques stressed by these respondents were behavioral techniques (68%), play therapy (58%), group therapy (21%), and crisis intervention techniques (6%). With parents, behavioral techniques (74%), parent counseling individual therapy (68%), and parent training (37%) were listed by respondents. A high percentage (79%) of the respondents also noted that family therapy was a treatment modality utilized. The most frequent outside consultations were to public and private schools (50%), outpatient pediatrics (44%), and psychiatry (44%). A large number of other consultation sites were listed at much less frequency.

The most frequent seminar topics provided by the facilities were clinical topics such as interviewing, pediatric psychology, handicapped child, and case presentation (68%), family, individual, and adult psychotherapy (26%), child development and psychopathology (21%), behavior therapy (21%), child assessment/psychodiagnostics (16%), psychosomatic disorders (5%), learning/behavior disorders (10%), behavioral medicine/behavioral pediatrics (10%), adolescent medicine (10%), pediatric neurology/neuropsychology (10%), child play therapy (5%), and Rorschach (5%). The kinds of clinical conferences listed included case conferences (47%), grand rounds (29%), staff conferences (18%), ward rounds (18%), team meetings (12%), and treatment conferences (6%).

The average number of predoctoral interns pediatric respondents accept is 2.7. On average, 1.9 postdoctoral interns and 1.3 postdoctoral fellows also are accepted. The average stipend for the predoctoral intern is $6711.46, $7666.67 for the postdoctoral intern and $10,608.33 for the postdoctoral fellow. The usual deadline for application of a training position is mid-January. Students are notified of acceptance into the program in the second week in February (thus most settings abide by the APIC guidelines). Most appointments are for one year (97%). The training year typically begins in September and ends in August. The average numbers of supervisors found in these training facilities are 5.7 PhD psychologists, 3.4 physicians (pediatricans), 1.3 social workers, and 2.1 other. Other disciplines trained include the wide range of health-related professions, but pediatricians are trained in largest number, as would be expected. Most pediatric psychology training facilities do not have APA-approval (63%) (an additional 25% did not respond to the question) as contrasted to 54% of clinical child psychology training programs having APA approval.

EMPLOYMENT OPPORTUNITIES

Where do pediatric psychologists work? One estimate comes from a survey of the members of the Society of Pediatric Psychology (Tuma & Cohen, in preparation) taken in 1980. Results indicate that most of the members work in child medical facilities and only a small percentage work in departments of psychology or traditional mental health settings. Seventy-five percent of the respondents work in medical schools, particularly in departments of pediatrics and departments of psychiatry, but some work in other departments. Surprisingly, 35% are employed in private practice and 16% in children's hospitals. Mental health centers account for 10%, but only 6% work in child guidance settings, and a few work in residential settings (2%) and state hospitals (less than 1%). Since respondents were permitted to respond to more than one category, these percentages are not necessarily indicative of the primary work setting, but they indicate the areas of involvement of pediatric psychologists. From these data, it may be concluded that the majority of all pediatric psychologists are employed within a medical setting for children, and only few work in traditional mental health or other kinds of settings.

The job market for pediatric psychology, then, is as we could expect from all the discussion in this book about roles, skills, training, and research application. All varieties of pediatric and family practice settings (Maguire & Asken, 1978) within and without the medical school are the primary targets for seeking employment following pediatric training. But what are the potentials for finding employment in these settings? Are they at capacity as far as being able to absorb psychologists? Are they interested in hiring pediatric psychologists? These questions can be answered from surveys throughout recent years.

In 1951–1952, Mensh (1953) found that 143 psychologists were employed in medical schools in the United States. In fact, 80% of the schools surveyed employed psychologists. Because of the practice of attaching all psychologists to departments of psychiatry at that time, most of these were probably in fact within these departments rather than pediatrics or other medical departments of the medical school. Another survey in 1960 showed that there were then 40 psychologists working in departments of pediatrics alone, never mind the more traditional hiring practices within psychiatry departments, of the 84 medical schools in the United States (Buck, 1961). This increased hiring of psychologists within departments of pediatrics has been attributed to the founding of the National Institute of Child Health and Human Development in 1962 (Routh, 1975). This institute has subsequently supported much medical and psychological training in pediatric psychology. In addition, in 1963, federal legislation established the network of University Affiliated Facilities for clinical training in professional fields related to developmental disorders (Routh, 1973). Two more recent surveys (Routh, 1970; 1972) show pediatrics departments of the 100 medical schools in the United States increased involvement with psychologists from 65 to 73 during the two-year period from 1968–1969 to 1970–1971. Much more recently, Lubin, Nathan, and Matarazzo (1978) reported an increasing number of psychologists involved in behavioral science education in university medical settings, indicating that the hiring of psychologists to work in medical settings is still on the upswing.

Other indications are, of course, the joint voices coming from medicine and psychology about the importance of the integration of psychology and medical care. The new medical model (Engel, 1977) and the new psychosomatic model (Lipowski, 1977) reflect the increasing acceptance of psychological principles and theories, and the movement toward increased involvement of psychologists in health care at all levels has created an excitement within both fields which should lead to increasing employment for psychologists for many years to come. Pediatric psychology appears to be a promising choice of a career in psychology.

SUMMARY AND CONCLUSIONS

In this chapter, an overview of how the training of the pediatric psychologist fits into the broader picture of training child psychologists is presented. The issues, confusions, and attempts at resolutions are outlined with the hope that the complexity of training will be appreciated. There are needs of the profession which will gradually be worked out as more of the issues and the variables contributing to the issues are ferreted out. Training issues are always difficult to grapple with in a field of endeavor as new as pediatric psychology. It is expected to happen, and it can be a fascinating process as the professionals involved in training approximate a workable format for training pediatric psychologists.

The various components that determine how training will proceed are then presented. Role functions, common denominators of training content and skills, and the locus of professional training are considered within the context of the variables which determine the direction of training activities. Following this presentation was discussion of the training components and sequence of training in pediatric psychology. The contributions of basic training, clinical training, medical psychology training, and child training to pediatric psychology preparation are outlined. General descriptions of the basic training, internship, and postdoctoral internship and fellowship training are then given along with the availability of that training. More detailed characteristics of training facilities and the training experience are presented from results obtained in a recent survey. Finally, considerations of employment availability is discussed.

It should be clear from this presentation that there exists a great need for pediatric psychologists. There is demand for them from both the medical discipline and the psychology discipline. To make the call for pediatric psychologists even stronger, federal deliberations concerning national health insurance and federal funding patterns which are supportive of psychology's involvement in the health care industry gain impetus every day. Many psychologists are responding to this call, and because it is the oldest, and pediatrics departments are among the busiest in the medical schools, as are family practice departments, pediatric psychology will continue to be one of the most popular of all the medical psychology groups. The potential both for serving children and for contributing to the new scientific thrust of the 1980s is unlimited. Pediatric psychologists have been, and will continue to be, at the forefront of the health psychology movement in American psychology.

REFERENCES

ADAMHA. *Manpower policy analysis task force report.* Rockville, MD: U.S. Department of Health, Education and Welfare, 1978.

American Psychological Association Task Force on Health Research. Contributions of psychology to health research. *American Psychologist,* 1976, **31,** 263–274.

American Psychological Association. Standards for providers of psychology. *American Psychologist,* 1977, **32,** 498.

Asken, M. J. Medical psychology: Toward definition, clarification and organization. *Professional Psychology,* 1979, **10,** 66–73.

Belar, C. D. Training the clinical psychology student in behavioral medicine. *Professional Psychology,* 1980, **11,** 620–627.

Buck, R. L. Behavioral scientists in schools of medicine. *Journal of Health and Human Behavior,* 1961, **1,** 59–64.

Cass, L. K. The training of clinical child psychologists. In G. J. Williams & S. Gordon (Eds.), *Clinical child psychology: Current practices and future perspectives.* New York: Behavioral Publications, 1974.

Denham, W. H. NIMH policy in relation to training for service delivery to children and youth: Implication for psychology and education. Presented at the meeting of the American Psychological Association, New York, 1979.

Drotar, D. Clinical psychology practice in a pediatric hospital. *Professional Psychology,* 1977, **8,** 72–80.

Engel, G. L. The need for a new medical model: A challenge for biomedicine. *Science,* 1977, **196,** 129–136.

Fischer, C. T. Graduate programs in clinical child psychology and related fields. *Journal of Clinical Child Psychology,* 1978, **7,** 87–88.

Fischer, C. T., Mannarino, A., & Magnussen, M. Interim report: Survey task force, education and training committee (Section on Clinical Child Psychology, Division 12, APA). Unpublished manuscript, 1979.

Fox, R. E. (Ed.) *Directory of internship programs in clinical psychology,* 4th ed. Columbus, OH: Association of Psychology Internship Centers, 1975.

Koocher, G. P., Sourkes, B. M., & Keane, W. M. Pediatric oncology consultations: A generalizable model for medical settings. *Professional Psychology,* 1979, **10,** 467–474.

Lipowski, Z. J. Psychosomatic medicine in the seventies: An overview. *American Journal of Psychiatry,* 1977, **134,** 233–244.

Lubin, B., Nathan, R. G., & Matarazzo, J. D. Psychologists in medical education. *American Psychologist,* 1978, **33,** 339–343.

Magrab, P. R. (Ed.) *Psychological management of pediatric problems,* 2 vols. Baltimore: University Park Press, 1978.

Maguire, P. H., & Asken, M. J. Psychological problems in family practice: Implications for training. *Journal of Clinical Child psychology,* 1978, **7,** 13–16.

Mensh, I. N. Psychology in medical education. *American Psychologist,* 1953, **8,** 83–85.

Mills, D. H., Wellner, A. J., & VandenBos, G. R. The national register survey: The first comprehensive study of all licensed/certified psychologists. In C. A. Kiesler, N. A. Cummings, & G. R. VandenBos (Eds.), *Psychology and national health insurance.* Washington, DC: American Psychological Association, 1979.

Olbrisch, M. E., & Sechrest, L. Educating health psychologists in traditional graduate training programs. *Professional Psychology,* 1979, **10,** 589–595.

Roberts, M. C. Clinical child psychology programs: Where and what are they? Presented at the meeting of the American Psychological Association, New York, 1979.

Ross, A. O. The clinical child psychologist. In B. B. Wolman (Eds.), *Manual of child psychopathology.* New York: McGraw-Hill, 1972.

Routh, D. K. Psychological training in medical school departments of pediatrics: A survey. *Professional Psychology,* 1970, **1,** 469–472.

Routh, D. K. Psychological training in medical school departments of pediatrics: A second look. *American Psychologist,* 1972, **27,** 587–589.

Routh, D. K. The psychologist in the University Affiliated Facility. *Pediatric Psychology,* 1973, **2,** 5–7.

Routh, D. K. What is a clinical child psychologist? *Clinical Psychologist,* 1977, **30,** 23–25.

Schwartz, S., & Tuma, J. M. Graduate training in consultation and liaison. *Journal of Clinical Child Psychology,* 1978, **7,** 47–49.

Sladen, B. Health care psychology and graduate education. *Professional Psychology,* 1979, **10,** 841–851.

Stabler, B., & Whitt, J. K. Pediatric psychology: Perspectives and training implications. *Journal of Pediatric Psychology,* 1980, **5,** 245–251.

Stone, G. C. A specialized doctoral program in health psychology: Considerations in its evolution. *Professional Psychology,* 1979, **10,** 596–604.

Swan, G. E., Piccione, A., & Anderson, D. C. Internship training in behavioral medicine: Program description, issues, and guidelines. *Professional Psychology,* 1980, **11,** 339–346.

Tefft, B. M., & Simeonsson, R. J. Psychology and the creation of health care settings. *Professional Psychology,* 1979, **10,** 558–570.

Tuma, J. M. Pediatric psychology? . . . Do you mean clinical child psychology? *Journal of Clinical Child Psychology,* 1975, **4,** 9–12.

Tuma, J. M. (Ed.) *Directory: Practicum and internship training resources in pediatric psychology.* Galveston, TX: Society of Pediatric Psychology, 1976.

Tuma, J. M. Practicum, internship, and postdoctoral training in pediatric psychology: A survey. *Journal of Pediatric Psychology,* 1977, **2,** 9–12.

Tuma, J. M. Proposal for a conference on professional training for clinical child psychologists. Grant application submitted to the National Institute of Mental Health, February 1, 1980. (a)

Tuma, J. M. (Ed.) *Directory: Internship programs in clinical child and pediatric psychology (including postdoctoral training programs)*, 2nd ed. Baton Rouge, LA: Society of Pediatric Psychology, 1980. (b)

Tuma, J. M., & Cawunder, P. Orientation and practice patterns of members of professional child psychology societies: A survey. In preparation.

Tuma, J. M., & Cohen, R. Pediatric psychology: An investigation of factors relating to practice and training: A survey. In preparation.

Tuma, J. M., & George, J. L. Feasibility of specialty training in clinical psychology: A survey of compliance to NIMH priorities. In preparation.

Tuma, J. M., & Grabert, J. Internship and postdoctoral training in pediatric and clinical child psychology: A survey. In preparation.

Tuma, J. M., & Pratt, J. M. A survey of clinical child psychology practice and training. In preparation.

Tuma, J. M., & Salcedo, R. A survey of training and practice characteristics of Division 37 members. In preparation.

Tuma, J. M., & Schwartz, S. Survey of consultation training at the internship level. *Journal of Clinical Child Psychology*, 1978, **7**, 49–54.

VandenBos, G. R. Personal communication. Washington, DC, January 15, 1980.

VandenBos, G. R., Nelson, S., Stapp, J., Olmedo, E., Coates, D., & Batchelor, W. *APA input to NIMH regarding planning for mental health personnel development*. Washington, DC: American Psychological Association, 1979.

Wellner, A. M. (Ed.) *Education and credentialing in psychology: Proposal for a National Commission on Education & Credentialing in Psychology*. Washington, DC: American Psychological Association, 1978.

Wenar, C. Personal communication. Ohio State University, Columbus, OH, November 29, 1979.

Wertlieb, D. A preventive health paradigm for health care psychologists. *Professional Psychology*, 1979, **10**, 548–557.

Wohlford, P. Clinical child psychology: The emerging specialty. *The Clinical Psychologist*, 1979, **33**, 25–29.

Wright, L. The pediatric psychologist: A role model. *American Psychologist*, 1967, **22**, 323–325.

Wright, L., Schaefer, A. B., & Solomons, G. *Encyclopedia of pediatric psychology*. Baltimore: University Park Press, 1979.

Index

Abused children, *see* Child abuse
Abuse/neglect, *see* Child abuse
Abusing parent, 180-183
 attitudinal variables, 182-183
 personality variables, 182-183
 potential, 181
Adaptive Behavior Scale, 84-85
Adoption, 271
Advances in Behavioral Pediatrics, 291
Algorithm, 256, 266, 275
 screening, 264
Allergies, 271
Ambulatory programs, 230
American Academy of Pediatrics, 253, 255
American Medical Association, 252
Anorexia nervosa, 130, 263, 267, 268, 303
Antecedents of illness, 11, *see also* Illness
Anticipatory guidance, 254, 274, 275
Anxiety:
 to hospitalization, 50-52
 to illness, 50-52
 see also Fears
Anxiety-reducing preparations, 272
Anxiety scales, 89
Anxiety-withdrawl, 297
APA Task Force on Health Research, 2, 4,
 5, 19, 22, 329, 336
Applied developmental psychology, 326
Assessment, 93, 240, 261, 262, 263, 326,
 341
 of chronically ill, 74-75, 80-83
 cognitive, 68-83
 diagnostic, 230, 254, 256, 259, 262
 future directions, 93-94
 of handicapped, 74
 of the high risk child, 70, 72, 73
 of infants, 69-75
 of intervention, 112
 neuropsychological, 78-79
 of the newborn, 69-70
 in pediatrics, 67-68, 93-94
 protocols, 266
 psychological, 84-93

 psychosocial, 84-93
 with special populations, 79-83
 strategies, 94
 techniques and scales, 70-71, 73-75, 341
 see also Behavioral assessment; Cognitive
 assessment; Neuropsychological
 assessment; Psychological
 assessment
Asthma, 268, 271
At risk children, *see also* Vulnerable
 children
Attachment, 29-30
Attention deficit disorder, 313
Audiologists, 263, 265
Audio-visual techniques, 266
Auditorily impaired infant, 74
Autism, 291, 313, 394

Babysitters, 276
Bathtub drownings, 275
Bayley Mental Development Index, 305
Bayley Scales of Infant Development, 71,
 74, 265, 275, 295
Bed-ridden children, 31
Bedtime problems, 268
Behavioral assessment, 21, 88-89
Behavioral medicine, 2, 5, 21, 252, 330
 behavioral sciences, 3
 behavior therapy, 3
 definition, 2
 vs. medical psychology, 2
 psychosomatic theory, 18
Behavioral Medicine Study Section, 314
Behavioral pediatrics, 165
Behavioral sciences, 3
Behavior disorders, 253, 254, 262, 267, 304
 in the physically ill child, 33-35
Behavior management, 17, 112
Behavior Problem Checklist, 89
Behavior rating scales, 68, 88-89
Behavior therapy, 13, 138, 139-151, 270,
 272, 341
Bibliotherapy, 270, 271, 272

Psychology and Psychiatry in Courts and Corrections: Controversy and Change
  by Ellsworth A. Fersch, Jr.
Restricted Environmental Stimulation: Research and Clinical Applications
  by Peter Suedfeld
Personal Construct Psychology: Psychotherapy and Personality
  edited by Alvin W. Landfield and Larry M. Leitner
Mothers, Grandmothers, and Daughters: Personality and Child Care in
Three-Generation Families
  by Bertram J. Cohler and Henry U. Grunebaum
Further Explorations in Personality
  edited by A. I. Rabin, Joel Aronoff, Andrew M. Barclay, and Robert A. Zucker
Hypnosis and Relaxation: Modern Verification of an Old Equation
  by William E. Edmonston, Jr.
Handbook of Clinical Behavior Therapy
  edited by Samuel M. Turner, Karen S. Calhoun, and Henry E. Adams
Handbook of Clinical Neuropsychology
  edited by Susan B. Filskov and Thomas J. Boll
The Course of Alcoholism: Four Years After Treatment
  by J. Michael Polich, David J. Armor, and Harriet B. Braiker
Handbook of Innovative Psychotherapies
  edited by Raymond J. Corsini
The Role of the Father in Child Development (Second Edition)
  edited by Michael E. Lamb
Behavioral Medicine: Clinical Applications
  by Susan S. Pinkerton, Howard Hughes, and W. W. Wenrich
Handbook for the Practice of Pediatric Psychology
  edited by June M. Tuma